John Milton Scudder

On the reproductive organs, and the venereal

John Milton Scudder

On the reproductive organs, and the venereal

ISBN/EAN: 9783337733490

Printed in Europe, USA, Canada, Australia, Japan

Cover: Foto ©ninafisch / pixelio.de

More available books at **www.hansebooks.com**

ON THE

REPRODUCTIVE ORGANS

AND

THE VENEREAL.

BY

JOHN M. SCUDDER, M. D.

PROFESSOR OF PATHOLOGY AND THE PRACTICE OF MEDICINE IN THE ECLECTIC MEDICAL INSTITUTE; AUTHOR OF THE ECLECTIC PRACTICE OF MEDICINE, DISEASES OF WOMEN, DISEASES OF CHILDREN, MATERIA MEDICA AND THERAPEUTICS, THE PRINCIPLES OF MEDICINE, SPECIFIC MEDICATION, THE USE OF INHALATIONS, ETC., ETC.

WITH COLORED ILLUSTRATIONS OF SYPHILIS.

"Honi soit qui mal y pense."

CINCINNATI:
WILSTACH, BALDWIN & CO., PRINTERS.
1874.

PREFACE.

THE author begs leave to introduce this work to the reader as a plain statement of facts which deserve careful consideration. It may shock the modesty of some, but it is to be hoped that the majority may see the necessity and the great good which may grow out of this study. Physicians have manifested a degree of *mock* modesty with reference to diseases of the reproductive function, which has prevented their investigation, and turned the many sufferers over to the hands of advertising quacks and charlatans. There may be some excuse for this in the "innate" modesty of man, but the time has now come when an intelligent knowledge is demanded. It will not now do for a physician to shrug his shoulders, and elevate his eyebrows at the mention of masturbation, spermatorrhœa, marital excesses, etc.

There are a great many wrongs in the sexual life of the people causing disease, which might be righted did the physician know, and should he exert his influence in a right direction. His relation to the public is not alone as a dispenser of drugs, he should be a teacher in addition. And to whom, if not to the profession, can the people turn for this information?

Some of the conclusions reached by the author may not suit the views or the prejudices of the reader, but all that is asked for them is a candid consideration. We live in a wicked world, and the millenium will hardly come in our time, and we have therefore to think of these sexual evils in the light of *greater* and *less*, and not as that which may be wholly eradicated. The writer has no desire to defend prostitution, but claims that the female prostitute is no whit worse than the male, and should receive the same treatment. Lastly, it has been the intention to point out that right education is the best means for the cure of these social wrongs, and that they can not be cured by the enactment of prohibitory laws.

The chapters on the venereal disease have been written with reference to the wants of the general practitioner, and not the specialist. The description of disease will be found plain, and the treatment one which will give success. The author has endeavored to study the therapeutics of these diseases without prejudice, and has presented his conclusions both for and against certain powerful remedies, used in the treatment of syphilis.

TABLE OF CONTENTS.

ON

THE REPRODUCTIVE ORGANS

AND

THE VENEREAL.

THE REPRODUCTIVE FUNCTION.

1. The reproductive function in man is so purely animal in its nature, and so little under the influence of the moral sentiments and the will, that we are surprised, not that diseases of these organs are found, but that they are not of more frequent occurrence. The intense passional feeling that prompts intercourse between the sexes, may be and is controlled by education in the majority, but in a minority it is so in excess that it must and will have gratification at any risk, moral or physical.

2. It is probable that this needs be to perpetuate the species, otherwise the cares of parentage, and the struggles necessary to provide for offspring, would so influence man that the race would soon be extinct. As it is, there is no condition so abject, no suffering so great, and no future so miserable, that men will not endure it to gratify this passion.

3. Society provides for its normal gratification, and for its legitimate uses, by the marital relation. The pairing of the sexes is a law of nature; how it shall be done is a law of society, and is the outgrowth, as a general rule, of the needs of the people. In different ages of the world and in different countries we find variations of the marriage relation. In the

early ages of mankind, this relation was, in all probability communistic, there being no bonds between individual males and females, the women of a tribe being held in common. This would place man on the plane of the animal and vegetable kingdom, and would give free play to the law of "natural selection," and the "survival of the fittest." Following this, came a division of women among the males, as a species of property; and as with other property, the stronger and more intelligent would secure the largest number, polygamy was the first result.

4. As men became organized into societies, and individual rights were recognized, the right of each man to a woman was conceded, and as the sexes became equal in numbers, monogamy was the necessary result.

5. If we are to study this subject intelligently, and especially with reference to the prevention of disease, it is necessary that we fully comprehend the nature of the reproductive function, the intense and sometimes uncontrollable passional attraction between the sexes, and the outgrowth from this of the marital relation and its laws as a means of protection against the abuse of the sexual organism. If any apology is necessary for the free discussion of the subject, this must be my apology.

6. THE MORAL ASPECT OF THE CASE.—We are met at the threshhold of this investigation by a class of moralists who say—"it is not wise to discuss the subject;" "it is impure and can but lead to impurity." Whilst it is patent to all that the "social evil," so called, runs riot, and that our whole people are influenced to some extent by sexual vice, these say that from its very nature it must not receive consideration from society or from law, and especially do they insist that no means looking to the modification of the evil shall be adopted, because that would necessitate its recognition—"there is only one way, enforce the commandment—Thou shalt not commit adultery."

7. Such teachers ignore the necessity of the reproductive function, the intensity and at times uncontrollable character of the passional desires of the sexes, and that it must and will have satisfaction, and that it may be controlled to the good of society or abused to its harm.

8. With these everything is good that is covered by the marital relation, everything is evil outside of it. Covered with the marital mantle, they give unbridled license to their own passions, frequently at the expense of the health, happiness and lives of their hapless wives, and yet they can not see that other men and women are of like nature with themselves. Such men are pious and religious withal, but their piety is pharisaical and their religion based upon precepts four thousand years old, which were given for the guidance of a peculiar and pastoral people. The commandment, "thou shalt not commit adultery," reads very differently in an age and to a people who practiced polygamy, and could have wives sufficient to satisfy their desires, to what it would in these times and to our people, when it is difficult to get and support one wife.

9. If those who dispense religion are to control popular opinion upon these subjects, and thus force law-makers and sociologists to ignore the evils that follow sexual vice, only in so far as they enforce the prohibitory law of Moses, then indeed we can not expect any relief. Experience has shown that no wrong of this character can be righted by prohibitory laws, and that it will not grow less by ignoring its existence.

10. The Christian religion *miscalled*, which enforces the harsh rule of Moses—"thou shalt not," instead of the gentle precept—"Come unto me all ye that labor and are heavy laden" of the Divine Teacher, stands to-day, as it has stood for a thousand years, in the way of *every* effort to control sexual wrong, and efface venereal disease. It stones the "woman taken in adultery," instead of saying, "Neither do I condemn thee; go, and sin no more."

11. With an education that postpones retribution to a

future state, and promises relief from the consequences of all wrong-doing by simple repentance, at that period of life, possibly, when the capacity for wrong-doing is lost, we can hardly expect that these wrongs will be righted. It might not be necessary to say this, it would not be necessary to speak of the moral aspect of sexual vice, did not the teachers of religion put themselves persistently in the way of all laudable efforts to control it.

12. If we must have the prohibitory laws of the Jews forced upon us, give us also their means of protection. Enforce circumcision as a means of lessening the libidinous impulse of the male, and the danger of contracting and communicating disease. Enforce the laws of purification of women; and above all, provide for the wants of women, and by years of Jubilee for an equalization of property. Give us all of the olden time or none.

13. Our civilization has within it, and as an essential part of it, the germs of prostitution and all sexual vice. Our education, habits, and methods of life, tend to the undue development of sexual passion, and of necessity entail prostitution when marriage is not possible or sufficient.

14. We fiercely denounce polygamy when practiced by Mohammedan or Mormon, yet wink at it when the use of many women is a vice of the wealthy in our midst. We forgive the man all sexual sins inside or outside of the marital relation, yet deny to the woman the chance of repentance and reformation, and to the child born out of wedlock, the name, protection, and support of its father.

15. PHYSIOLOGY A BETTER GUIDE THAN RELIGION.—Physiology is the best guide to a correct understanding of this subject. If we can understand clearly the demand made by the reproductive instincts, how they may be exercised for the good of the individual and the species, how they may be controlled by calling into action other functions of body and mind, we will be in a better position to guide and control them.

16. The first law of our being, always operative, and unchanging as the "laws of the Medes and Persians," is, *that as any function of the mind or body is exercised, it gains strength.* If by education, dress, association, public spectacles, etc., we excite sexual feeling, we may expect it to grow. If on the contrary the child is educated and trained to work, the sexual instinct remains in abeyance, until such time as it may have legitimate use.

17. If one would train children to avoidance of these evils, he would call into activity other functions of the mind, strengthen the will, develop the body, and give no food to sexual desire. Chastity was a necessary result of the full development of man in the olden time. The mental and physical gymnast of Greece or Rome had abundant procreative power, and yet we do not learn that it was ever abused, as in our time. We do not learn in the history of the memorable voyage of the Trojan chief Eneas, that Dido or other of womankind had to suffer from their libidinous desires.

INNERVATION OF THE SEXUAL ORGANS.

18. THE reproductive organs in male and female receive their nervous supply from three sources—the sympathetic nervous system, spinal cord, and brain. By the first they are intimately associated with all the vegetative functions; by the second they are associated with other automatic functions, and they are to some extent independent of the will; and by the third they are associated with certain functions of the mind, and are to a certain extent controlled by the will.

19. FROM THE SYMPATHETIC. — The innervation from the sympathetic is very important, especially in the female. The procreative act is cerebro-spinal because muscular, but the life of the new being, its development and growth, is purely vege-

tative, and must be controlled by the vegetative system of nerves. We have marked examples of this in gestation, during which, there are frequently sympathetic lesions of the digestive apparatus, deranging the processes of digestion, blood-making, nutrition, waste and secretion. We have other examples in lesions of the circulation, temperature, etc.

20. In some diseases of the female reproductive organs, the sympathetic nervous system suffers, and all functions controlled by it are impaired. Thus in apparently slight disease of the cervix-uteri, or displacement, we sometimes have marked loss of appetite, impaired digestion and blood-making, with a wrong of the circulation, nutrition and waste, that seem out of all proportion to the cause.

21. We find similar manifestations of disease in the young female, from disturbance of the menstrual function alone. In some cases the impairment of the vegetative functions is such as to cause the most extreme marasmus, as in chlorosis.

22. And thus we find, also, that abuse of the reproductive function in women will give rise to most serious general disease. One has but to look at the married women he meets, to find examples of this, and to see its manifestation in almost every direction. The ill health of married women is, to a very considerable extent, far more, I am sure, than is usually thought, attributable to this.

23. In diseases of the reproductive function in man, we observe the same sympathetic relations. Among the train of symptoms following onanism, and attending spermatorrhœa, are lesions of digestion, blood-making, nutrition and waste. So in some structural diseases, as in chronic orchitis or prostatitis we find that degeneration of tissue is a very common result.

24. In disease of the reproductive organs or functions, then, attention to the sympathetic system of nerves becomes a most important part of a rational therapy. Indeed, those means which prove most successful in the cure, act upon and through this system of nerves. All function is dependent

upon structure—as is the structure, and the force acting upon it, so is the function. There are two factors in the problem of healthy or diseased action—the structure of the organ, and the nervous force applied to it. To get normal structure, we want normal sympathetic innervation, which controls the renewal of tissue, and with a proper supply of blood, and normal use, we get a right condition of the organism. Now let nerve force be rightly applied, and we can but have normal function.

25. As the physical development and life of the species must be, to a considerable extent, dependent upon the integrity of the procreative function, and its right use, we can see how society at large has a right of inquiry into those evils, and the use of means for their correction. If sexual vice only influenced the person sinning, it might be claimed that it should pass unnoticed, as a part of that individual freedom we prize so much. But as it influences the physical life of the man, and at times of associate women, and perpetuates itself in the offspring for generations, society has just claims to give it consideration, and devise means for its prevention.

26. SPINAL INNERVATION.—The reproductive apparatus in both male and female is abundantly supplied with spinal nerves, its various parts being thus associated in action, and the function, to a certain extent, rendered automatic. These nerves are both sentient and motor, and we have the most marked examples of reflex action, impressions being conveyed to the spinal cord, and the impulse sent from it, without the cognition of the brain.

27. The reproductive act is, in its principal part reflex, or determined by the spinal cord. The mind may, from desire, determine the copulative act, and the will may influence the voluntary muscles to that end; but the erythism of the organs, and the final ejaculation in the male—venereal spasm in male and female—are purely automatic, and from the spinal cord.

28. This is clearly proven in some diseases of these organs.

An irritation of the prostatic urethra will determine an erection, the same as an influence of the mind. So will an irritation of the *bas-fond* of the bladder, in some cases of phosphuria and uric acid deposits; and occasionally ascarides of the rectum, or disease of a distant part of the urinary apparatus. Not only will these causes determine the turgescence of the organs, but will also through the sentient spinal nerves induce the venereal orgasm, without the copulative act, or anything to simulate it.

29. In some cases of spermatorrhœa, we find the emissions distinctly epileptiform in character from the beginning. There has been no erotic impulse of the mind, possibly no sexual thoughts or desires, the venereal orgasm being purely reflex, and unconsciously performed. Again, we find that a certain action often performed, becomes automatic, and thus onanism frequently develops this reflex action, and though the mind be kept free from sexual excitement, emissions continue to occur.

30. This is particularly the case with women, and is not unfrequently the cause of the impaired health of widows. The sexual organs have been accustomed to frequent excitement, and the spinal cord to this reflex action. The venereal orgasm relieves the nervous system from excitement, and so long as it is complete the health does not suffer. If now the sentient nerves of the reproductive apparatus are periodically excited, the sexual stimulus withdrawn, there being nothing to determine the completion of the reflex movement, the nervous system must eventually suffer severely.

31. We find occasional instances of a similar character in men. Under the marital relation they have for years been accustomed to the frequent and regular performance of this act. The spinal cord becomes accustomed to it, as much as it does to defecation and urination, and if now from death or some other cause, there is an arrest of its performance, the health suffers.

32. INNERVATION FROM THE BRAIN.—The reproductive function is not only vegetative and automatic, as we have seen, but in man it is intimately associated with certain operations of the mind, and may have its representative organ in the brain. In the lower forms of animal life it is vegetative alone, in the lower vertebratæ it is reflex or automatic, in the higher vertebratæ it is instinctive as well as automatic, and in man it is promoted and influenced by the mind. In all, so far as we know, the instinctive prompting is pleasurable; in most the act is one of exquisite pleasure, though it may be followed by pain or entail death.

33. Certain operations of the brain are in part instinctive, and among those are sexual attraction, the desire for progeny, and the love of children. In the old scheme of phrenology, in which the brain was mapped out, and the function of its several parts designated, we had the organs of *amativeness* and *philoprogenitiveness*—the one giving sexual love, and prompting to the reproductive act, the other the desire for and the love of children. Whether the phrenologist has well located his organs, or can determine their development by cranial bumps, we will not stop to inquire, but there is abundant evidence that these functions of the mind do exist, and must be represented in the structure of the brain.

34. Any consideration of this subject, therefore, that should ignore the function of the brain, would be imperfect, if not erroneous, for we have our conscious life in and through the brain; and as it is, to a considerable extent, is the development and function of the body at large.

35. Let us assume as granted that the sexual organs are designed for the reproduction of the species alone, and for no other purpose. That in so far as the instinct toward the venereal act, or pleasure derived from it, is concerned, they are but wise provisions of nature to this end, and are not objects of the action. Nature provides an incentive that insures the perpetuation of the species, and the man is wise who accepts the pleasure as the result and not as the end.

36. We may say that the reproductive instinct is associated with two groups of mental functions—the one moral the other purely sensual—the one leading to its right use, the other to its abuse.

37. In the first it is associated with love of country, love of home, love of children, love of use, "and the love of women which passeth understanding." In the second it is impelled by animal sensibility, with which it is so intimately related, and is associated with the love of display, the love of rule, the love of self, and of sensuous gratification. Associated with the first, the function is controlled to the good of the individual and the species; associated with the second, and it is used for sensuous gratification, without regard to the rights or well-being of others.

38. If the time ever comes when the world is freed from sexual vice, it will be when the education from youth up is in the right direction. When children are trained to love of country, home, their species, children, use, and to the higher and purer love of man for woman, then we need not fear that the sexual function will be abused. Such training is possible, such training is surely profitable, and in so far as physicians can influence the people, the influence should be in this direction. If the girls of a family are thus educated, and these functions called into action from youth up, there will be little danger of their lapse from virtue; the ranks of prostitutes will have to be replenished from other sources. If boys are thus trained, these functions of the mind having vigorous growth, they will have respect and regard for women, and will be chaste in thought, word and deed.

39. If on the contrary children are raised to regard the pleasures of sense as the highest good; if fine houses, clothing and people are the subject of thought and desire; if associated with persons who are lax in morality, and manifest it by dress, look, word, or deed; if the sexual passions are unduly stimulated by reading the fictions of the day, by the semi-obscenity of the leg-drama, and other popular plays, and by

much of the amusement of "society," then we will probably get a crop of what we have sown—"ye have sown the wind, and ye shall reap the whirlwind."

40. In so far as society attempts to control or overcome the "social evil," it must be done in this way. Laws for repression are useless. It is of no avail to say, "thou shalt not steal," when the education of a portion of the people is dishonest—steal they will, though the punishment, as in the olden time, was death. It is of no use to say, "thou shalt not covet," when children are trained from youth up to covetousness. It is of no use to say, "thou shalt not kill," when we train that portion of the mind that puts "murder in the heart." And it is of no avail to say, "thou shalt not commit adultery," when we so train our children as to develop the love of pleasure, and the sexual desires. Theft, covetousness, murder, adultery, are fruits of a vicious education, and we will reach the "millenium" when we have learned this lesson, and have trained our children rightly.

41. "It is never too late to mend," and it is never too late to commence a good education to amend a bad life. If we would educate and train our criminals to the use of the better functions of the mind, and to a proper control of those which have become criminal, we might redeem them from vice and make them useful members of society. The sinner is sick, let him have that care and humane attention that we give to physical sickness.

42. The prostitute of either sex may be classed with monomaniacs or with the intemperate. The sexual wrong can be controlled by some, by others it can not. When the will is sufficiently powerful, all that is necessary for redemption is, that the person be placed in such circumstances that he can exert it in freedom; if the will is not sufficiently strong at first, then such safeguards should be thrown around the person, as will give protection until the mind is trained by orderly use.

THE SEXUAL ORGANS.

A BRIEF description of the anatomy of the sexual organs may refresh the mind of the reader, and give a better understanding of some of the subjects we will discuss.

In both sexes, the sexual organs are alike surmounted by an eminence of cellular tissue enclosing fat, and covered with stout capilli or hairs. The integument receives an abundant supply of sensory nerves, which associate it with the organs of copulation. This elevation, called the *mons Veneris* in the female, in some persons possesses sexual sense in very high degree, and anything which excites it calls forth an increased circulation to and turgidity of the erectile tissue.

43. The sexual organs of both sexes may be divided into the external or copulative, and the internal or reproductive. The copulative organs are formed in part of erectile tissue, and are very abundantly supplied with nerves of sensation from the spinal-cord and brain. The reproductive organs proper are principally supplied from the sympathetic nervous system.

IN THE MALE.—The organs of generation are the penis, the prostate gland, vesiculæ seminales, and the testes.

44. The penis is composed of two erectile bodies, the *corpora cavernosa* and the *corpus spongiosum*. The first forms the upper or larger portion, the second the lower and smaller portion and the extremity or glans penis, and contains within it the canal of the urethra. The penis has a very firm attachment to the bones of the pelvis, and is supported from above by a strong ligament. It is covered with a delicate integument, loosely attached to the body of the organ by fibrous tissue, and terminating in a fold—the *prepuce*—which has an attachment to the body of the organ behind the glans. The penis is abundantly supplied with blood, and by the peculiar situation of a pair of muscles, the *erectores penis*, the veins

are compressed, the organ made turgid with blood, and thrown in a state of erection.

45. The *prostate gland* situated at the commencement of the urethra properly belongs to the sexual organs, furnishing a secretion to be admixed with that of the vesicalæ seminales and testicles.

46. The *vesiculæ seminales* are situate between the base of the bladder and rectum. They are two lobulated membranous pouches, which probably serve as reservoirs of semen, though they furnish a secretion peculiar to themselves.

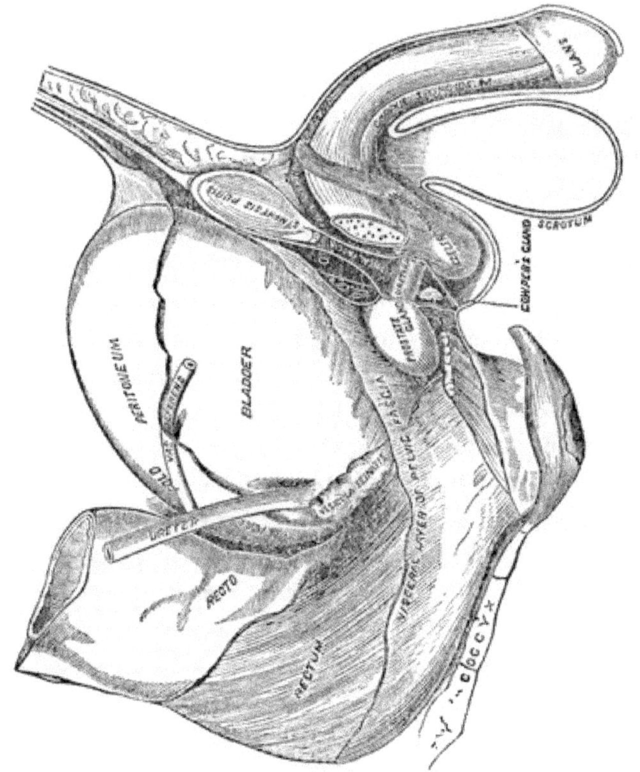

Side View of the Pelvic Viscera of the Male Subject, showing the Pelvic and Perineal Fasciæ.

47. The *testes* are contained in a cutaneous pouch—the *scrotum*, which is divided into two lateral halves by a septum. They furnish the male sperm for the fertilization of the ovum, and discharge their secretion during copulation by ascending

ducts, the vasa deferentia, which passing upward through the inguinal rings, descend on the wall of the bladder to the vesiculæ seminales.

48. IN THE FEMALE.—The external organs in the female are the *mons Veneris* already described, the *labia majora* and *minora*, the *clitoris*, the *meatus urinarius*, and the entrance of the *vagina* the introitus to the reproductive organs proper.

The internal organs are the *uterus*, *Fallopian tubes*, and *ovaries*.

49. The *labia majora* are two more or less prominent cutaneous folds extending from the mons Veneris to the perineum, containing areolar tissue, fat, and erectile tissue. Their prominence depends, in most women, on the amount of adipose tissue, though in some the erectile tissue is in such proportion as to give prominence when the organs are excited. Externally the skin is covered with hair, and supplied with nerves from the same source as the mons Veneris. Within the fissure, the lining membrane gradually loses the character of the skin and assumes that of mucous membrane.

50. The *labia minora* are lesser folds of the lining mucous membrane, extending from the clitoris backward for three-fourths the extent of the opening. They contain a plexus of vessels, forming a species of erectile tissue, and vary very greatly in prominence and extent in different persons.

51. The *clitoris* is thought to be the analogue of the male penis, and to possess the sexual sense in greatest degree. The truth is, probably, that it is a rudimentary organ, very like the male mammæ. In some women it is large, and composed of erectile tissue, it is erected during vascular excitement, and being freely supplied with nerves, adds to the voluptuousness of coition. But in others it can scarcely be detected, even during excitation, though they possess the sexual sense as fully developed as the others.

52. The *meatus urinarius* is found immediately behind the clitoris, and from it may be traced the urethra, about an inch

and a half in length, imbedded in the vesico-vaginal wall. The urethra has an erectile coat, in some women remarkably developed, and it also is in a turgid condition during sexual excitement.

53. The *vagina* is a membranous canal, between five and six inches in length along its posterior wall. It is composed of an external muscular coat, a middle layer of erectile tissue, and an internal lining of mucous membrane. The muscular coat consists principally of longitudinal fibres, continuous with the superficial layer of the uterus. The amount of

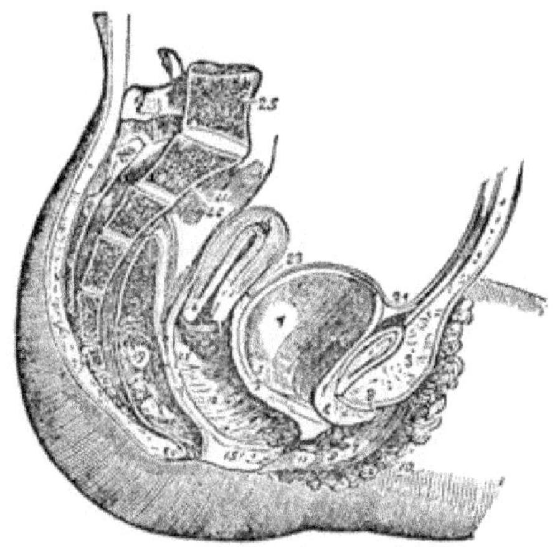

A SIDE VIEW OF THE VISCERA OF THE FEMALE PELVIS.

1. The symphysis pubis; to the upper part of which the tendon of the rectus muscle is attached. 2. The abdominal parietes. 3. The collection of fat, forming the prominence of the mons Veneris. 4. The urinary bladder. 5. The entrance of the left ureter. 6. The canal of the urethra, converted into a mere fissure by the contraction of its walls. 7. The meatus urinarius. 8. The clitoris, with its præputium, divided through the middle. 9. The left nymphæ. 10. The left labium majus. 11. The meatus of the vagina, narrowed by the contraction of its sphincter. 12. 22. The canal of the vagina upon which the transverse rugæ are apparent. 13. The thick wall of separation between the base of the bladder and the vagina. 14. The wall of separation between the base of the bladder and the vagina. 15. The perineum. 16. The os uteri. 17. Its cervix. 18. The fundus uteri. The cavitas uteri is seen along the center of the organ. 19. The rectum, showing the disposition of its mucous membrane. 20. The anus. 21. The upper part of the rectum invested by the peritoneum. 23. The utero-vesical fold of peritoneum. The recto-uterine fold is seen between the rectum and the posterior wall of the vagina. 24. The reflection of the peritoneum, from the apex of the bladder upon the urachus to the internal surface of the abdominal parietes. 25. The last lumbar vertebra. 26. The sacrum. 27. The coccyx.

erectile tissue varies in different persons, and is most abundant at the lower part of the vagina. The mucous membrane shows an anterior and posterior ridge or raphe, and between them it is thrown into numerous transverse ridges or rugæ.

The mucous membrane of the vagina is reflected upon the dependent portion of the uterus (the cervix uteri), giving it an investment, and reflected in the os, being continuous with the mucous lining of the cavities of the uterus. In its entire extent it is abundantly supplied with nerves of sensation, but possesses the sexual sense in highest degree at its inferior and superior portions.

54. The *uterus* is a pyriform organ, resting upon and partly depending in the vagina. In the unimpregnated state it measures about three inches in length, two in breadth at its widest part, and an inch in thickness, and weighs from an ounce to an ounce and a half.

It is divided into *fundus*, *body* and *cervix*—the first being the superior portion above the Fallopian tubes, the second the portion between this and the neck, and the third the lower and constricted portion, principally dependent within the vagina.

The walls of the uterus are thick, the cavity being quite small, and are composed of three coats—an external of peritoneum investing the fundus and body, a middle coat of muscular tissue, which forms its chief bulk, and an internal lining of mucous membrane.

The muscular coat is composed of layers of fibres so arranged that there will be equal contraction upon the cavity from all directions toward the outlet. In the cervix their arrangement is such, that they can both open and close the os, and cause a vermicular movement from below upward. It has been thought that this muscular tissue was only called into action for the expulsion of the ovum, or some foreign body which by its presence and growth had aroused the development of the uterine muscular fibre. This, however, is very certainly a mistake, for, as we shall see presently, it is called into action during sexual excitement, and is active during the venereal orgasm.

The circulation of the uterus is peculiar and closely resembles erectile tissue, in the tortuous course of the vessels, their free anastomosis, and direct communication of many arteries and veins without the intervention of capillaries. The increased vascularity of the organ during the excitement of ovulation, has long been noticed, and we will call attention to the fact that a similar state is produced by sexual excitement, though not to the same degree.

55. The *Fallopian tubes* lead from the uterus to the ovaries, and are the conduits for the ova. Each tube is about four inches in length, and is terminated by an expansion—the fimbriated extremity—which is applied to the ovary during ovulation.

56. The *ovaries* are to the female what the testes are to the male, furnishing the germ of the future being. The ovary shows some fifteen or twenty ova in various stages of development, though in the tissue may be seen the germs of many others. They are discharged at each menstrual period, from puberty until it ceases at the "change of life." The nerves are principally from the vegetative system, though a branch from the uterine system (sexual) passes upward and along the Fallopian tubes.

GENERATION.

57. So far as we know, there is no such thing as "spontaneous generation" in the age we are living in. Man, as well as all living things, vegetable or animal, is begotten of parents having the same structure and functions. All living organisms have one typical form—a cell—and from the

multiplication and adaptation of these come every form and function.

58. In the economy of nature, the new birth springs from the contact of two cells, a "sperm cell" and a "germ cell," the one communicating reproductive life to the other. Some species of plants and animals are hermaphrodite or bisexual, each individual possessing both male and female organs, and producing both sperm and germ cells. In other species the individual is unisexual, and it requires a conjunction of the two, male and female, for generation.

59. Nature makes wonderful provision for the perpetuation of species. In the case of vegetables, she gives wings to the sperm cells of some, to others motion, to others an attraction to bee or bird that animal life may aid in bringing the two together.

60. In the higher animal life, we find the sexual sense and a passional attraction, which brings the sexes together and effects such conjunction that the object is accomplished.

61. Whilst the generative function is pleasurable in all animals, and this is the exciting cause of the copulative act, it is not essential to it in all cases, at least on the part of the female. If intromission on the part of the male is possible without pleasurable sensations, then the sperm cells may be brought in contact with the germ cells, and reproduction effected without this element.

62. In the female we find this is frequently the case. In many species, and in some women, we find a repugnance to the embrace of the male, which requires much solicitation to overcome, and in some it is quite certain the copulative act is never pleasurable, may be in fact painful, and yet the intercourse be fruitful. We may account for this by regarding the essential elements of coition on the part of the female as reflex and vegetative, and if the purely sensitive nerves are not active, there may not be even the ordinary sexual sense.

63. COITION.—Though reproduction of the species may be the end of coition, it is not usually the object. The intense pleasure that attends the act is the exciting motive, and is partly instinctive and in part a function of the mind. Thus direct excitation of the sexual organs will develop the desire and impulse, as will the thought of the pleasure to be obtained, whether stimulated or not by sight or touch. We will find it necessary to keep this in mind whilst studying lesions of this function, for a disease may equally have its origin and continuance in disease of the organs, or of the brain.

64. In most species the sexual instinct is strongest in the male, and nature provides him with the requisites for its gratification. In some it is increased strength, in others a brilliant plumage, or similar attraction for the female, in all sufficient for the purpose. In man both sexes seem equally provided with the elements of attraction. Whilst the man has strength, and powers of persuasion, the woman has the beautiful plumage, and solicits with fine clothing, and many an art calculated to excite the sexual sense.

65. In our civilization the marital rite is necessary to the free and iawful exercise of this passional attraction, and we may regard it as the one impediment to the free play of the sexual instinct. Our laws recognize coition under the marriage relation, condemn it outside of this; and as they are but the outgrowth of our social life, society recognizes it in marriage, condemns it outside.

66. ACTION OF THE MALE.—Excited by touch, or sight, or the thought of female charms, there is an increased nervous and vascular flow to the organs of generation. The erectile tissue becomes turgid with blood, and the penis erected and its sensitiveness increased. Introduced into the female organs, its play backwards and forwards, by friction upon the rugose walls of the vagina increases the excitement, until at last it becomes so intense as to call forth a reflex action from

the spinal cord, and a contraction of the muscles which surround the vesiculæ seminales and the ejaculator muscles, and the semen is ejected with some considerable force. The completion of the act is most intensely pleasurable, though the sensation is but momentary, and is followed by a corresponding degree of depression.

67. Most physiologists have thought that the discharge during a coitus was wholly of the semen in the reservoir of the vesiculæ seminales, with the secretion of this gland and the prostate. I think this an error, for in many men a distinct vermicular movement will be noticed in the epididymis and the course of the spermatic cord, and a contraction of the scrotum upon the testes which are drawn upwards. This is very marked immediately preceding and during the venereal orgasm. We also find that persons with a lax and thin scrotum, and dependent testicles, have feeble sexual power. From these facts we may conclude that the discharge is in part directly from the testes, and it may be wholly from these.*

---

*The physiological explanation of the pleasure attendant on the sexual act is, perhaps, as follows:—"Accumulation of blood," says Kobelt, "causes, whenever it occurs in the body, a gradual augmentation of sensibility; but in this case the glans penis, in passing from a non-erect state to the condition of complete turgescence, becomes the seat of a completely new and *specific sensibility*, up to this moment dormant. All the attendant phenomena react on the nervous centers. From this it appears that, in addition to the nerves of general sensibility, which fulfill their functions in a state of repose and also during erection, although in a different manner, there must be in the glans penis *special nerves of pleasure*, the particular action of which does not take place except under the indispensable condition of a state of orgasm of the glans. Moreover, the orgasm once over, the nerves return to their former state of inaction, and remain unaffected under all ulterior excitement

"They are, then, in the same condition as the rest of the generative apparatus; their irritability ceases with the consummation of the act, and, together with this irritability, the venereal appetite ceases also to be repeated, and to bring about the same series of phenomena at each new excitation."—*Kobalt*, "*Die mannlichen und weiblichen Wollust-Organe des Menschen und einiger Saugethiere*," p. 35.

68. In some persons the act is performed in a sluggish, methodical way; there having been no cause for the full excitation of the organs, the sense of pleasure is very slight. In others again, it is so intense that considerable time is required for the nervous system to completely recover from it.

69. The power of procreation is usually attained at the age of fourteen to sixteen years, at the period of puberty, and is marked by a change in the bodily constitution. The

---

*To the use of the sexual organs for the continuance of his race, Man is prompted by a powerful instinctive desire, which he shares with the lower animals. This Instinct, like the other propensities, is excited by sensations; and these may either originate in the sexual organs themselves, or may be excited through the organs of special sensation. Thus in Man it is most powerfully aroused by impressions conveyed through the sight or the touch; but in many other animals, the auditory and olfactive organs communicate impressions which have an equal power; and it is not improbable that, in certain morbidly-excited states of feeling, the same may be the case in ourselves. That local impressions have also a very powerful effect in exciting sexual desire, must have been within the experience of almost every one; the fact is most remarkable, however, in cases of Satyriasis, which disease is generally found to be connected with some obvious cause of irritation of the generative system, such as pruritis, active congestion, etc. That some part of the Encephalon is the seat of this as of other instinctive propensities, appears from the considerations formerly adduced; but that the Cerebellum is the part in which this function is specially located, can not be regarded as by any means sufficiently proved. The Instinct, when once aroused (even though very obscurely felt,) acts upon the mental faculties and moral feelings; and thus becomes the source, though almost unconsciously so to the individual, of the tendency to form that kind of attachment toward one of the opposite sex which is known as *love*. This tendency can not be regarded as a simple passion or emotion, since it is the result of the combined operations of the reason, the imagination, and the moral feelings; and it is in this engraftment (so to speak) of the psychical attachment, upon the mere corporeal instinct, that a difference exists between the sexual relations of Man and those of the lower animals. In proportion as the Human being makes the temporary gratification of the mere sexual appetite his chief object, and overlooks the happiness arising from spiritual communion, which is not only purer but more permanent, and of which a renewal may be anticipated in another world—does he degrade himself to the level of the brutes that perish. Yet how lamentably frequent is this degradation!—*Carpenter's Physiology.*

sexual organs are now more fully developed, hair appears on face and pubes, and the voice becomes rougher and stronger. The procreative power may last the allotted age of man—three-score years and ten, if not abused, but with the majority it fails at sixty or sixty-five years.

70. ACTION IN THE FEMALE. — The woman may be, and frequently is, entirely passive during the act of coition. The sexual sense is dependent upon an increased flow of blood to and turgidity of the erectile tissue, and unless this is effected by excitation of the organs, or a mental influence, there will be neither pleasurable sensation nor venereal orgasm, at least of the external organs.

71. When excited, we find that there is an increased flow of blood to the entire reproductive organs, and the erectile tissue becomes filled with blood, the perineal muscles contract, the vulva and vagina are firmer, and the mucous membrane much more sensitive. In some rare cases this excitation and contraction is so great that penetration is difficult or painful.

72. The friction of the male organ upon these sensitive surfaces increases the excitement, until at last there is a reflex action from the spinal cord, and consequent contraction of the perineal muscles, and the muscular fibre of cervix uteri and vagina, with increased discharge of mucus, and the secretion of the glands of Bartholine.

73. It has been supposed that the uterus was wholly passive during coition, and many theories have been advanced to account for the passage of spermatozoa to the uterine cavity and ovaries. The old idea of a gaseous emanation from the semen — *halitus seminis*—becoming untenable, the movement was attributed to the spermatozoa alone, which by some special affinity or instinct moved upwards through the cervical canal, uterine cavity and ovarian tubes, until they reached the female egg. A still later theory imagined that the fertilization was accomplished by means of a mucous plug filling the

canal of the cervix, which during copulation was extended to receive the spermatozoa, and was then drawn back with them, thus affording a trap to catch them or a convenient ladder for their ascent.

Want of knowledge here is due to imperfect observation—to a want of facilities for observation. Yet I think it can be clearly shown, that the cervix uteri is a prominent actor in fruitful coition, and has in its structure the means to insure the reception of the male sperm, and transmit it upwards. In July, 1871, I published a brief article on this subject, from which I will quote.

74. "ERROR 1st.—*That the sexual sense is located in the clitoris and the entrance of the vagina.* We are taught that the clitoris is the analogue of the male penis, is formed of erectile tissue, is extremely sensitive, and in the sexual act is in a state of erection; that the vagina is also erectile, and is supplied with the same nerves of sexual sense.

"To complete the analogy, these parts should be freely supplied from the ovarian nerves, associating the external with the internal organs. But so far as we know, they do not receive a single filament. On the contrary, the entire nervous supply is from a nerve of common sensation—the *internal* pudic, which is also distributed to the skin of the labia and the *mons Veneris*.

"The clitoris is very variable in size, and in ninety-nine out of one hundred cases is rudimentary like the male mammæ. It is *not* in a state of erection during sexual excitement, and in women who have the strongest sexual feelings and enjoyment the finger will hardly detect it on examination. In forty-two women examined with reference to this point—most of them public women—but six had a good development of clitoris, and of these four were not passionate.

"In seven cases of extreme sexual excitation, simulating active spermatorrhœa in the male, (nymphomania), that have come under the writer's notice, but one had an enlarged clitoris. The complete extirpation of the clitoris, root and branch, *a la* Spencer Wells, did not in the least lessen the trouble, nor the gratification obtained from sexual intercourse.

"Writers on diseases of women uniformly agree that disease or irritation of the external sexual organs is rarely if ever the cause of that severe nervous disturbance which so frequently occurs in the male, but that such disturbance invariably grows out of disease of the cervix uteri.

"I wish to call the reader's attention next to the fact, that the larger number and some of the most intractable diseases of women we meet with, are diseases of the sexual function, and not of the sexual organs. These manifest themselves as lesions of innervation—of the functions of the brain and spinal cord—and lesions of the vegetative functions, through the sympathetic nervous system. Some of these diseases are very severe. In the one case the functional lesions of the brain assume the form of hysteria, monomania or insanity. In the other, there is an impairment of digestion, blood-making, nutrition, and waste, giving rise to loss of flesh and strength, to depravation of tissue, and at last to structural lesion.

75. "ERROR 2.—Locating the sexual sense in the clitoris may be called an error of *commission*. We wish now to refer to one of *omission*.

"In tracing the nerves of the uterus we find that the larger number of spermatic branches pass from the ovaries to the uterus, and a dissection of the gravid uterus will very clearly show their distribution principally to the cervix. We also find it abundantly supplied from the hypogastric plexus, with mixed spinal and sympathetic nerves, which are also freely distributed to the vagina in its upper two-thirds.

"If now we make a dissection of the cervix-uteri we find it composed principally of a tissue that is truly erectile, with but very few muscular fibres which are clearly continuous with the longitudinal fasiculæ of the uterus. That which is known as the *os-internum*, and closes the cavity of the uterus, is the true muscular wall of the organ.

"In sexual excitement there is an unusual fullness and elasticity of the cervix, a true condition of erection. Such excitement not unfrequently attends the making a vaginal examination by touch or speculum, and in many women the condition of erection is such as to prevent the introduction of the uterine sound, an examination of the canal of the cervix, or the introduction of a sponge-tent.

"The venereal orgasm is followed by complete relaxation of the cervix, and such dilatation of its cavity, that a finger can frequently be passed into the os—a large sound passes freely to the os-internum, and its cavity can be freely inspected.

"Diseases of the ovaries and cervix-uteri uniformly correspond, and the one will produce the other. Structural disease of the cervix uniformly affects the sexual and reproductive functions, showing the closest relationship between them.

"The venereal organism of the female then is, the vaginal canal, the cervix uteri and the ovaries; as it is the corpus spongiosum (glans penis) and cavernosum and testicles in the male.

"It would seem to be hardly worth while, and yet it is necessary, to point out that the sexual function is one of the mind, as well as of certain organs called sexual, and that this function of the mind may become diseased.

76. "Spermatorrhœa is more a disease of the mind than of the sexual organs; very frequently is wholly a disease of the mind, and must be so treated. So in women, the disease is very frequently of the mind in part, and may be wholly of it. In this the diseases of the two sexes do not differ, but in their course and history they do differ. Spermatorrhœa is developed by self abuse, and is frequently perpetuated by it. The disease of the woman is produced by the abuse of the husband, and is perpetuated by this.

"A right use of the sexual organs in the male is never fol-followed by disease, even though such use is excessive. It is the abuse of the sexual function, and the imperfectness of its gratification, that produces disease

"It is just the same in the female. If the sexual act is complete, so that both the mind and the sexual organism are satisfied, no disease arises even though there be excess in frequent repetition. But if the act is incomplete on the part of the female, the sexual organs being irritated merely, and the mind not gratified, then disease will surely follow.

"I wish next to call the reader's attention to the diseases of the sexual function—as a function of the mind. The physical lesions of the cervix-uteri are frequently grown from this, they are always rendered more intractable by it, as are the derangements of the menstrual function.

"I am satisfied that a very large number of these nervous lesions are grown from frequent excitation of the sexual organs, without gratification of the sexual instinct. That is, there is frequently repeated sexual irritation, impairing the nervous system—both brain, spinal cord and sympathetic—until we have a condition closely approximating spermatorrhœa in the male—it is one of excitation with exhaustion.

77. "For this I have prescribed with very great success Staphysagria and Pulsatilla. Sometimes they are given singly, sometimes together or alternately. If there is undue excitation of the reproductive organs, Aconite with Macrotys, and *rest*, will be the treatment. If the reproductive organs are exhausted, with an enfeebled circulation of blood, then we use Hamamelis, Tincture of Phosphorus, and Ergot.

"The remedies first named, are *par excellence*, the remedies for the disease of the sexual function, and the various nervous disturbances that flow from it. And not unfrequently what seems to be a persistent structural lesion will disappear under their use.

"All writers on diseases of women agree that diseases of the cervix-uteri are among the most frequent met with, and that it is these that so impair the general health. But no one, so far as my reading has extended, has pointed out the relation between the disease of the sexual function and the structural disease of the cervix. No one, I think, has pointed out the true cause of these lesions. They do not arise from pregnancy or parturition, nor are they inflammations from cold. On the contrary, in ninety-five out of one hundred cases they are very certainly grown from sexual abuse.

"These structural diseases manifest themselves in various forms. From simple excitation with determination of blood, to a condition of true inflammation with deposits. From a slightly enfeebled and congested condition, to that persistently tumid congested state, in which the cervix has increased to twice or even five or six times its natural volume. And with these we have altered secretion from the cervical canal, erosion, and ulceration of varying degrees of severity.

"In the olden time I treated these lesions of the cervix with local remedies. The cervix was frequently cauterized with Nitrate of Silver, Iron, or Carbolic Acid, in the milder cases; with Potassæ cum Calce or Caustic Potash in the severer. Now I never think of using such means, but depend upon direct remedies for the relief of the disease of the sexual function, and to restore normal innervation and circulation to the affected parts.

"Rest from sexual excitation is absolutely essential to a cure in some cases. But in others a cure is obtained more quickly by a full gratification of the sexual instinct two or three or four times during the lunar period. In those cases where the husband is persistent, in season and out of season, in satisfying his libidinous appetite, with corresponding feebleness in the act, a cure is impossible, and the life of the woman too frequently pays the penalty of the sins of the man.

"Many cases of severe and long continued ulceration have been treated with internal remedies alone. Many with only the employment of the five remedies, Pulsatilla, Staphysagria, Macrotys, Phosphorus and Hamamelis, and with a success never obtained with the older means."

I have no doubt others have made similar observations, but feared to publish because the facts seemed contrary to the statements of physiologists, or from modesty—a failing peculiar to physicians. The opinion I have held is corroborated in a case reported by Dr. Beck, of Fort Wayne, Indiana, which I append:*

---

*Mrs. H. L., aged thirty-two years, of strongly-marked nervous temperament, blonde, married eight years, has one living child, son, seven years old; has had one abortion; last pregnancy was six years ago; commenced to menstruate at fourteen years of age; present illness has existed six years, dating evenly with abortion; symptoms which have been apparent during its course were dragging and weight in pelvis, more or less pain in back and loins, slight vesical and rectal irritation, inability to walk without great fatigue, inability to lift weight of any moment, slight leucorrhœa, and a sinking sensation referred to the epigastric region—supposed cause to be a "falling of the womb;" present condition as regards menstruation, menstruates regularly every twenty-eight days, normal as to amount and suffers no pain of any moment; leucorrhœa very slight as to amount, exists all the time, is white, glairy, and unmistakably uterine; pain is intermittent, by no means severe, and is referred to the back, loins, inguinal and sacral regions; locomotion is impeded to a great extent by the consequent fatigue; as to other symptoms, she is usually constipated, and has a copious eruption of acne upon the face; of physical signs, the touch shows the os uteri just inside the vulvæ, the speculum was not used; the probe shows the pelvic-uterine axis to be changed considerably, but no flexion of uterus, and probe enters cavity two and one-half inches. Diagnosis, prolapse of the uterus in the second stage; treatment, mechanical support to the uterus by means of McIntosh's stem pessary, and internally ferruginous tonics, iodide of potassium, and liq. potass. arsenit. This much for the history of the case, as compiled from an office examination.

Calling at the residence of the patient next day for the purpose of adjusting the uterine supporter, I made an examination by the touch, and, upon introducing my finger between the pubic arch and the anterior lip of the prolapsed cervix, I was requested by her to be very careful in manipulating those parts, as she was very prone, by reason of her passionate nature, to have the sexual orgasm produced by very slight contact of the finger. Indeed, she stated that this had more than once occurred to her, when making digital investigation of herself. Here then was an opportunity never before afforded any one to my knowledge, and one not to be lost upon any consideration. Carefully separating the vulvæ with my left hand, so that the os uteri was brought clearly into view in a strong light, I swept the right forefinger across

78. DURATION OF THE ACT.—The duration of the act is very brief in healthy persons—but a few minutes—though we find considerable variation in different persons of both sexes. In some men the excitation is so extreme that penetration is hardly effected before the venereal orgasm occurs. In others there is a tardy and not complete turgescence of the erectile

---

the cervix two or three times, when, almost immediately, the orgasm occurred and the following is what was presented to my view:

The os and cervix uteri had been firm, hard, and generally in a normal condition, with the os closed so as not to admit the uterine probe without difficulty; but immediately the os opened to the extent of fully an inch, made five or six successive gasps, drawing the external os into the cervix each time powerfully, and at the same time becoming quite soft to the touch. All these phenomena occurred within the space of twelve seconds' time certainly, and in an instant all was as before; the os had closed, the cervix hardened, and the relation of the parts had become as before the orgasm.

Now I carefully questioned my patient as to the nature of the sensations experienced by her at the period of excitement, and she is very positive that they were the same in *quality* as they ever were during coition, even before the occurrence of the prolapse; but admits that they were not exactly the same in *quantity*, believing that during coition the orgasm had *lasted longer*; although not at all or in any respect different as to sensation. I had almost forgotten to make mention of the intense congestion of the parts during the "crisis," and introduce the statement here.

When, in connection with the statement of the patient, who is a very intelligent and appreciative lady, I add my own observation to the effect that there was no inflammation of any kind present either in the os or cervix uteri, the vagina, bladder, or rectum, and that the parts were in an entirely normal condition except as to position, I think we had the phenomena before us which are always present during coition; and the passage of the spermatic fluid into the uterus was explained fully, satisfactorily, and beyond the shadow of a doubt.

I do not doubt that many of my readers have seen in streams of water, sometime during their lives, a species of fish known as the "sucker," which has a very peculiar shaped mouth. These fish, when at rest in the water, pass the water through their mouths and out at their gills as all other fish do, but, in doing so, they make a peculiar suction motion with their mouths, in which the mouth is inverted into itself. Precisely such a motion does the uterus make during the period of sexual excitement. This is a homely illustration, I am aware, but I know of none other in nature which answers so well.

tissue, and necessarily there is a want of sensitiveness in the penis, and coition is prolonged and the venereal orgasm obtained with difficulty. This is especially the case where the organs are exhausted by sexual excesses.

79. As has been already remarked, women have less desire, a more tardy turgescence of the erectile tissue, and less sensitiveness of the sexual organs. Probably the venereal orgasm is not complete, in the majority of women, once in ten times, and I have been informed by intelligent married women, that they had never experienced it, and had rarely felt any pleasurable sensation. In some it is experienced just after a menstrual period, and not at other times, or when there has been long abstinence.

80. In some the excitation of the female organs is so slow, that the man completes the act before the sexual nerves have been sufficiently aroused to call forth reflex action. Many cases of disease are produced in this way. The husband has strong desires, and has frequent connection for gratification, but each time he only arouses sexual excitement in the wife without gratification, and the female organs are left in a state of turgescence without natural relief.

81. It may be remarked that coition produces less exhaustion, and conduces to the health of the parties, when the act is complete with both. That it may be so, the sexual organs should not be abused, and the sexual act should be performed as well for the satisfaction of the opposite party, as for self-gratification. We may notice further that the imperfect coitus leads to abuse of the sexual organs, especially upon the

---

This then is the explanation of the passage of the spermatozoa to their destination: the act of coition arouses some special nervous action in the uterus which causes it to act in the manner above described, when the "crisis" arrives. I do not believe that the operation is either purely physical, or simply mechanical, but feel sure that the great nerve-centers have more or less the control of the matter, although perhaps this is not now demonstrable.—*St. Louis Medical and Surgical Journal.*

part of the male, for the vasa deferentia not being fully relieved, there is continued desire.

82. THE IMMEDIATE EFFECT OF THE ACT.—The immediate effect of the act is a temporary exhaustion and languor, and in many persons a desire to sleep. In some rare cases the excitation during the venereal spasm is so extreme as to cause death. Thus cases are reported in which men have died suddenly on their wedding night, and more frequently we have coroner's inquests on men found dead in houses of ill-fame, without any trace of ill-usage or poison.

83. In the majority of persons, where connection is not too frequent, it is followed by a sense of self-satisfaction and fresh vigor. Lallemand remarked, "When connection is followed by a joyous feeling, as well as fresh vigor; when the head feels more free and easy, the body more elastic and lighter; when a greater disposition to exercise or intellectual labor arises, and the genital organs evince an increased vigor and activity, we may infer that an imperious want has been satisfied within the limits necessary for health. The happy influence which all the organs experience is similar to that which follows the accomplishment of every function necessary to the economy."

There is no doubt but that the proper gratification of the sexual function is conducive to health and longevity; and if so we very reasonably conclude that the abuse of the function predisposes to disease and shortens life.

84. REPETITION OF THE ACT.—We are frequently asked, when cautioning persons against the abuse of the sexual organs, "how frequently should connection be had?" The quotation from Lallemand, just given, is a very good answer. When the individual feels buoyant and vigorous after its performance, it is not too frequent; when languor persists for some time, or there is a sense of feebleness of the organs, it is too frequent.

Some persons might for a time have connection every night without exhaustion, and I have known men who kept it up for many years. In rare cases the rutting propensity is so great that coition is had several times in one night. In others, and probably the majority, once or twice a week will be the extent of full capacity.*

---

*In Jeremy Taylor's rules for holy living we find the following advice for married persons: "In their permissions and license, they must be sure to observe the order of nature and the ends of God. *He is an ill husband that uses his wife as a man treats a harlot*, having no other end but pleasure. Concerning which our best rule is, that although in this, as in eating and drinking, there is an appetite to be satisfied, which can not be done without pleasing that desire, yet since that desire and satisfaction were intended by nature for other ends, they should never be separate from those ends, but always be joined with all or one of these ends, *with a desire of children, or to avoid fornication, or to lighten and ease the cares and sadnesses of household affairs, or to endear each other*; but never with a purpose, either in act or desire, to separate the sensuality from these ends which hallow it.

"Married persons must keep such modesty and decency of treating each other that they never force themselves into high and violent lusts with arts and misbecoming devices; always remembering that those mixtures are most innocent which are *most simple* and *most natural, most orderly* and *most safe*. It is the duty of matrimonial chastity to be restrained and temperate in the use of their lawful pleasures; concerning which, although no universal rule can antecedently be given to all persons, any more than to all bodies one proportion of meat and drink, yet married persons are to estimate the degree of their license according to the following proportions:—1. That it be moderate, so as to consist with health. 2. That it be so ordered as not to be too expensive of time, that precious opportunity of working out our salvation. 3. That when duty is demanded, it be always paid (so far as in our powers and election) according to the foregoing measures. 4. That it be with a temperate affection, without violent transporting desires or too sensual applications. Concerning which a man is to make judgment by proportion to other actions and the severities of his religion, and the sentences of sober and wise persons, always remembering that marriage is a provision for supply of the natural necessities of the body, not for the artificial and procured appetites of the mind. And it is a sad truth that many married persons, thinking that the floodgates of liberty are set wide open, without measures or restraints (so they sail in the channel), have felt the final rewards of intemperance and lust by their unlawful using of lawful permissions. Only let each of them be tem-

If sexual intercourse is too frequent the man suffers in two ways—from the drain upon the system by the forced secretion of semen, and by the exhaustion of the nervous system from over-excitation. The woman more frequently suffers from nervous exhaustion, if the coition is complete, and from nervous irritability if there has been excitation without the venereal spasm.

MASTURBATION.

85. During childhood, the sexual organs are immature, and the sexual sense should be in complete abeyance. It is true that the child possesses sexual sensibility, and it need but be called into exercise to develop rapidly. Hence in the training of children all such causes of excitement, whether of the sexual organs, or of the mind, should be avoided.

86. With the majority of children there is entire ignorance in this respect, and here very surely "ignorance is bliss." But children are very imitative and learn rapidly, and sometimes the seeds of future ills will be sown by careless parents or servants; and in some cases accident teaches the child that excitation of the sexual organs gives pleasure.

87. I have known cases, as young as two years, where it required much care upon the part of the mother to break up the habit of exciting the sexual organs to erection. The little fellow had found by accident or otherwise that handling

---

perate, and both of them be modest. Socrates was wont to say that those women to whom nature had not been indulgent in good features and colors should make it up themselves with excellent manners, and those who were beautiful and comely should be careful that so fair a body be not polluted with unhandsome usages. To which Plutarch adds, that a wife, if she be unhandsome, should consider how extremely ugly she should be if she wanted modesty; but if she be handsome, let her think how gracious that beauty would be if she superadds chastity."—*Bell and Daldy Edition*, 1857.

the penis, or rubbing it, was pleasant, and would persist in doing it. If continued, it very surely impairs the health—the child loses flesh and strength, and the nervous system suffers.

88. In the majority of cases the habit is readily broken up by careful attention. In very young children the clothing may be so arranged, that the hands can not reach the organ; in all, the mother should endeavor to control the habit by persuasion and judicious reproof.

89. Boys will learn the practice of masturbation as early as six or eight years, if thrown in company with older boys who are addicted to the habit. It seems like a good joke to the older ones, and they frequently gratify their prurient imagination in this way. Parents can not be too careful, even of young boys, and especially is it impolitic to let them associate with, or sleep with those who may be suspected of masturbation.

90. The health of young boys frequently suffers more than when the habit is acquired at a later age. It is noticed that the child is not as free and open as before, is bashful and timid, the hands involuntarily seek the sexual organs in sleep, and sometimes in the day. They become nervous, are easily startled, the sleep is broken, and finally we have loss of flesh and strength, impairment of the mind, and it may be convulsions.

91. In the majority of cases the habit may be broken up, by careful attention on the part of parents. The nobler faculties of the mind should be called into play, prompt him to be "manly," and withdraw him from the society of those who would lead him astray. Such a boy should be carefully guarded, and for weeks or months should be constantly under surveilance, though without his knowledge. In the majority of cases, it does not require a very long time, if there is a complete suspension of the habit, and forgetfulness of it as well.

92. In some cases the nervousness that is so prominent

may be arrested by—℞ Tincture Pulsatilla, gtts. v.; Water, ℥iv.; a teaspoonful every four hours. If there is irritation of the bas-fond of the bladder and urethra—℞ Tincture Eryngium, gtts. xxx.; Tincture Pulsatilla, gtts. v.; Water, ℥iv.; a teaspoonful four times a day; or ℞ Santonine, grs. xx.; Sugar, ℨij. Mix, and make forty powders—one three times a day.

93. In some rare cases, the evil has become so fixed, that masturbation is performed involuntarily, or at least the sufferer has no power to withhold his hands. So serious does it become at times, that the excitation is effected with the legs, when the hands can not be used. Here it becomes necessary to make such application to the penis as will make excitation of it impossible. Acetum Cantharides, Cantharidal Collodion, or Dupy's Cantharidal Oil, will serve this purpose—a very small portion being applied in two or three places whilst the boy is sleeping. He need not know but what this soreness is natural, indeed it is better that he should think so, and attribute it to the practice of masturbation.

94. The general treatment will be that indicated for the relief of the nervous suffering as above, and such restorative medication as may be indicated. If the habit is once arrested, we will see a marked improvement in a few weeks, and with careful surveilance, it may be completely broken up within the year. When epileptic symptoms show themselves, or there is a marked impairment of the mind, the Bromide of Ammonium in the usual doses, will be found the most effective remedy.

95. From the age of twelve to eighteen masturbation is a common vice, few boys escaping wholly. It is learned by association with others, whether in school or in company for play, or wherever or whenever boys are brought together. At the age of puberty the sexual organs have an increased development, and become more sensitive to excitement both local and mental. The youth feels the attraction of the opposite sex, and the sexual organs respond readily to sensuous

thoughts. Intuitively he is conscious of their pleasurable use, and it needs little prompting from others to gratification in this way.

96. In all right minded boys this gratification is at first followed by a sense of disgust, and they repeat it with hesitation. But after a time they are no longer affected in this way, prurient thoughts take prominent place in the mind, and prompt to self-abuse. It is a repetition of Pope's couplet:—

"Vice is a monster of such hideous mien," etc.

97. Masturbation is most frequently commenced where boys are associated together, but the habit is most destructive when its practice is continued alone—"solitary vice." As the victim goes on, he has less and less power to resist, even though he may know that it is injurious, and may have the desire to quit it.

The unnatural drain upon the system impairs the general health, and the abnormal excitation injures the nervous system. The youth loses energy, is sluggish in his movements, his shoulders droop forward, looks down, and bends forward when he sits; evidently there is impairment of nutrition and loss of tone. His character has also changed, he is no longer open and free even with his associates, seeks solitude, and is diffident and bashful when in the company of women. In some cases they become irritable and fretful, have little courage, are easily startled, and do not sleep soundly.*

---

*"However young the children may be, they get thin, pale, and irritable, and their features become haggard. We notice the sunken eye, the long, cadaverous-looking countenance, the downcast look which seems to arise from a consciousness in the boy that his habits are suspected, and, at a later period, from the ascertained fact that his virility is lost. I wish by no means to assert that every boy unable to look another in the face, is or has been a masturbator, but I believe this vice is a very frequent cause of timidity. Habitual masturbators have a dank, moist, cold hand, very characteristic of great vital exhaustion; their sleep is short, and most complete marasmus comes on; they may gradually waste away if the evil passion is not got the better of; nervous

98. In rare cases the condition becomes pitiable. In addition to loss of flesh and strength, and the ability to work, play, or study, the nervous suffering becomes extreme. The sufferer is haunted by the fear that he will lose his mind, or that something unpleasant, he knows not what, may happen to him. His mind dwells constantly on his unpleasant condition, and his morbid fancies run riot over all the unpleasant things he may have heard of. Sometimes the mind is permanently impaired, or epilepsy is induced.

99. The habit of masturbation is sometimes persisted in through life. Recently a case was reported, in which the party confessed to its practice almost every night from boyhood up to the age of sixty-nine. Yet he was a married man, had raised a large family, and did not seem to suffer from the excessive drain. Such instances are very rare, for usually, the onanist fails of success in life.

100. In persons of mature years it is singular to what experiments prurient thoughts will prompt. In my earlier practice I had a ludicrous example. A man, some forty years of age, rang me up one night. He had something covered up in front of him and seemed to be suffering severely. A brief explanation and inspection showed that he had inserted his penis, when flaccid, through the neck of a bottle and was fast. There was nothing to do but break the neck of the bottle, which was accomplished with but slight injury to the organ. Our surgical authorities report many similar cases. Among these, the man who fitted his wedding ring over the penis, another who employed a napkin ring, and others who employed rings of other kinds. The operation of filing or cutting them off, was not a very pleasant experience. Probably one of the most ludicrous cases was the man who, taking a bath, fancied the opening of the stop-cock would afford "a

---

symptoms set in, such as spasmodic contraction, or partial or entire convulsive movements, together with epilepsy, eclampsy, and a species of paralysis accompanied with contractions of the limbs."—*Lallemand.*

good opening for a young man." His cries brought assistance, and he was found suspended to it by his penis.

101. Self-pollution is the cause of many of the chronic diseases of the reproductive organs, especially of prostatorrhœa, spermatorrhœa, and sexual debility. The undue stimulation of the organs and prurient thoughts lead to nocturnal emissions, which persist even after the sufferer sees the evil effects of masturbation, and ceases to abuse himself. And from this involuntary excitation may grow all the lesions which we will have to study.

102. As a general rule, we find that the habit of masturbation may be readily broken up, if proper measures are taken. A full explanation of the evil consequences that are likely to ensue if it is persisted in, and an appeal to their better instincts, will frequently be sufficient. If there is any one thing that a man values more than another, it is the capacity of a man sexually. Let the youth know that self-abuse is followed by impaired health of body and mind, and sexual debility and disease, and you present the strongest argument for continence.

103. It is true it requires a strong effort to break up the habit, when it has been followed for a length of time. Quite as much, probably, as to stop drinking, opium eating, or other habits of intemperance. It requires a strong motive, but this subject may be so presented as to offer the strongest inducement to quit forever the pernicious habit.

104. Breaking up associations with idle and dissolute young men, and bringing the youth into the society of the opposite sex, is very important in many cases. Rarely do we find self-abuse in either sex, in our public schools, or where there are mixed classes. Free association with the opposite sex of the same age is almost a sure protection against this vice, as it may also be a means of cure. This is a strong argument in favor of the education of the youth of both sexes together, and one that should not be overlooked. Add to this the fact that youth educated in mixed classes are less

likely to sexual excesses when they have reached adult years, having better control over the sexual instinct, we conclude that as the world grows wiser, it will find safety at least in this regard in our public school system.

105. Active employment is an excellent means of breaking up the habit. If a boy is employed from morning until night, both mind and body being engaged, there is less disposition to prurient thought or sexual excitement, indeed in many cases the desire is wholly in abeyance. Lallemand remarks, "The urgent necessity of recruiting each day the great waste occasioned by varied and progressive gymnastic exercise diminishes in an equal proportion the secretion of semen ; for the economy only occupies itself with the reproduction of the species when it has provided for the conservation of the individual, as I stated when speaking of the influence of nutrition on generation.

106. In those cases in which the sufferer has become convinced of his error, and has stopped the habit, but being alarmed by the possible results, allows his mind to dwell constantly on the subject, we may employ remedies to advantage. He is nervous and timid, has a fear of impending danger, with sometimes unpleasant sensations of fullness in the head or dizziness; of tightness in the chest and præcordial oppression.

Occasionally functional heart disease springs from this nervous trouble, and there is palpitation or irregular action. In some the nervous excitation assumes an epileptic character, or epilepsy may be fully developed, and run its usual course.

107. For the head symptoms I have been in the habit of prescribing Pulsatilla, as — ℞ Tincture of Pulsatilla, ʒss.; Water, ℥iv.; a teaspoonful four times a day. If there is prostatic irritation with discharge, or the patient is morose and irritable, we may add the Staphysagria in the same proportion. For the epileptic tendency I have obtained better results from the Bromide of Ammonium ʒss. to Water ℥iv.; a teaspoonful three or four times a day. Bromide of Potassium

may be used when patients are full blooded, and excitement of the sexual organs present, and Bromide of Lime at bed-time when the sleep is broken and not refreshing.

108. If the general health is impaired, we treat the patient according to special indications. If the indications for any medicine are pronounced, we will sometimes find that it will be a remedy for the nervous and mental lesions as well as the physical. Thus in a recent very severe case, the violet coloration of tongue, nails, etc., indicating Nitric Acid, it gave rest and strength to the nervous system, good sleep, and there was a rapid recovery.

MASTURBATION IN WOMEN.

109. Whilst our older authorities have almost wholly ignored the fact of self-pollution in women, some recent writers have given it undue prominence. We have already seen that the sexual sense was less developed in women than in men, and the desire for sexual gratification very much less. With most women the desire is only associated with *love*, and is probably as much or more for the pleasure of the loved one as for self-gratification. In the majority the sexual sense requires stimulation from mental impressions and emotions, and is developed by loving caresses, which by reflex action excite the sexual organs. The majority of women are, therefore, wholly free from this vice.

110. In some, however, from disease, or from a wrong mental organization, or an undue sensitiveness of the sexual organs, strong sexual desires are awakened, and as they can not have natural satisfaction, masturbation is resorted to. It is, probably, more frequently a vice of female boarding schools, especially where the pupils sleep together and are not under proper restraint. The cases must be very rare when

the sexes are educated together, and they are also rare in convent education.

111. There are two periods in the life of women when there is the greatest tendency to self-pollution. The first is from the first appearance of the menstrual discharge to the full development of the body; the second from the age of twenty-seven to thirty-five, especially in those who have been disappointed in love. At those ages also we find the greatest tendency to lapse from virtue, and the ranks of prostitutes are recruited from those ages.

112. There is not only the less imperative desire on the part of the female, but there is also less gratification from masturbation. Thus a girl may be persuaded by an associate to commit the act, but finding little gratification from it, and this little more than compensated by the loss of self-respect and disgust which follows, she never repeats it again. I am satisfied that these statements are correct, as I have them from ladies who have had a large experience as educators of women.

113. When once habituated to masturbation, the girl or woman exercises much ingenuity in finding objects to gratify her desires. Anything that is moderately smooth and of proper size answers the purpose, and if nothing can be had, the hand is made to answer the purpose. In some cases the excitation of the urethra is found more pleasurable than the vagina, and thus we have numbers of cases reported in which hair-pins, pencils, etc., have escaped into the bladder, and have been removed by dilatation, or an operation. I have had one case where a piece of turned wood, acorn-shaped, the ornament of an old-fashioned bed-post, was employed, and being fully introduced into the vagina could not be withdrawn by the woman. It required the use of the forceps, and considerable effort for its withdrawal.

114. Women suffer from masturbation in a similar manner to men. The undue excitement stimulates the emotions at the expense of the will, and the sufferer becomes hysterical,

and at times very despondent. She finds that her memory is impaired, she can not think clearly, loses her ambition, and the ordinary pursuits of life become burdensome. The general health also suffers, and the various vital functions are impaired.

115. In addition to this, the abnormal excitement of the sexual organs leads to local disease, and may produce any of the many lesions to which women are subject. The more common diseases are vaginal and cervical leucorrhœa, disease and flexions of the cervix, and prolapsus uteri.*

116. The treatment of these cases will be similar to that named for the other sex. When the injurious results are pointed out, and probably proven by the patient's present sensations, the habit will generally be abandoned. Parents

---

*Perhaps the present is the most suitable time I shall find for alluding to a practice, unfortunately of not very rare occurrence, which, while it destroys the health of the body, if persisted in, impairs in no less a degree the powers of mind, and which is nearly always accompanied by leucorrhœa—I allude to masturbation. I do not believe all I have heard as to its great frequency, but that it is practised by many females is too true. In some, I have no doubt, it has been the result of uterine disease, the habit having been contracted accidentally in the first instance, in the efforts to procure alleviation from the irritation which so often exists about the orifice of the vagina; but, be the cause what it may, it is soon accompanied by vaginitis and endo-cervicitis, manifested by the presence of the well-known glairy cervical discharge. Beware, however, of charging a patient with being addicted to this degrading habit, because suspicious symptoms present themselves; the dilated pupil, the downcast look, the uncontrollable excitement, which a vaginal examination causes, generally tell the tale; added to this, there is often a severe lancinating pain complained of immediately over the pubes, and in several cases I have noticed that vomiting *at night* has been a prominent symptom. These distressing cases can be cured by moral means alone; local treatment is useless, and generally injurious, for it attracts the patient's attention to the genital organs, the very thing we should be most anxious to avoid. I can not find words sufficiently strong to condemn, as I would, the barbarous practice of mutilating the patient by the removal of the clitoris. This operation is as useless as it is disgusting, for there is no truth in the idea that in the clitoris alone is seated the nervous expansion which subserves the sexual orgasm.—*Athill.*

must never forget, however, that girls should never be exposed to such influences as will lead to self-pollution.

117. The nervous system may be relieved by the use of Pulsatilla, Macrotys, Staphysagria, and the Bromides, as has been described. A restorative treatment may be necessary, with bathing, out-door exercise, and especially some regular occupation. All disease of the sexual organs may be treated in the usual manner. In these cases frequent examinations, by touch or speculum, is much to be deprecated, and local applications should be used as sparingly as possible.

MARITAL EXCESSES.

118. It is a common opinion that the marriage rite gives entire freedom in sexual congress, and few persons ever think that it may be abused. The man believes that now he may legitimately gratify the sexual instinct, and the woman thinks she is bound by the marital tie to yield to his solicitations. In sleeping together, (a very bad habit of married people), there is cause for undue excitement upon the part of the husband, and abundant opportunity for its gratification.

119. Men have most absurd ideas of the marital demand. They think that the good impressions they may have made on the wife, and the affection they have won, may be lost, unless they show that they have abundant ability to *consummate* the marriage rite. Probably this is one cause of marital excess at first, and a fear of impaired virility may be a cause for its continuance.

120. As Acton well remarks, "This feeling of *virility* is much more developed in man than is maternity in woman. Its existence, indeed, seems necessary to give a man that consciousness of his dignity, of his character as head and ruler, and of his importance, which is absolutely essential to the well-being of the family, and through it, of society itself. It

is a power, a privilege, of which the man is, and should be, proud—so proud that he should husband it, and not squander or deprave it. Too many a man, with a recklessness that can only be attributed to ignorance of its value, exhausts or defiles this noblest prerogative of his manhood, a possession as precious in its own way as that of chastity."

But as we have already seen, the husband may be disabused of the idea, that frequent coition is expected by the wife. Her passions are not urgent, and she is satisfied with occasional intercourse. Neither can virility be increased by this frequent use; indeed we find that the contrary effect ensues, and the virile power is frequently weakened, and sometimes lost by marital abuse.

121. Marital excess is the rule, a moderate and legitimate gratification the exception. None know this better than the physician, yet how rarely are they willing to state the facts, even though this may be a cause of severe disease, and may endanger life.*

---

*It is a common notion among the public, and even among professional men, that the word *excess* chiefly applies to *illicit* sexual connection. Of course, whether extravagant in degree or not, all such connection is, from one point of view, *an excess*. But any warning against sexual dangers would be very incomplete if it did not extend to the excesses too often committed by married persons in ignorance of their ill-effects. Too frequent emissions of the life-giving fluid, and too frequent sexual excitement of the nervous system are, as we have seen, in themselves most destructive. The result is the same within the marriage bond as without it. The married man who thinks that, because he is a married man, he can commit no excess, however often the act of sexual congress is repeated, will suffer as certainly as the unmarried debauchee who acts on the same principle in his indulgences—perhaps more certainly, from his very ignorance, and from his not taking those precautions and following those rules which a career of vice is apt to teach the sensualist. Many a man has, until his marriage, lived a most continent life; so has his wife. As soon as they are wedded, intercourse is indulged in night after night; neither party having any idea that these repeated sexual acts are excesses which the system of neither can bear, and which to the man, at least, is absolute ruin. The practice is continued till health is impaired, sometimes permanently; and when a patient is at last obliged to seek medical advice, he is thunderstruck at

122. The wife suffers far more frequently than the husband. Sometimes in the first weeks of married life, the excesses of the husband are sufficient to impair her health, and he is forced to moderate or suspend sexual intercourse. In others the bloom slowly leaves her cheeks, she experiences aches and pains to which before marriage she had been a stranger. The vegetative functions are impaired, and she slowly loses flesh and strength, and in a year or two is prematurely aged.

123. This cause is supplemented by the cares and over-exertion incident to housekeeping, for which probably she is unfitted by age or education. Add to this the still further drain on vitality of child-bearing and nursing, and we need not wonder at the poor health of our wives and mothers.

124. Whilst it is true that moderate indulgence in sexual intercourse is conducive to health, in both sexes, it is certain that the marital relation is followed by an abuse by the majority. In some instances the husband suffers in his general health, whilst the wife grows vigorous. In others, and far more frequently, the wife suffers, the husband enjoying robust health. In rare cases, both parties suffer equally.

125. It may be said that sexual intercourse is not injurious to either party, when the act is fully complete in each. Even when frequent, we find the ill effects but slight, when compared with the imperfect sexual orgasm. This is well illustrated by the cases of some prostitutes, who enjoy excellent health when they enjoy free intercourse with stout, virile men, but suffer when they are kept by one who lacks virility. I have known instances of this in married life—women who

---

learning that his sufferings arise from excesses unwittingly committed. Married people often appear to think that connection may be repeated just as regularly and almost as often as their meals. Till they are told of the danger the idea never enters their heads that they have been guilty of great and almost criminal excess; nor is this to be wondered at, since the possibility of such a cause of disease is seldom hinted at by the medical man they consult.—*Acton.*

enjoyed excellent health with one husband, but had poor health with another, though all other conditions were the same.

126. Prostatorrhœa and spermatorrhœa may result from marital abuse, as well as from masturbation, and the symptoms will not materially differ in the two cases. The condition of the female, analogous to spermatorrhœa in the male, is most frequently produced by marital excess.

127. Acton remarks, "Since my attention has been particularly called to this class of ailments, I feel confident that many of the forms of indigestion, general ill health, hypochondria, etc., so often met with in adults, depend upon sexual excesses. The directors of Hydropathic establishments must, probably, hold some such opinions, or they would not have thought it expedient to separate married patients when they are undergoing the water treatment. That this cause of illness is not more widely acknowledged and acted on, arises from the natural delicacy which medical men must feel in putting such questions to their patients as are necessary to elicit the facts."

128. Bedding married persons together is a very bad habit at best. Outside of the sexual abuse that springs from it, it frequently proves injurious, the feebler party losing life by simple contact. Add to this the absorption of the exhalations from the body, inhaling the breath, or a vitiated atmosphere, and we find frequent cause for prescribing single beds, if not separate rooms.

129. The wife should not lose control of her person by the marriage rite. It is hers to say when the husband shall have intercourse, his to gain the end by endeavors to please. This is a law of animal life, and in no species is it violated but in man.

130. As a general rule there is little difficulty in rectifying these marital wrongs, when once they are determined. If a man has a true affection for his wife, and learns that he is causing disease by frequent intercourse, he will moderate his

passions, consent to single beds, or to absolute continence, for a time, if it is necessary. When a man is so brutish that he will gratify his desires at the expense of the health, happiness, or life of the wife, there is no marital bond that should compel her to submit.

131. I have had occasion to prescribe single beds very many times, and it has been pretty uniformly followed by better health, and greater happiness to both parties. It does not prevent normal sexual gratification, but it is a means of preventing abuse. The husband is necessarily placed in his proper relation, and must solicit the favor of the wife, and she will not be inclined to submit too frequently to injure the health of either.

PROSTITUTION.

132. As we have already seen, the sexual instinct in man is very strong, and under some circumstances, will have gratification. Entire continence through life is possible to some; continence to complete maturity, is possible to a large number, though, as Acton remarks, it requires "a strong influence of the will, and a courageous self-rule." Proper training from childhood up will have strengthened the will, whilst at the same time the sexual instinct has not gained strength, by avoidance of those circumstances calculated to call it forth.

133. In the earlier ages of man, he was governed to a very considerable extent by purely animal instincts. And this function in all probability was exercised in a manner similar to that we observe in the higher mammalia. In our higher civilization there is no animal so libidinous as man, but as we descend toward barbarism we find there is less and less tendency to sexual excesses. Primitive man had women in common, and sexual selection was governed by the same laws as in the animal kingdom. The desire of the female

would be strongest at such periods as would render intercourse most fertile, and at these times the solicitations of the male would be most successful. As the female had the choice of a father for her children, she would most likely select the strongest and most attractive, and thus the condition of the race would be improved.

134. With an improvement of race and condition, would come better provision for the animal wants—shelter, food, clothing, and an idea of ownership—which would soon extend to women. As each individual would endeavor to obtain as much of all the goods as possible, men would strive for the possession of women, and the stronger and more highly developed men would obtain a plurality.

135. Nature wisely provides for her creatures in all circumstances of life. To a people practicing polygamy, a larger proportion of female births would be essential, otherwise a portion of the males would be deprived of wives. In those rare cases where a people practice *polyandria*, one woman having several husbands, a larger number of male births would be necessary.

136. It would have seemed that in those periods when polygamy was constantly practiced, prostitution would have been unnecessary. Yet we find it existing in the midst of and practiced by the much married, as well as by those who were restricted to one wife. Thus we read in Genesis that when Judah, going up to the sheep-shearing, saw Tamar sitting in an open place, "he thought her to be a harlot." "And he turned unto her by the way and said, Go to, I pray thee, let me come in unto thee. And she said, What wilt thou give me?" This may be taken as the earliest record of prostitution, though the reason is doubtless from want of record rather than from absence of prostitution.

137. In every age of the world since we have written history we find that prostitution has prevailed to a greater or less extent. There have been times when it was recognized and protected by law, and again periods when it was prohib-

ited and severe punishments meted out to the outcast women, but through all it has maintained its existence, and continually renewed its votaries. No stronger evidence could be adduced that it is an absolute necessity of our present social existence, and that it would be the part of prudence to recognize it, and by judicious laws so regulate it that the least evil may grow out of it.

138. It is not necessary for our purpose to trace the history of prostitution, as it is the same in all countries and among all peoples. The *lupanaria* of Rome were not materially different from the bawdy-houses of the present day, both loving darkness better than light. Yet a truth is forced upon us by the examination of this history—the evil becomes less as it is allowed more liberty, and is not forced to seek the cover of darkness, and the by-ways of great cities.

139. There was a period in ancient Greece and Rome when prostitution was not considered disgraceful, and when Thais, Lais, Aspasia, Phyrne, and many others were noted for their graces of body and mind, and held a desirable social relation. If history is to be believed, we would reach the conclusion, that chastity or unchastity has little influence in woman's degradation, as compared to the public ban which forces her to hide herself from all that is good in the world.

140. When we come to study prostitution in our day, we are surprised at its extent, and the powerful hold it has upon the people; living and prospering, though prohibited by law and condemned by religion and social usage. It shows itself in many phases, from the common street-bawd, who sells her favors to whoever will buy, to the woman of education and refinement, who finds pleasure, support and gratification of her love of dress and luxury in it. Of the common prostitute we have about one to each one thousand inhabitants; and of those who do not make it an entire means of support, probably twice this number.

141. Prostitutes who lead regular lives do not suffer in health as many imagine; but the larger number add intem-

perance to sexual excess, and from this, and disease of the reproductive organs, the larger number die young, the average duration of prostitution being but about six years. Kept women, or those who see but few men, are usually healthy, and quite frequently live to a good age.

142. Diseases of the reproductive organs are frequent among prostitutes. The simplest forms are acute inflammations of the uterus and ovaries from excess and intemperance, vaginitis and vaginal leucorrhœa, displacements of the uterus, and urethral and vesical irritation. In the majority there is a strong love of social pleasures, and a kindly feeling for others hardly surpassed in other classes. Insanity is of rare occurrence, and one is surprised at the knowledge of men and things shown by mere girls in age.

143. In large cities many women moving in good society visit houses of prostitution and assignation for the gratification of the sexual appetite. These most frequently confine their favors to one man, but sometimes exceed the common-bawd for promiscuity. These are not to be regarded as sinners *par excellence*, for in many cases they are women of most kindly feelings, and with this exception are inclined to do right. We may, indeed, regard it as a disease, as is intemperance, and we pity more than we blame, and use remedies to cure, rather than means to punish. Surely the fact that they are women should not cause us to lose sight of our common humanity and the commands of charity.

144. Private women, or kept mistresses, will probably number as many as the regular prostitutes. Many causes are operative to replenish their ranks. Seduction possibly stands first, as it does in furnishing inmates of houses of prostitution. Following this comes the love of dress, of ease, of luxury, without labor; strong sexual desires that must have gratification; and last, though not least, the difficulty in procuring work that will yield a decent support, and that is regarded as respectable.

145. Society might and should provide means for the pro-

tection of these women. Let the law punish seduction as a penitentiary offence (surely the crime against society is gross enough); let it legitimatize children born out of wedlock, that they may bear the father's name, and inherit in common with those born in wedlock, and the first cause will be to a considerable extent removed.

146. Let a people honor habits of industry and thrift, condemn over-dress and display, regard men and women for their intrinsic worth rather than for the clothes they wear, and you will have removed the second cause. Man is an imitative animal. If fine clothes and accessories make fine people—and people are constantly planning and striving for this. If for it they risk their good name for honesty and fair dealing, take advantage of the neighbor, sell sons or daughters in marriage—why should we blame the woman who sells her favors for what society thinks so desirable?

147. Make labor honorable, and pay women for the work they do, and we will have removed the last cause. We have made the honorable work of caring for a household *servile*, and treat the woman who aids the mother in her cares, as if she was of a different species. We complain of the scarcity of servants, of their incompetence, and forget that we have made both by lowering the character of the employment.

148. Can you prevent prostitution by legal enactments?*

*"It (the report) states that the women in the several places subject to the Acts attended with regularity throughout the year, and that in a few instances only was it necessary to take proceedings before a magistrate. The Acts have exercised a repressive influence in several ways. Notwithstanding, we are told, the continued influx of common women from unprotected districts, the total number in the several districts on the 31st of December last had been reduced. The beneficial working of the Acts is, however, more clearly demonstrated by the reduction in the number of juvenile prostitutes; and this is very striking The number of prostitutes in the different districts under the age of seventeen on the 31st of December last was nine; whereas in 1866, when the Acts were first put in force, there were three hundred and seventy-seven under that age. Again, on the 31st of December last, those under the age of eighteen were sixty-seven; whereas in 1866 there were five hundred

No. You can not even lessen it; indeed, many times it seems to gain strength by prohibitory laws. Laws against prostitution only cause it to seek by-ways, and hide itself from those who are not interested in it, but never from those who want it. They give secrecy—that which many men desire, and breed disease both moral and physical because there is nothing to control it. The laws are enforced against the women, never against the men. When a house of prostitution is "raided," the women are exposed to the jeers and contumely of the crowded court room, are heavily fined, and sent to the work-house. The men taken with them are privately discharged—and yet we call this a Christian country?

149. Lastly, male prostitution is regarded as rather honorable than otherwise. A fast life is spoken of as rather a good antecedent in a man—and sowing wild oats as rather an agreeable divertisement. Such a man moves in good society, is received in moral families, is intimate with virtuous women, is courted by the church, and marries. But the woman who has sown wild oats, God help her, can never return to society, can never earn bread by honest labor, is of necessity an outcast.

---

and ninety-five! The number of brothels has been reduced by eighty-six during the past year, many of those suppressed being of the lowest description: seventy-one young creatures between the ages of twelve and seventeen, and one hundred and thirty-five women between the ages of seventeen and thirty-one, who were known to have commenced immoral practices, gave up that course of life upon being spoken to by the police; and the Assistant-Commissioner's Report contains individual instances of many girls and married women who owe their rescue from a life of sin and misery to the well-directed and humane efforts of the officials engaged under these Acts."—*Report on the effects of Acts regulating Prostitution.—Lancet.*

PROSTITUTION THE CAUSE OF VENEREAL DISEASE.

150. In prostitution we have the cause of venereal diseases, and it has been supposed that laws for its suppression would eventually eradicate these. Thus, whilst ridding the world of a moral evil, we would get rid of the fearful disease which seems to follow it as a punishment.

But the history of prostitution shows that the influence of prohibitory laws is the reverse of this. We have already seen that laws against prostitution are only partially enforced, can be but partially enforced. Their operation causes the social evil to hide itself in by-ways, and the very secrecy necessary serves as a cause for the propagation of infection, by preventing cleanly habits and proper hygienic surroundings. The woman under the ban of the law, and liable to arrest and punishment at any time, loses that regard for her own health and others, that she would have with better surroundings.

151. It has been denied that laws regulating prostitution diminished the venereal diseases, and we are pointed to the statistics of Paris and some German cities as proof. It is my opinion, however, from the facts that have come to my knowledge, that it is possible to so enforce sanitary laws, as to greatly diminish the danger of infection, and eventually to get rid of the severest types of these diseases.*

---

*Captain McDonough, Chief of Police in St. Louis, in an official report says: "I will recapitulate a few of the moral effects produced by the St. Louis social evil law in this city, which, in my opinion, far outweighs any moral objections which have been, or can be, alleged against it.

"1. By this report it is shown conclusively that the number of public women has uniformly decreased each year.

"2. That they are more decorous in their manner in public.

"3. That the plying of their wicked trade upon the public streets has been almost entirely discontinued.

"4. That a considerable number of abandoned women have been reclaimed and restored to respectable life, and, in several cases, married.

152. As we can trace prostitution through the entire written and traditional history of man, so also can we trace the venereal disease. David doubtless suffered from this when he said:—"My sore ran in the night; there is no rest to my bones, because of my sin. My wounds stink, and are corrupt, because of my foolishness, for my loins are filled with a

---

"5. That clandestine, or private prostitution, which often develops into open vice, has been materially checked, through fear of the legal consequences of such indulgence, when brought home to the offender.

"6. That juvenile prostitution has been greatly diminished, if not wholly removed. * * * That the results have so far been encouraging, is beyond doubt.

"The most enthusiastic promoters of the measure could not have hoped for a larger or more beneficent success than has attended its workings during the two years in which it has been in force. * * * The young and the heedless have been warned by the police of the consequences of entering a life of shame. The number of bawds has largely decreased, and the deaths, formerly very numerous, in consequence of diseases concomitant on a life of shame, have in a great measure been prevented.

"Under the law, this evil has been removed, as it were, from the exclusive domain of the moralist and intrusted to practical heads and practical hands to give it shape and form, in order that, if possible, some good might result from a vice so stupendous and so mischievous; one which has existed and flourished in all nations and all countries from the time whereof the 'memory of man runneth not to the contrary.' St. Louis alone, on this continent, has grappled with the monster; and while it is not claimed that the authorities have suppressed it, or even expected to do so, nevertheless, by the intervention of the strong arm of the law and strict police surveilance, it has been stripped of some of its worst features, and great reductions have been made in the ranks of its votaries, as you may observe from the records of this office, and which are a part of this report."

The Mayor of St. Louis has said: "As many are of the belief that the fact of legally regulating houses of prostitution causes an increase of the evil, I am happy to state that such is not the fact. There has been an actual decrease in the number of these houses and their inmates since the establishment of this law, and the decrease in disease is fully fifty per cent. If this be the case, we think we have all just cause of congratulation that the cause of humanity is being benefited by the social evil ordinance, and that, looking at past results, it can scarcely longer be called an experiment, but a success in all that its most sanguine advocates claimed for it.

loathsome disease, and there is no soundness in my flesh." Probably this is the earliest written account of the venereal, and it may be that this was not the infectious disease with which we are acquainted.

153. The earlier medical writers refer to disease of the reproductive organs, but their descriptions are not very clear, and it has been doubted by some whether syphilis was known, until about the time of the siege of Naples in 1494. Dr. Good in his Study of Medicine remarks:

"It appears to have been known to the world from an early age, as I have remarked in the running comment to the volume of Nosology, that acrimonious and poisonous materials are, at times, secreted by the genitals, capable of exciting local, and perhaps constitutional affections in those who expose themselves to such poisons by incontinent sexual intercourse. Celsus enumerates various diseases of the sexual organs, most of which are only referable to this source of impure contact; but the hideous and alarming malady which was first noticed as proceeding from the same source toward the close of the fifteenth century, and which has since been called almost exclusively *venereal disease*, has suppressed till of late, all attention to these minor evils, in the fearful contemplation of so new and monstrous a pestilence, to various modifications of which most of the anterior and slighter diseases of the same organs seem to have been loosely and generally referred; as though there was but one specific poison issuing from this fountain, and consequently but one specific malady. On which account, much confusion has arisen in the history and description of the disease; and syphilis, its most stinking species, though commonly admitted, as we shall see presently, to be of comparatively recent origin, is by writers of considerable eminence, regarded as of far higher antiquity."

154. The fifteenth century was noted for its immorality, and syphilis may be regarded as the natural result of the venereal excesses of that period. At the siege of Naples referred

to, both the besiegers and besieged seem to have lost all the better instincts of manhood. A venereal delirium was added to the other excesses of the period, and whilst the camps were filled with a multitude of female camp followers, the utmost license was allowed the soldiery. The bloody sorties from the city, hunger and thirst, numbers decimated by disease, and the innumerable woes attending war in that age, were inoperative to check the evil—indeed, served but to stimulate it. In the city, where the sufferings from the siege were still greater, there was the same venereal insanity, and the historians seem at a loss to know whether the disease originated within or without.

155. At this period Columbus returned from his second voyage to America, and it was claimed some years afterwards, that the venereal disease was introduced into Europe by his crews, and was supposed to be the result of their intercourse with the natives. But Fracostoria, who was an eye witness of the entire progress of the disease, claims that it had made its appearance some weeks previously, and had already spread over Auvergne, Lombardy, and Italy.

156. From this period at least, we have a complete history of the malady, and whilst there are undoubtedly periods of special virulence, and of comparative mildness, the general character of the disease has remained the same, and it has presented the same acute and chronic symptoms.

157. These periods of virulence and mildness are too marked to be mistaken, and if we examine into their causes, we may learn an important lesson. In all periods of social turbulence, whether from war or other causes, the venereal disease has been virulent. It is associated with want and suffering, whether from bad harvests, unpropitious seasons, bad hygienic surroundings, or epidemic influences. It grows milder in periods of profound peace, when a people are well fed, well clothed, and well housed; and especially when peace of mind is added to comfort of body.

158. Noticing these facts, we would conclude, that as a

people grow in intelligence and wealth, the comforts of life being pretty equitably distributed, the venereal poison will be less virulent. That as those addicted to prostitution are more kindly cared for by the government, and sanitary laws are enforced, the disease will be less frequent and less virulent. That just in proportion as prostitution is made criminal, and is forced to seek darkness, and to be secure forced to neglect cleanliness and good hygiene, the disease will be more common and more virulent.

159. An army in the field is an excellent illustration. If badly "policed," and sanitary measures neglected, it will suffer severely from disease. But place it in charge of a medical chief, who will strictly police the encampment, and enforce the observance of hygienic laws, and good health is restored. We conclude, therefore, that a strict sanitary police of all houses of prostitution is one of the most important means of prophylaxis against venereal disease.

160. The necessity of personal cleanliness is so obvious, that it need but be alluded to. When this is strictly attended to, persons may escape contagion even though exposed. Atkins remarks, "From what has been written, it must appear clear that the only chance of preventing infection, alike on the male and female is personal cleanliness after sexual intercourse with strangers. The good that has resulted from pelvic inspection of females, as in Paris, Brussels, and other places, has been greatly attributed to the greater attention to personal cleanliness which such inspections have brought about. If a man have sexual intercourse with a strange woman, let him wash the penis immediately after the act, taking care to cleanse the folds of *prepuce*, especially near the frænum, and in the sulcus of the *corona glandis*. If a woman shall have sexual intercourse with a strange man, let her use a syringe with hot water, to wash out the vaginal surface, taking care to cleanse the folds of mucous membrane at the orifice of the canal, and of the *labia pudenda*."

161. Parkes recommended a wash of Sulphate of Zinc.

Others have recommended Carbolic Acid, Sulphurous Acid, and Permanganate of Potash. But if we think for a moment that these agents, if strong enough to destroy the specific character of the virus, will excoriate the organs, we will not attribute prophylactic virtues to them. Certainly the best agents are water and soap. When the tissues are abraded, or delicate, it is probable that absorption takes place during copulation, and in such cases washing is of no benefit, for the most minute portion of virus absorbed is sufficient to infect.

IMPOTENCE IN THE MALE.

162. Of all the faculties of mind or body, there are none that seem to be so highly valued as sexual power. Men will cheerfully endure bodily suffering, or the misfortunes of life, but let them once get the idea that sexual power is failing, or is likely to be lost, and they are most miserable. We hear much about "manhood" and "its loss," as the crown of life, and its most serious misfortune, as if the soul of man resided in his penis, and his chief occupation was the begetting of children. All men seem to think somewhat alike in this respect. A man need not be a Sybarite to have these feelings, for it is the case with the youth devoted to pleasure, as with the parson in gown and bands, or the grave and reverend senior who, from appearance, we would think had passed the period of care in this respect.

163. Whilst, as men, we might laugh at the absurdity of these feelings and this fear, as physicians we are called upon to give relief in these as in other cases. And whilst we may not place the exaggerated estimate upon those powers that others do, we can not fail to recognize the mental suffering that follows their impairment.

164. True impotence is very rare, and one may not see an

example of it in a long practice. The most common forms for which we have to prescribe are from wrong innervation, undue excitation, and impaired innervation.

165. UNDUE EXCITATION.—In some cases the sufferer complains that the venereal excitement is such that the orgasm occurs before penetration can be effected. In others the excitement will culminate without a complete erection. In both the organs may be in normal condition, and erection may be normal except in company with a woman. In some cases it is very certainly a lesion of the mind—the imagination is so active in this direction that the organs are unduly stimulated. In others the over-excitation is from exalted sensibility of the reproductive organs.

166. Doubtless many men have suffered in this way for months, on first getting married, without complaint, until finally the undue exaltation of the nervous system wore off, but sometimes we are asked to give relief. I may give two cases as examples:

L ——, æt. 30, of temperate habits, steadily pursuing his occupation of carpenter, not addicted to masturbation, became so excited at the near prospect of marriage that he had nocturnal emissions, and finally erections during the day with partial emission. He strove to control the feeling, and finally consulted a specialist who prescribed large doses of Bromide of Potassium, with the effect to control the excitement for the time being, and advised the consummation of the marriage. Some weeks afterward he applied to me for aid. His countenance was haggard, step unsteady, appetite poor, tongue furred, bowels constipated, and mind bordering on insanity. The story was clear—though laboring under intense sexual excitement he had not been able to have connection.

I assured him of relief, if he would follow my directions, and volunteered to make such explanations to the wife as would be satisfactory. Absolute continence for ten days was enjoined. A cold salt water sponge bath to spine and pelvis recommended every morning; the bowels were gently moved with a saline cathartic; a single dose of Acetate of Potash to be taken in the evening; Tinct. Nux Vomica, gtts. ij. in the morning; and for the nervous symptoms: ℞ Tincture Pulsatilla, ʒss.; Water, ℥iv.; a teaspoonful four times a day. I need but say, that after the ten days, there was no trouble, and within the year I was called to assist in the delivery of the first child.

B ——, æt. 24, has been married a week, and has not yet been able to consummate the marriage. He is of jovial temperament, and laughs it off, saying that so far as he is concerned he cares very little, but he is grieved on account of his wife. Emission is almost instantaneous upon erection, when the organ becomes flaccid and useless. Ordered: Bromide of Potassium, grs. xxx., two hours before retiring, and a local application to the penis of: ℞ Tannic Acid, ʒss.; Water, ℥iv.; continuance for a few days, when the act was comfortably performed.

167. The treatment of these cases is thus pretty clearly outlined. Allay the patient's fears, and advise continence for a time. For excesssive venereal excitement, Bromide of Potassium. For the peculiar nervous fear, Pulsatilla. For the excessive sensibility of penis, a solution of Tannic Acid, or of Permanganate of Potash.

168. IMPAIRED INNERVATION.—Persons who have suffered from spermatorrhœa frequently have difficulty in copulation. In some cases the erection is incomplete, in others it is so brief as not to give time for the act, in others the sexual stimulation is not sufficient to cause emission. In all of these cases we will find impaired innervation as a principal cause, and its restoration will give relief.

169. TREATMENT.—If there is impairment of the general health, the basis of treatment will be a judicious tonic and restorative course. Occasionally we will find this sufficient.

The special remedies we employ to strengthen the reproductive functions are Nux Vomica, Ergot, Iodine, Phosphorus and Belladonna. These are employed in the usual doses, and associated with the tonics and restoratives. I have been in the habit of prescribing for the simpler of these cases; ℞ Extract of Nux Vomica, Iodine, aa. grs. vj.; Hydrastine, ʒss. M. Make thirty pills, and give one four times a day. The Prussian Phosphuretted Oil, in doses of five drops three times a day, is a valuable addition to this. In one bad case I administered this in combination with Cod Oil and solution of Strychnia with the most gratifying results.

I generally direct the salt water bath to the spine, abdomen, perineum and genitals, to be used on rising in the morning, with brisk friction. Instead of directing that he experiment with the virile member to determine whether he is getting well, I have him live a life of absolute continence, if unmarried, and but occasional intercourse if married. This I deem of the greatest importance.

In those exceptional cases where the organs have been exhausted by excess, and where the person wishes medicine by which he may continue his sexual pleasures, good morals would suggest that we withhold our aid; yet, as medicine is an article of merchandise, and he will get it of some one else, if not of us, we may prescribe the Iodine pill as above.

It is necessary that the patient should have the disease so explained to him, that the morbid fear that is so frequently noticed shall be removed, and for this purpose we will try to gain the patient's implicit confidence. If this is not done, we will frequently find our remedies unavailing. The patient should be directed to take exercise in the open air, to use a daily bath, confine himself to a nutritious and not stimulating diet, and sleep on a hard bed. An entire abandonment of masturbation, and sexual excitement, as far as possible, is imperative, and he should likewise be cautioned not to let his thoughts turn to these subjects. There is no doubt but that the will can materially aid in controlling this unnatural excitation, and if possible it should be made to assist in the cure.

170. STRUCTURAL IMPEDIMENTS.—Among the lesions preventing the sexual act, or causing sterility, we may study the structural diseases of the sexual organs which serve as impediments. These might be grouped in two classes—lesions which prevent penetration, and lesions which prevent ejaculation.

171. Among the first, we may notice those cases in which the penis is congenitally attached to the abdominal wall, or inflammatory adhesions have been formed from ulceration of the skin. Three cases of this kind have come under my observation, in two of which a surgical operation freed the member for legitimate use; in the other the malformation was associated with imperforate urethra and hypospadias.

172. Congenital *chordee*, from shortening of the corpus spongiosum has proven a bar to copulation, and a cause of sterility. Whether it is susceptible of cure will be a question for the surgeon, and would have to be decided by the condition of the individual case.

173. Chronic *chordee* from gonorrhœa may persist for months or years. It is evidently caused by the organization of exudative material in the corpus spongiosum and mucous lining of the urethra. In one case of this kind, the continued application of Tincture Veratrum, and the internal use of Iodide of Ammonium was sufficient for a cure. In another case, under the care of a friend, the patient was advised to get a fresh clap, when the discharge was allowed to continue, sedatives being continually taken and applied, until a natural cure was effected. The treatment was a success, though I should not advise it. In 1871 a gentleman from California consulted me with regard to a difficulty of this nature, which had been a source of annoyance to him for some seven years. So great was the pain from connection, that for the five years preceding he had not known a woman

Examination of the organ showed no lesion, and I advised a trial—time had cured the case without his knowledge.

174. An *irritable urethra* may prove an impediment to copulation or to emission. The erection is painful, and as the turgescence of the organ becomes greater before the orgasm, the pain becomes so excessive that it can not be borne. In other cases, though the orgasm occurs, the erythism of the urethra is such that there is no emission, until the erection passes off, when it slowly oozes away.

For these cases I would advise the internal use of Veratrum with the alkaline diuretics. The Tincture of Veratrum might be applied over the course of the urethra once or twice a day, and a hot bath used in some cases. For an injection, a solution of Sulphate of Hydrastia will prove the best remedy. In some cases, the symptoms would suggest Pulsatilla, Staphysagria, or Hamamelis.

175. *Stricture* of the urethra rarely prevents the sexual act, though it may prevent emissions, and thereby be a cause of sterility. For treatment the reader is referred to the article on this subject.

176. *Hypospadias* and *Epispadias* may be causes of impotence. In some cases the urethra may be restored and the fistula closed. If not, and the man is virile, it is proposed to receive the semen from the fistula, and artificially impregnate the woman.

177. The *frænum* of the penis is sometimes so short as to incurve the organ and prevent copulation; or it may be so attached to the meatus as to prevent emissions. Clipping with a pair of scissors gives relief, care being taken to avoid hemorrhage from the little artery found in this fold.

178. *Phimosis* may be an obstruction to copulation, or may prevent emission. In some cases the opening in the prepuce is very small and not in front of the meatus, and in these we very frequently find more or less structural disease—ulceration, thickening of the prepuce, calculus formations, etc. Circumcision is the better treatment in these cases, but if the

patient will not submit to it, let the prepuce be slit up on a grooved director, or with probe-pointed scissors, and the glans exposed. Cullerier recommended several of these incisions. Dress the part with cold water.

179. In some rare cases a paraphimosis becomes a source of trouble. There is no difficulty at ordinary times, but in the increased turgescence before the orgasm the glans becomes strangulated, and emission prevented. An incision at one or more points, with the edges kept apart whilst the process of healing is progressing, will give relief.

180. *Enlargement* of the *prostate* from chronic inflammation, hypertrophy, fibroid or cystic growths, may prove a cause of impotence. A careful examination of the organ will detect the lesion, and in some cases it may be relieved.

181. Hemorrhoids may cause impotence. Possibly from pressure upon the vesiculæ seminales, or doubtless in some cases from an impairment of the pelvic circulation. The hemorrhoidal condition, with relaxation of the perineal tissues, frequently impairs virile power, and may cause entire impotence. In some of these cases a well adjusted elastic support to the perineum, in addition to the usual treatment of hemorrhoids will give relief.

182. Acton claims that the use of the common truss for hernia, occasionally proves a cause of impotence. "When a case of the kind comes under my care, and the patient complains of want of sexual power, I always examine how the truss pressess. If I see any reason to suppose that it can by any possibility be the cause of the symptoms, I attempt in the first place by diet and abstinence from certain articles to cause absorption of fat in the mesentery and omentum; this being done I attempt, but with great caution, to reduce the size of the truss. It is singular how often this can be done with safety. I find that not only are the sexual powers often recovered when the pressure is thus relieved, but that the penis, when it is no longer thrust aside, regains its natural size when that has diminished."

183. *Non-descent of the Testes* is always a cause of impotence. The man may seemingly have full virile power, the copulative act well performed, and emissions that seem natural, yet there is sterility. On examination the semen is found to contain no spermatozoa.

184. *Varicocele* may be a cause of impotence. In this case a well adapted suspensory bandage will give relief, but if very bad, an operation should be had for the radical cure.

185. *Pendulous scrotum*, the testes having no support, and dragging on the spermatic cords, may prove a cause of impotence. In most cases of this character virile power is feeble, and the copulative act is imperfectly performed. The use of a suspensory bandage, stimulant and astringent baths with friction, and especially Hamamelis, may be employed with good results.

186. Structural diseases of the testes, preventing the secretion of the seminal fluid, or obstructing its emission, prove causes of impotence. Some of these are amenable to surgical treatment. Even hydrocele will arrest the secretion, and prevent its discharge.

IMPOTENCE IN THE FEMALE.

187. I have already called attention to the fact that women have much less venereal excitement than men, and that it is not necessary in many cases for reproduction. Many women never have a pleasurable sensation in sexual commerce; in others the venereal orgasm is slight, and of rare occurrence; in some it is well marked and intensely pleasurable, and in the very few the sexual sense has as much development as in man.

188. We find cases, in which there is no reciprocity in the sexual act. The man is very excitable, and has the venereal orgasm before the female organs are in a condition to re-

spond, and the woman never has any enjoyment from the act. In such cases the woman's health will sometimes suffer severely, and the nervous symptoms of spermatorrhœa will be developed.

189. In some cases there is a natural coldness on the part of the woman; it may be from enfeebled innervation, which can be remedied by medicine.* This want of sexual power may be but the expression of imperfect ovulation, and we then direct our means to an improvement in this respect.

---

*With seeming diffidence she entered upon the recital of the old, old story, so familiar to physicians, the aggregate of which points to "uterine difficulty." As the story progressed, our mutual bashfulness diminished, and by mutual hitches we intensified our propinquity to each other. The peroration accomplished, I found myself feeling her pulse, examining her tongue, etc. I now informed her in one rigidly formulated sentence, that a perfect diagnosis of her difficulty would involve a vaginal examination. She did not faint nor go into "hysterics," but gracefully and piously assented. As she prepared for the ordeal, I noticed a certain nervousness about her, different from that which results from genuine modesty, and my perceptions were put on the *qui vive*. Her excitement increased as the moment for the final act drew near, and when I touched her genitalia, a quiver went through her frame. [I will say in this connection that although I am not religiously careful in my avoidance of the clitoris, I did not touch hers. My observation has convinced me, contrary to the dicta of early teachings, that clitorises, as a class, are not as explosive as nitro-glycerine.] When I introduced my finger, her actions became such as to convince me that she was in the thrills of the venereal orgasm. Here was a pickle indeed, and all my assurance, added to my full sense of innocence, were scarcely sufficient to prevent a well-defined feeling of sheepishness. Observing my embarrassment, she broke out in a flood of apologetic protestations, ending in a confession of her "great weakness," viz.: uncontrollable sexual desires. She acknowledged that she had practiced onanism many years, not by titillation of the clitoris, nor by the introduction of her finger or anything else into the vagina, but by *friction across the mons Veneris*, effected with the palm of her hand. She stated furthermore, that very many of her sisters in Zion were in a condition similar to hers, and that almost all of them were afflicted with prolapsus uteri, caused as she believed by standing and dancing so long at a time. The reader may draw his own conclusions touching the wisdom of those doctrines which involve the violation of natural law, and which consign its devotees to lives of mental slavery and physical wretchedness.—*Dr. Cooper, Eclectic Medical Journal, March*, 1873.

The use of those restoratives that may be indicated, among which are the Hypophosphites, Cod-Oil, Arsenic, in some cases Lime-water, with the special stimulants, Iodine and Nux Vomica, as heretofore named, will frequently prove beneficial.

190. In some cases the habit of onanism has been the cause of a want of pleasure in sexual congress, and possibly of sterility. Acton gives a case of this kind.*

---

*A gentleman came to ask my opinion on the cause of want of sexual feeling in his wife. He told me he had been married four years. His wife was about his own age (twenty-seven), and had had four children, but she evinced no sexual feeling, although a lively, healthy lady, living in the country. I suggested several causes, when he at last asked me if it was possible that a woman might lose sexual feeling from the same cause as men. "I have read your former edition, Mr. Acton," said he, "and though you only allude to the subject incidentally, yet from what I have learned since my marriage, I am led to think that my wife's want of sexual feeling may arise, if you can affirm to me that such a thing is possible, from self-abuse. She has confessed to me that at a boarding-school, in perfect ignorance of any injurious effects, she early acquired the habit. This practice still gives her gratification; not so connection, which she views with positive aversion, although it gives her no pain." I told him that medical men, who are consulted about female complaints, have not unfrequently observed cases like that of his wife. It appears that, at last, nothing but the morbid excitement produced by the baneful practice can give any sexual gratification, and that the natural stimulus fails to cause any pleasure whatever. A similar phenomenon occurs in men, and this state is seldom got the better of as long as self-abuse is practised. I feared, therefore, that his surmises were correct, and that the lady practised self-abuse more frequently than she was willing to admit. So ruinous is the practice of solitary vice, both in the one and other sex, so difficult is it to give it up, that I fear it may be carried on even in married life, where no excuse can be devised, and may actually come to be preferred to the natural excitement. Venereal excesses engender satiety just as certainly as any other indulgences, and satiety is followed by indifference and disgust. If the natural excesses of masturbation take place early in life, before the subjects who commit them have arrived at maturity, it is not surprising that we meet with women whose sexual feelings, if they ever existed, become prematurely worn out Doubtless sexual feeling differs largely in different women; and although it is not my object to treat otherwise than incidentally of the sexual economy in women, yet I may here say that the causes which in early life induce abnormal sexual excitement in boys operate in a similar manner on girls. This

192. *Vaginismus* may prevent sexual congress. The sexual organs are so excitable that the thought of the act causes intense congestion, and contraction of the muscles of the perineum; or the slightest touch is sufficient to occasion the spasm of the muscles and intense sensibility of surface. In some cases this spasm of the structures is most intensely painful, and lasts long after the cause has subsided.

The milder cases that I have seen have been readily relieved by the internal administration of Gelseminum, and rectal injections of Lobelia and Tincture of Opium. Should this fail, forcible dilatation under Chloroform, or a division of the sphincter vaginæ is recommended.

193. *Stricture of the vagina* is readily recognized, and the canal being continuous to the cervix uteri, dilatation with graduated bougies, offers a successful treatment of the difficulty.

194. *A fleshy or fibrous hymen* may offer an obstruction to sexual congress which can not be overcome, but the knife and finger readily break it down.

195. Physical inability to perform the sexual act is very rare, but the mental repugnance is not uncommon. Such women should not marry, if the condition is known before, and it should be just cause of divorce, if developed after marriage. Two cases of the latter kind have come to my knowledge, and rendered the lives of both husbands and wives very unhappy. It is possible, sometimes, that remedies may relieve the peculiar sensitiveness of the nervous system upon which this occasionally depends. I have seen one case in which very marked relief came from the use of Pulsatilla and Macrotys; the remedies not only relieving the mind, but rec-

---

tendency may be checked in girls, as in boys, by careful moral education in early life. But no doubt can exist that hereditary predisposition has much to do with this, independently of education and early associations. It is publicly maintained by some credible persons that there are well-known families, for instance, in which chastity is not a characteristic feature among the females.

tifying a wrong of the menstrual function, which was followed by conception and a cure, though the patient had suffered for some ten years, and was sterile.

196. In some cases, where the fault is in the reproductive organs, remedies may be directed to these. Stimulating when there is want of normal excitement; sedative when the excitement is too great. Electricity will, no doubt, prove a valuable remedy in many of these cases.

197. *Sterility* is not dependent, in most cases, upon inability to perform the sexual act in either sex. As we have already seen, the reproductive function in the female is to a considerable extent independent of any sexual feeling, and conception will occur when the woman has been wholly passive, and has had no sensation of sexual orgasm. To a more limited extent this is true of man, and he may beget children without the marked pleasurable sensations that the majority experience.

198. In the female, sterility is most frequently dependent upon imperfect ovulation, rather than structural wrong in the reproductive canals, though this is the cause in some cases. This imperfection may or may not be marked by menstrual irregularities: if these are present, they serve to point out the remedies for the case. Imperfect ovulation may be divided into three classes: 1st. Where there is undue excitation of the ovarian nerves, and determination of blood; 2d. Where there is impaired innervation and congestion; 3d. Where there is impaired nutrition, neither of the previous conditions being present.

199. In the first class of cases, Macrotys and Pulsatilla are favorite remedies, and during the menstrual mollimen Veratrum. If there is undue excitement of the mind, with reference to this function, I would give Pulsatilla; or if there was undue nervous excitation of the organs. Macrotys is a remedy when the nervous excitation is associated with determination of blood. Veratrum and Macrotys are associated when the general circulation shares in the excitement. In

plethoric persons, these means are associated with cooling purgatives, saline diuretics, and a spare diet.

In the second class, we would think of Cannabis Indica, Hamamelis, Staphysagria, Tincture of Phosphorus, and Ergot, with such general restorative means as may be indicated.

In the third class of cases, we employ a general restorative treatment, as may be indicated, which will embrace the bitter tonics, Iron, Hypophosphites, Cod Oil, Arsenic, and animal foods. Here as elsewhere success will be to a considerable extent dependent upon a careful examination for special indications for remedies. I would rather trust for success, upon one remedy, when clearly indicated, than upon the entire list of restoratives as generally used.

200. *Dysmenorrhœa* is not an uncommon symptom in sterility of women. It may be dependent upon stricture of the os internum or cervical canal, but in most cases it is a functional lesion. There is undue excitement of the sympathetic and spinal nerves distributed to the uterus, and in most cases this is associated with an erythism of the semi-erectile tissue of the organ, which prevents the free escape of the menstrual blood. This condition may be remedied in a large majority of cases by the use of: ℞ Tinct. Pulsatilla, Tinct. Macrotys, aa. ʒss.; Water, ℥iv.; a teaspoonful four times a day. Commence four or five days previous to the menstrual period, and continue until the discharge is free and painless, repeating the treatment every month until a cure has been effected.

201. The opposite condition, *congestion* of the lower segment of the uterus, may or may not be associated with pain, and yet be a cause of sterility. Examination shows the cervix enlarged, with the peculiar tumid, waxy appearance of tissue and enfeebled circulation, whilst the touch gives a sense of fullness with impaired circulation and nutrition. The os may be patulous and open, with free secretion from the cervical canal, or it may be constricted. These cases are benefited by the use of Pond's Hamamelis, Tincture of Phos-

phorus and Staphysagria, and associated with a good general treatment a cure may be anticipated.

202. This brief consideration of the causes of sterility would be incomplete without an allusion to the most common of all causes, *incompatibility of temperament*. In every locality instances may be observed of healthy couples who have no children. Both husband and wife have healthy reproductive organs, and there are neither physical nor functional reasons why they should not be fertile. In many cases, a prior or second marriage has been fruitful in both parties, proving conclusively that the wrong is of neither party as an individual, but an incompatibility of the two. Prof. Powell first called attention to this fact, and pointed out the means by which such incompatibility might be determined. The simple statement "that persons of absolutely the *same* temperament are sterile," expresses the fact; and that as they approximate this *sameness*, the offspring will be non-viable.*

*LAW I. When the constitutional similitude of the respective sexes is such that a qualified observer can not detect an appreciable difference, sterility will be the result of their marriage. *Illustration:* Washington and his wife were, respectively, sanguine, and it is known that sterility was the result. Between Gen. Jackson and his wife there was a nominal difference of constitution; he was bilious sanguine, and she was bilious: nevertheless they were physically the same, both being exclusively vital, and it is known that sterility was the result. The first Napoleon and Josephine were, in person, greatly different, and in constitution they were nominally as different, and in constitution they were nominally as different, and yet there was no physiological difference. He was sanguine encephalo-bilious lymphatic, and she was bilious encephalic; consequently they were, respectively, compounded of equal varieties of vital and non-vital conditions, and it is known that sterility was the result of their alliance.

LAW II. When the constitutional similitude of the respective sexes is less than complete, or is appreciably different, progeny will result, but it will be dead-born, imbecile, scrofulous, deaf, blind, or in some otherwise imperfect. *Illustration:* I can furnish three hundred examples of this law, but as they are not historically known, they would be of no value in this relation. I can cite one, however, which is historically known, viz.: the first Napoleon and his second wife. Her temperament was bilious encephalo-sanguine, and his

SALACITAS.

203. We employ the old designation of Dr. Mason Good to designate a class of diseases characterized by inordinate sexual passion or lust, including as it does the disease in male and female. Like other affections it varies in intensity, from the passion that is under control at ordinary times, to the lascivious madness to which the names satyriasis and nymphomania have been given.

---

temperament I have indicated. There was between them an appreciable difference of constitution, and the result of this difference was one son; but the difference was too small to secure to him a normal viability, for he died of a scrofulous affection of the lungs, at the age of eighteen years. It is most indisputably the fact, that a considerable difference of constitution must obtain between the respective parties to a marriage, to secure to offspring a soundly viable constitution. To discover the least difference consistent with a physiological marriage was indispensable, but before discovering this the conviction became forced upon me that my discovery could not become of general utility without the discovery of a law of universal application. By a great amount of observation and study, I succeeded in discovering the desired law, and it is of easy application, and will universally secure a physiologically legitimate offspring, and the greatest possible happiness to the parents. Those, therefore, who make domestic happiness, and a really useful progeny, conditions of marriage, must observe the following law:

LAW III. One of the parties must be exclusively vital—that is, must be either sanguine, bilious, or sanguine-bilious (the last being a compound of the two former, is also vital), and the other party must as certainly be more or less non-vital, that is, more or less lymphatic or encephalic. All marriages, in contravention of this law, are physiologically incestuous, and the consequences will be vicious in proportion to the delinquency.

LAW IV. The greatest dissimilitude of constitution that can obtain between the sexes, when they are respectively of the same species, is that which obtains between a vital and a non-vital temperament—and this is the most favorable to progeny. But marriages of this character are greatly impracticable in any country. It is a very remarkable fact in the physiology of human procreation, that a high degree of constitutional dissimilitude is about equally unfavorable to progeny. It has been seen that a high degree of similitude entails a scrofulous diathesis, and a high degree of dissimilitude, as when one party is white and the other negro, the progeny is invariably scrofulous, I believe.—*Scudder's Domestic Medicine.*

"In a state of health and civilized society there are two reasons why mankind are easily capable of restraining within due bounds the animal desire that exists in their frame from the period of puberty till the infirmity of age: the one is of a physical, and the other of a moral kind. The natural orgasm of men differs from that of brutes in being permanent instead of being periodical or dependent upon the return of particular seasons; and on this very account is less violent, more uniform, and kept with comparative facility within proper limits. This is a cause derived from the physical constitution of man. But the power of habit and the early inculcation of a principle of abstinence and chastity in civilized life, form a moral cause of temperance that operates with a still stronger influence than the preceding, and lays down a barrier, which, though too often stealthily broken into, yet, in the main, makes good its post and serves as a general check upon society.

"As man rises in education and moral feeling, he proportionally rises in the power of self-restraint; and, consequently, as he becomes deprived of this wholesome law of discipline, he sinks into self-indulgence and the brutality of savage life. And were it not that the very permanency of the desire, as we have already observed, torpefies and wears out its goad, the savage, destitute of moral discipline, would be at all times as ferocious in his libidinous career as brutes are in the season of returning heat; when, stung with the periodical ardor, and worked up almost to fury, the whole frame of the animal is actuated with an unbridled force, his motions are quick and rapid, his eyes glisten, and his nerves seem to circulate fire. Food is neglected; fences are broken down; he darts wild through fields and forests, plunges into the deepest rivers, or scales the loftiest rocks and mountains, to meet the object that is ordained by nature to quell the pungent impulse by which he is urged forward."

Dr. Good's classification was a good one, dividing it into

four classes, as met with at the period of puberty, in old age, in full habit, and as the result of a debauched life.

204. At the period of puberty, the development of the sexual organs and sexual functions being rapid, we occasionally find a condition of disease characterized by the term *salacity*. It is of more common occurrence in those who have not been educated to self government and industrious habits. The mind is badly controlled at best, and habits of self-gratification have been indulged through life. At this period comes new feelings and desires, and as the mind dwells upon them they increase in strength, until they influence the entire life. In some of these cases the sufferer is of full habit, but in the majority they are spare and delicate, and have had a rapid growth. When the excitation is greatest, especially in the latter class, there are not unfrequently epileptic symptoms.

205. The treatment in these cases will vary. When the patient is of full habit, cooling purgatives, saline diuretics, and the cold bath, are among the most important means. In the opposite class of cases, we think of the Hypophosphites—the Compound Syrup with Hypophosphoric Acid is a favorite of mine—Iron, Nitric Acid, with a nutritious diet. In all cases, Bromide of Ammonium, ʒss. to Water, ℥iv.; a teaspoonful four times a day, seems to exert the most direct influence in controlling the sexual feeling.

Where there is local disease to account for it, this should be removed if possible.

"The salacity of age is a very afflictive malady, and often wears away the hoary form to the last stage of a tabid decline by the frequency of the orgastic paroxysm, and the drain of seminal emissions without enjoyment. It is usually the result of some accidental cause of irritation in the ovaria, the uterus, the testes, or the prostate gland; and has sometimes followed upon a stone in the kidneys or bladder; and is hence best removed by relieving or palliating the local irritation by a warm hip bath, anodyne injections, or cataplasms of hemlock or the other umbellate or lurid plants in common use."

206. Occasionally cases are met with where the sufferer has led a regular and orderly life, but finds the sexual power growing stronger and stronger, until it is with difficulty that it can be controlled. Most of these cases are of married men, in which from disease or loss of the wife, they have been deprived of the usual gratification of the passion. As an example, I give the case of a clergyman of most exemplary character, who applied to me for relief, saying, "that unless this passion could be controlled by medicine, he would become insane, or commit some grievous crime." This is not an exceptional case, and the facts being so well established should lead us to have charity for some who "are tempted beyond what they can bear."

207. I can not omit to notice here the influence of *obscene* literature which is widely distributed throughout our country. Commencing with the popular weeklies, which contain nothing but exciting novelettes, that unfit the reader for the duties of life, stimulating the passions in place of educating the mind, until we reach the lowest depths of human degradation in vicious and obscene books and pictures, we have every stimulus to sexual vice. This vile stream reaches every nook and corner of our country, works its way into the haunts of the vicious, and the houses of respectable Christians, into the cottages of the poor and the mansions of the wealthy, and wherever it goes pollutes the minds of its readers. The extent of this evil is shown by the following letter from Anthony Comstock: (see note.)* We are glad to notice that the presentation of these facts to Congress has closed the mails to a part of this vicious traffic.

BROOKLYN, January 18, 1873.

DEAR SIR: I have the honor to acknowledge the receipt of your favor of the 12th inst., in which you ask for a statement from me in reference to the traffic in obscene literature. In reply, I have been engaged in the suppression of this business since about one year ago. At that time I knew only one

208. The treatment in this case will consist in the use of cooling purgatives, a farinaceous diet with fruits, the cold sitz bath, and steady occupation. Physical labor or exercise to the full capacity is frequently sufficient to control the desires. As remedies we may use the Bromide of Ammonium, or the Bromide of Potassium, or Lime, if the rest is broken. To allay the excitation of the reproductive organs, especially

---

place where this business was carried on. The dealer was arrested, his papers "pigeon-holed," and he continued on in the same business, even letting out these vile books at ten cents per week to the youths and children of our public schools. In seeking to procure the arrest of this man again, I was betrayed by a policeman, who has since been dismissed from the service upon my preferring charges against him to our Police Commissioners. After this the Sunday Mercury came out against me, and said, "if I was the Christian man I professed to be, I could find plenty of these men in Ann and Nassau streets and elsewhere." Accordingly, profiting by this hint, and by aid of the numerous advertisements in this same paper, the Day's Doings, the New Varieties, and the Illustrated Police Gazette, I have succeeded in unearthing this hydra-headed monster in part, as you will see by the following statement which, in many respects, might be truthfully increased in quantity. These I have seized and destroyed.

Obscene photographs, stereoscopic and other pictures, more than 182,000; obscene books and pamphlets, more than 5 tons; obscene letter-press in sheets, more than 2 tons; sheets of impure songs, catalogues, handbills, etc., more than 21,000; obscene microscopic watch and knife charms and finger-rings, more than 5,000; obscene negative plates for printing photographs and stereoscopic views, about 625; obscene engraved steel and copper plates, 350; obscene lithographic stones destroyed, 20; obscene wood-cut engravings, more than 500; stereotype plates for printing obscene books, more than 5 tons; obscene transparent playing cards, 5,500 to 6,000; obscene and immoral rubber articles, over 30,000; lead moulds for manufacturing rubber goods, twelve sets, or more than 700 pounds; newspapers seized, about 4,600; letters from all parts of the country, ordering these goods, about 15,000; names of dealers in account books seized, about 6,000; list of names in the hands of dealers, that are sold as merchandise, to forward catalogues and circulars to, independent of letters and account books, seized, more than 7,000; arrest of dealers since Oct. 9, 1871, over 50; publishers, manufacturers and dealers dead since March last, 6.

With the exception of one arrest, this has all been done since the 2d of last March; and with the exception of about three arrests, the whole work has

where there is an unpleasant sensation of warmth in the urethra or ardor urinæ, Gelseminum is an excellent remedy.

209. With regard to the salacity of a *debauched* life Dr. Good well remarks: "It can only be cured by a total change of habit: which is a discipline that the established debauchee has rarely the courage to attempt. Exercise, change of place and pursuits, cooling laxatives, and a less stimulant diet than

---

been accomplished by myself, or under my own supervision, so that I know whereof I speak.

There are various ways by which this vile stuff has been disseminated. First, by advertising in the above named papers. Some weeks there is not a single advertisement in some of the papers that is not designed either to cheat or defraud, or intended to be a medium of sending out these accursed books and articles. For instance, I have arrested a number of persons, one in particular, who advertised a musical album, to be sent for fifty cents. I sent the fifty cents, and received back a catalogue of obscene books, with the following card attached:

"The album is only a pretense to enable us to forward you a catalogue of our fancy books. Should you order any of these books, your fifty cents will be credited."

It is needless to say, I ordered, then arrested him, locked him up in the New Haven jail, and he has been indicted by the Grand Jury in the United States Court of Connecticut, and now is held in bail for trial. In the same way, by advertising beautiful views or pictures of some celebrated place or person, these men receive answers from innocent persons for these pictures, and among the pictures sent will be one or more of these obscene pictures, and catalogues of these vile books and rubber goods. For be it known that wherever these books go, or catalogues of these books, there you will ever find, as almost indispensable, a complete list of rubber articles for masturbation or for the professed prevention of conception.

Secondly. These abominations are disseminated by these men first obtaining the addresses of scholars and students in our schools and colleges, and then forwarding these circulars. They secure thousands of names in this way, by either sending for a catalogue of schools, seminaries and colleges, under the pretense of sending a child to attend these places, or else by sending out a circular purporting to be getting up a directory of all the scholars and students in schools and colleges in the United States, or of taking the census of all the unmarried people, and offering to pay five cents per name for lists so sent. I need not say that the money is seldom or never sent, but I do say that these names, together with those that come in reply to advertisements, are sold to other parties; so that when a man desires to engage in this nefa-

he will commonly be found accustomed to, may assist him in the attempt; but in general the mind is as corrupt as the body, and the case is hopeless. He perseveres, however, at his peril, for with increasing weakness, he will at length sink into all the miserable train of symptoms which characterize that species of marasmus which is usually expressed by the name of tabes dorsalis, and which we have described already."

---

rious business, he has only to purchase a list of these names, and then your child, be it son or daughter, is as liable to have thrust into its hands, all unbeknown to you, one of these devilish catalogues.

You will please observe that this business is carried on principally by the agency of the United States mails, and there is no law to-day by which we can interfere with the sending out of these catalogues and circulars through the mail, except they are obscene on their face; and there are scores of men that are supporting themselves and families to-day by sending out these rubber goods, etc., through the mails, that I can not touch for want of law. There are men in Philadelphia, in Chicago, in Boston, and other places, who are doing this business, that I could easily detect and convict, if the law was only sufficient. There was one year ago published in and about New York and vicinity, 144 different obscene books. I have seized the stereotyped plates, steel and copper plates, etc., for 142 of these books. There were four publishers on the 2d of last March; to-day three of these are in their graves, and it is charged by their friends that I worried them to death. Be that as it may, I am sure that the world is better without them. One man, since the year 1842, (according to his account book that I have), has published some eighteen or twenty different books, and has never, to my knowledge, been arrested, but has for years been the victim of black-mail by the detectives of New York city, and in this manner has been practically licensed by them to do this business.

It is with great pleasure that I state, that the refusal of President Grant to pardon those who have been convicted of this offense in the United States Courts, and of Gov. Hoffman those who have been convicted in this State in the State Courts, has sent dismay into the camp of these men, and will go very far toward checking this business. The district-attorney and his deputies are ready to prosecute any and all cases when they are brought to their notice, and there is no question about these men having justice done them if convicted before any of our judges; so that all we want to break up this nefarious business, is a broader law. I present these facts for your consideration

I have the honor to be, with great respect, Sir, your obedient servant,

ANTHONY COMSTOCK

HON. C. L. MERRIAM, House of Representatives, Washington.

210. *Satyriasis* and *Nymphomania* are of very rare occurrence, and will most usually be treated at Insane Asylums.

"The pulse is quick, the breathing short, the patient is sleepless, thirsty, and loathes his food; the urine is evacuated with difficulty, and there is a continual fever. In women the disease is often connected with an hysterical temperament, and even commences with a semblance of melancholy; and I once had an instance of it, from local irritation, shortly after child-birth. The child having suddenly died, and there being no more demand for a flow of milk, the fluid was repelled from the breasts with too little caution, and the uterine region, from the debility it was yet laboring under, became the seat of a transferred irritation. Among females the disease is strikingly marked by the movements of the body, and the salacious appearance of the countenance, and even the language that proceeds from the lips. There is often, indeed, at first some degree of melancholy, with frequent sighings; but the eyes roll in wanton glances, the cheeks are flushed, the bosom heaves, and every gesture exhibits the lurking desire, and is enkindled by the distressing flame that burns within."

211. Probably this madness is of more frequent occurrence in the female, and arises from a suspension of marital intercourse from death or other causes. The only marked case that I have seen, however, was in an unmarried woman of thirty-five years, but this was the result of a broken engagement of marriage.

212. Baker Brown lost his good name and business by recommending and practising clitoridectomy, for the cure of this lesion. But it was not original with him, for many years before the eminent Surgeon Dubois wrote, "The organ was removed by a single stroke of the bistoury, and all hemorrhage prevented by the actual cautery. The wound healed easily, and the patient obtained a radical cure of her distressing affection." Leveret performed the operation at a still earlier day, and though it is not to be recommended in all cases of excessive sexual excitement, there is no reason why

it should not be resorted to, when the organ is found enlarged and extremely sensitive.

213. Widows sometimes suffer severely from ungratified sexual excitement. In some cases the vegetative processes suffer. The appetite is variable and impaired, digestion and blood-making enfeebled, nutrition poor, and the surface assumes a peculiar blanched, sallow appearance, and the tissues lose their normal elasticity and hardness. In others the reproductive organs suffer. She has irregular menstruation, congestion of ovaries and uterus, neuralgia, leucorrhœa, ulceration, displacement, etc. But in the majority the nerve centers suffer most, and we find an unnatural depression of spirits, absence of mind, enfeebled memory, and the class of symptoms usually attributed to "softening of the brain."

214. Of course the treatment of these cases will vary, according to the lesions, yet in many we will find most benefit from special remedies. Of these I think Bromide of Ammonium stands first, giving marked relief to the spinal and sympathetic systems. When stimulation is desirable, this may be alternated with the Iodine Pill, heretofore named. In others still, when the mind is much involved, Pulsatilla alone, or with Macrotys, will prove the remedy.

SPERMATORRHŒA.

215. As we have already seen, the abuse of the sexual organs by masturbation or excessive venery will lead to an increased sexual desire, which may be under the control of the will, or independent of it. The first we have studied under the name *salacitas*; the second we purpose to study under the name spermatorrhœa.

216. The disease may be divided into three stages. In the first the sexual instinct can be controlled, and the involuntary action of the sexual organs is but occasional, and has not yet

impaired the general health. In the second, the sexual excitation and emission is markedly automatic, and though partially or completely under the control of the will, when the mind is active during the day, shows especial aberration when the will is suspended during sleep. In the third, the will has entirely lost command of the procreative function, and the venereal orgasm is wholly automatic and involuntary.

217. Whilst the common cause of spermatorrhœa is *self-abuse*, we find many cases in which masturbation has not been practiced, or if so, suspended long before the development of this disease. One of the severest cases that I have had to treat was wholly the result of irritation of the base of the bladder, from venereal disease and uric acid deposits, the patient having lived a continent life until marriage, and had then been moderate in his indulgence. It is not of frequent occurrence wherever the sexual function has had legitimate exercise, yet we will find cases of this kind in the married, and especially when sickness or loss of the wife has prevented ordinary indulgence. As we have already seen, the sexual function may assume undue proportions from causes over which the patient has had little control. The emotional faculties predominating, salacious thoughts may repeat themselves, even though the person strives against it, and in the end, growing by repetition, they finally exert a controlling influence upon the organism. In some of these cases there is undoubtedly disease of the brain, and a careful examination may detect this.

218. When we come to examine the condition of the reproductive organs, we find occasional causes of spermatorrhœa. It is true that in the majority of cases these have been developed by self-abuse, but in some the structural lesion of the reproductive organs was primary, and the only source of trouble.

219. Among these may be mentioned the irritable urethra, especially the prostatic portion; irritation of the prostate and of the base of the bladder; rectal irritation; eczema with

pruritus; balanitis; phymosis; sub-acute orchitis; cystic disease of testes; pendulous scrotum; varicocele; irritation of kidneys. Most of these are but exceptional causes, yet one should never overlook their influence.

220. When we study masturbation as a cause of spermatorrhœa, we can readily see how it is developed. Salacious thoughts frequently repeated, give strength to this function of the mind, and at the same time impair the will. The sexual instinct congenitally strong, grows by exercise, and the will-power, at best but sufficient for mental control, gradually loses its influence. Other functions of the mind may be so employed as to increase the wrong. Music, the love of the fine arts, and especially the love of the beautiful in dress, and social arts connected with women, may all serve to excite sexual emotions, when the mind has already this bias. The abnormal excitation of the organs in masturbation tends to develop an undue sensibility of the spinal and sympathetic nerve centers, which eventually serves as a cause of the involuntary emissions.

221. The disease is usually developed slowly, and two or three years may elapse before the sufferer thinks it necessary to apply for relief. In rare cases, it comes on rapidly, and in a few months, the patient will show the marked symptoms of the lesion.

222. In the majority of cases we have little difficulty in diagnosing spermatorrhœa, though it is not so easy to determine the special lesion upon which it is dependent. Here as elsewhere, we want to know that the spermatorrhœa is but a symptom, and we must know the character of the lesions if we expect success from remedies.

223. There is something in the appearance of the patient that tells the story of sexual wrong, before he has opened his mouth. The downcast countenance, the inability to look you fairly in the eyes, the unsteadiness of the eye, peculiar contraction of the *levator labii superioris*, and *orbicularis oris*, foreshadow to you the story of sexual abuse continued until

the sexual orgasm is involuntary. As a general rule, the sufferer tells his story clearly and without prevarication. He realizes the character of the disease, and its dangers, and probably has made it a study, and read what he could obtain in relation to it, for months back. The only trouble many times is, that he knows too much, and the story is prolix.

224. In the first stage of the disease, we have the story of strong desire with difficulty controlled by the will. Of frequent erections, especially when excited by company, by sight or conversation, or in female society. Then there are *nocturnal* emissions, once or twice a month, then every week, and finally oftener than this. Associated with this excitement, we have an increased secretion from the prostate, Cowper's glands and canal of the urethra, which is discharged after micturition, defecation, upon lifting, and when the penis has been in a state of erection.

225. As the sufferer learns the nature of the disease, the mind becomes troubled. He learns to watch for the symptoms, feels depressed after each nocturnal emission, is excessively annoyed by the prostatic discharges, for which he is constantly on the outlook. As the mind broods over the trouble, the impairment becomes greater. He is forgetful, loses interest in the common affairs of life, cares little for society, and shuns women. Presently comes unpleasant sensations in the head of tightness, dizziness, inability to command the muscles, *tinnitus aurium*, *muscæ volitantes*, etc.

226. As yet, the vegetative functions may be but little impaired, but presently his appetite is variable, bowels inclined to constipation, urine "badly concocted," secretion from the skin sticky, unpleasant, sour, the pulse shows want of power, and irregularity, the tongue incurved, pointed and slimy, the facial expression characteristic, the movements unsteady and without energy, etc. Going further, blood making is impaired, the tissues are soft and relaxed, he loses flesh and strength rapidly, and the nervous symptoms are greatly increased. Now in some cases we will find commencing symp-

toms of phthisis, tabes dorsalis, structural disease of the brain, atrophy or tubercular or cystic disease of testes, atrophy of penis, phosphatic urine with disease of the bladder, etc.

227. The mental affection is a marked feature in every case, and eventually leads to structural disease of the brain. The first recognition of disease will frequently come in an unpleasant sensation of vertigo, associated with a fear of some impending danger. Soon the mind dwells upon the reproductive lesion, and the fear of "loss of manhood," or permanent impairment of mind, becomes a source of constant annoyance. This is especially the case where the sufferer has possessed himself of the secret circulars of advertising specialists, who use every means to increase the alarm.*

---

*In the first edition of my work on "Diseases of the Urinary and Generative Organs," I wrote a chapter entitled Syphiliphobia, in which I collected together a variety of complaints that presented many of the characteristics of true disease. Since then, a wider knowledge of these subjects has sprung up. Hypochondriacs and a large class of patients who have leisure to dwell on their morbid thoughts and feelings have, by reading the books so freely advertised in the quacks' corner of the newspapers, come to the conclusion that they are suffering under spermatorrhœa—a word with which they are familiar. In this corner formerly five or six such advertisements directed public attention to the so-called disease; the headings of "Manly Vigor" and "Secret Diseases" have disappeared, and are replaced by the term "Spermatorrhœa," the form of sexual disease now in fashion; and as, in such hypochondriaco-misanthropic persons, the sexual feelings are generally more or less affected, the conclusion is arrived at that every one who, with a bad conscience, feels himself out of sorts, is suffering from spermatorrhœa. There is a fashion in diseases, just as there is in amusements or occupations. Patients come to us, half persuaded that they suffer in the way described, but still in doubt whether what they complain of is fancy or the real disease. In such cases we have to deal with ignorance, irritability of temper, and sometimes with true symptoms, though magnified by great exaggeration, and no inconsiderable alarm about the consequences. Conscience tells many that their previous lives have been far from faultless, and these pseudo-medical books exaggerate their indiscretion and predict the most awful consequences, describing trains of symptoms enough to frighten the most courageous. It is not difficult for my readers to surmise what must be the effect on the ignorant, the weak-minded, and those already depressed by their fears, with no friend

As the disease progresses, he finds difficulty in concentrating the mind on any object, and is listless and with difficulty interested in the daily affairs of life. This impairment will frequently be periodic. For some days he will feel bright and active, but from change of weather, slight indigestion, social surroundings, or a nocturnal emission, he will suffer this depression for some time. It is usually associated with some dizziness, and want of nerve power, and not unfrequently with præcordial oppression, and irregular circulation.

229. In the advanced stage, the memory becomes impaired, the mind receives impressions with difficulty, and fails to retain them, reasoning power is defective, and above all is the brooding fear, that finally the past and present will fade from consciousness, and permanent idiocy result.

230. Short of insanity or idiocy, and atrophy or structural disease of the testes, the prognosis is favorable. Of course the cure will require a longer time, and be more difficult the further the disease has advanced. There is, however, one pre-requisite to success: the patient *must* leave the care of the disease to the physician, and have a reasonable confidence in the success of the physician. Without this, medicine will do but very little good.

231. TREATMENT.—It is well to notice first that we may have two distinct and opposite conditions of the sexual organs and of the nerve centers. In the one there is a condition of hyperæsthesia, with hyperæmia, in the other there is an enfeebled circulation and nutrition. The first class numbers but few cases, the last a large number in the advanced stage.

232. Recognizing the disease as associated with hyperæmia, the patient being full blooded and vigorous, we prescribe

at hand to confide in or to calm their excited feelings. Too many throw themselves into the meshes of these harpies, and the consequence is that they are fleeced to an amount that is almost inconceivable, except to those familiar with the swindling transactions of the class.—*Acton.*

as follows: ℞ Tinct. Veratrum, gtts. xx; Tinct. Gelseminum, ʒij.; Water, ℥iv.; a teaspoonful every three or four hours. The bowels are moved occasionally with a saline diuretic and Sulphur, regular evacuation being insisted on; if the urine is scanty and irritant, Acetate of Potash, in abundance of water. With this, if necessary, we prescribe Bromide of Potassium, grs. x. to grs. xxx., at bed time. The patient should live temperately, keep good hours, and have his time constantly occupied—hard labor, or exercise in the open air, being the best.

233. In cases where atony is a marked feature, we pursue the opposite course. The patient has Phosphorus in the form of the Hypophosphites, Phosphuretted Oil, Pills of Phosphorus, with Nux Vomica, Iodine, Ergot. The Compound Iodine pill answers a very good purpose, and will frequently prove the best stimulant. If the bowels are very torpid, they may be stimulated with equal parts of Sulphur and Cubebs taken at night, and Tincture of Nux Vomica, gtts. j. or ij. in a glass of water in the morning. The general electrical sponge bath is sometimes an important means of cure, the positive pole being placed at the coccyx, and the negative carried over the surface of the body, and especially up and down the spine.

In the more common cases, we have neither the one nor the other condition described above, the lesion being wholly functional. There are two features of the disease which especially attract our attention—the head symptoms, and the spermatic and prostatic discharge.

234. For the unpleasant cerebral symptoms I most commonly prescribe Pulsatilla in the proportion of ʒss. to ʒj., to Water, ʒiv.; a teaspoonful every four hours. If this loses its influence, it may be alternated with Tinct. Cactus in the same proportion: this is especially a good remedy when heart-symptoms have been developed—a not unfrequent complication. If the disease assumes an epiliptic form, we may use: ℞ Bromide of Ammonium, ʒss.; Water, ℥iv.; a teaspoonful four times a day.

235. In many cases the prostatic discharge has caused the greatest alarm, and it is regarded as an involuntary seminal emission—described by specialists as a dangerous feature of the disease. For this I usually prescribe the single remedy, Staphysagria, and with very marked success. The proportion is usually: ℞ Tinct. Staphysagria, ʒj.; Water, ℥iv.; a teaspoonful four times a day. If this should lose its influence, it is alternated with Tinct. Phosphorus, Hamamelis, or Eryngium. Frequently the discharge is entirely arrested within twenty-four hours, by the Staphysagria, and though it may return from indiscretion, the remedy maintains a controlling influence.

236. As the patient feels relief from the unpleasant head symptoms, and increased mental freedom from the stimulus of the Pulsatilla, and he finds the unpleasant discharge is arrested or modified, he becomes hopeful, and this reacting on the vegetative functions, every process of life is improved. I do not allow the occasion to pass unimproved, in confirming the patient's belief that he is getting well, and his faith in the doctor and the medicine; and many times I have seen the case progress without a single untoward symptom to a radical cure. But frequently the patient has backsets from various causes, and we will have to encourage his hope and faith to enable him to persevere to the end.

247. It may be well in this connection to point out the special indications for some additional remedies, which may be substituted for, or associated with those already named. Here, as in other diseases, I believe in giving anything that is pointed out by special symptoms, and if the indication for the remedy is sufficiently strong, trust the patient to the one alone.

Belladonna is especially indicated where there is marked dullness and hebetude, with disposition to sleep, expressionless face, dull eye with dilated or immobile pupils.

Ergot may be used in similar cases, but especially if there is impairment of muscular power of the legs, with tendency to drag them, and a sensation of fullness and weight in the perineum.

Hamamelis is especially indicated where there is an enfeebled venous circulation with fullness and relaxation of the perineum, congestion of the prostate, mucous membrane of the rectum, and hemorrhoids.

Collinsonia, where there is an acute hemorrhoidal condition, with determination of blood to the pelvis. The dose is always small: ℞ Tinct. Collinsonia, gtts. x. to ℨss.; Water, ℥iv.; dose, one teaspoonful.

Eryngium, when the patient complains of pain in the bladder, irritation of urethra, and difficult or painful micturition.

Apis, when the patient complains of superficial burning or itching, either within the bladder, the mucous membrane of urethra, or the glans or prepuce.

Erythroxylon Coca is a valuable remedy when the nocturnal emissions are persistent and exhaustive. It will sometimes effect a radical cure, there being no further trouble after its administration is commenced.

Rhus, when the burning is more intense, and erythematous spots show themselves on scrotum, perineum, genitals or abdomen. Orbital pain with flushed cheeks, especially on left side, is an important indication for the remedy.

Bryonia, where there is pain in the envelop of the testes, pubic pain, with pain and soreness of the back part of the head.

Macrotys, when the patient has muscular pains, lumbago, deep seated pain in body of penis or testes, with sense of fullness and occasional deep soreness of head.

Santonine, where there is a tendency to retention of urine, but without the evidences of muscular atony.

Iron, where the tongue shows solid blueness, the glans penis is continuously blue.

Nitric Acid, where there is a marked violet coloration upon a rose-red tongue, or the same violet color of the glans penis.

Thuja Occidentalis, where there is tearing, throbbing pain, sense of ulceration and rawness, and in the urethra as if drops of water were running along; pain in the crown of the head, and sense of tension about the nasal bones.

Arsenic, where the skin is dirty and parchment-like, with impaired elasticity.

Lime, where there is a tendency to suppurative inflammation of connective cellular tissues.

Stramonium, when the patient complains of tensive pains in the bladder, and extreme tenesmus in passing urine or feces. When the patient has become habituated to the use of Opium.

Phytolacca, where there is a tendency to orchitis, enlargement of the testes, with deep, tensive, dragging pain.

Chelidonium, where the skin has a leaden, sallow appearance, the tongue full, and of a dull, leaden color, urine very pale.

Lobelia, if there is full and tumid mucous tissues, with enfeebled circulation.

There are other remedies which might be of occasional use in these cases, but I have pointed out the more important of them. The hygienic means, and appropriate diet, will be suggested by each individual case. There are but few which require a spare or low diet; the majority want good food, for the better digestion, blood-making and nutrition are, the more rapid and permanent the cure.

238. When we come to study the *topical treatment*, we find great diversity of opinion. Lallemand regarded the disease as having a local origin in the majority of cases, and he pointed out the tenderness of the prostatic urethra as the cause of the sexual alteration. For this trouble he proposed cauterization with Nitrate of Silver or the Potassæ Cum Calce. To introduce it he devised a special instrument, the *porte caustique*.* Acton prefers the syringe with long urethral tube,

* *Lallemand's Plan.*—A catheter should be passed in order to empty the bladder, and to judge of the length of the urethra. This, the Professor recommends, should be done by stretching the urethra, and, as the catheter is withdrawn, watching the moment when the water ceases to pass. Having thus

and a solution of Nitrate of Silver, grs. x. to the ounce of water. I like Acton's method best, and would advise it

---

discovered the length of the canal, if the finger be placed on the instrument at the point just beyond the glans penis, the exact depth to which the porte caustique should be subsequently introduced may be accurately ascertained. On the instrument which goes under Lallemand's name, there are means for measuring this distance which can be fixed by the slide seen in the woodcut.

When I was in the habit of employing Lallemand's porte caustique, I did not find it necessary to pass a catheter, as I usually enjoined a patient not to drink on the day I propose applying the instrument, and requested him to empty the bladder immediately before its introduction. It is a good precaution, moreover, to previously relieve the bowels by Castor Oil, or of an enema. The porte caustique must be prepared in the following manner:—"Fuse some broken pieces of Nitrate of Silver in a watch-glass held over a spirit-lamp by means of a pair of forceps, taking care to apply the heat at first at some distance, otherwise an explosion may take place; when fused, the caustic should be poured into the little cup, allowed to dry, and the projecting portions removed by a file, the canula must then be returned into the closed instrument, which, after being oiled, may be passed down into the bladder, the patient being in bed or lying on a sofa; a surgeon at all in the habit of passing instruments is able to distinguish when the instrument enters that viscus. The diseased part is at once known to the patient (so Lallemand states) by the instrument causing some pain. This once ascertained, the surgeon will withdraw the outer canula to the extent of half an inch, and at the same time give a rotatory motion to the inner canula containing the caustic. By this means the diseased surface is slightly cauterized, eschars are not necessarily formed, nor are any passed in the urine, and the internal canula, being drawn within the external one, cauterization is confined to the morbid structures only. Rest in the horizontal position must be enjoined, and the patient desired not to make water for some hours. If pain comes on, a good dose of Laudanum, or an enema with Opium may be prescribed. For the few following days there is some pain in making water. The discharge increases, and is mixed with a little blood; but by attention to diet and rest, together with moderate doses of Copaiba or Cubeb capsules, these symptoms abate, and with them the emissions, although in some cases the cauterization may induce one or two escapes of semen during the following nights. Sexual intercourse must be strictly prohibited, and any cause which may originally have produced spermatorrhœa must be studiously avoided. In some cases it may be necessary to have recourse to a second or third application of the caustic; but at least ten days should elapse between each cauterization, and any accidents which may arise must be treated on general principles.

where there was marked and persistent irritation of the urethra not relieved by the remedies named.* I have also used

* *Cauterization.*—In passing an instrument as above described, one of two conditions usually exists: either the instrument passes down to the veru-montanum without pain, when all at once excessive sensibility is felt in one or more spots; or the urethra is found large, patulous, and insensible, hardly seeming to feel the presence of the instrument; the former condition is, however, the one most frequently met with. Having explored the urethra, the surgeon should leave the patient quiet for that day, the only precaution taken being that of administering a mild aperient, and desiring him to abstain altother from stimulants or coffee. The sufferer usually prefers that the operation be performed at the surgeon's residence, and I have never found any objection to the patient returning home in a cab if the distance is not great. On the morning of the operation the patient may be allowed to eat a simple breakfast of bread, butter, or meat, but he must be strictly enjoined to abstain from fluid of any kind.

Before proceeding to perform the operation, I desire the patient to completely empty the bladder. I employ a syringe which is made entirely of stout glass, to obviate breakage, and to avoid all decomposition of the solution of Nitrate of Silver. When put together and charged with fluid (containing a solution of ten grains of nitrate of silver to the ounce of distilled water), the instrument is passed down the urethra, the patient standing against the wall. No oil should be used, as it will interfere with the action of the caustic. The surgeon should take the precaution of folding a towel between the legs, in order to protect the trousers of the patient from being stained. The piston of the instrument is then to be forced down, at the same time that the finger and thumb of the operator's left hand compress the lips of the meatus firmly against the instrument, so as to prevent the fluid escaping from the urethra until the syringe is withdrawn, which is done as soon as the injection has been forced out of the instrument. I may mention here that the syringe usually holds about two or three drachms. The pressure of the fingers on the urethra is then withdrawn, and the whole of the injected fluid passes out into the vessel which is placed to receive it. The patient may now sit or lie down in an arm chair, and remain there a quarter of an hour. The first result of the operation is to produce a warm pricking sensation at the end of the penis, which soon, however, subsides, and usually in ten minutes disappears gradually. In some cases an urgent desire to make water may come on, but as the bladder has been previously emptied, this is a fictitious want, and rapidly passes off, the patient being told to restrain the desire as much as possible. As to the pain felt after the operation, I have been over and over again assured that the suffering consequent on the application of the

with excellent results in these cases, a solution of Sulphate of Hydrastia, grs. iv. to Water, ℥j.; filling the urethra from the long tube, and holding the injection for some minutes.

---

caustic has been much less than the patient anticipated, and in some instances it has been so slight that the patient doubts if any caustic can have reached the affected parts.

Other patients say they have experienced none of that shock to the nervous system which interested individuals had led them to believe was sure to follow the injection of a solution of nitrate of silver, and which they had read that medical men had understated, in order to induce patients to submit to the operation. The first effect of the operation is to produce an oozing from the urethra, caused by the escape of a drop or two of caustic mixed with mucus, and hence a piece of linen or a folded handkerchief should be placed around the meatus to absorb the moisture, and protect the shirt from becoming stained. The patient within half an hour may be allowed to return home, but must not walk at all that day, and should swallow a copaiba capsule directly, repeating it every eight hours. Too strict injunctions can not be given to abstain from drinking fluid of any kind until after making water, and not to pass urine until absolutely obliged. Some men can easily remain twelve hours without passing water; a space of time which allows the caustic solution to act on the mucous membrane. When the patient is no longer able to resist the desire of making water, say twelve hours after the operation, he may drink as much weak tea, soda-water, or diluents as he pleases Immediately after the operation he may take his usual meals, abstaining, as before said, from fluid, and confining himself to an easy chair or sofa. During the few following hours some slight whitish discharge, like mucus, will flow from the urethra; but there will be little or no pain. When the patient first makes water there is some scalding, but the urine passes without difficulty. In some few cases, where I have reason to suppose there is an extra amount of irritability of the bladder, I have prescribed opium after the operation, but this is very rarely necessary. When the patient has made water once, he may do so as often as he likes, and each time the slight scalding will diminish, until it wholly disappears. On the day following, a tinge of blood is sometimes noticed attending the last drops of urine, but this disappears in a day or two, the urine becoming again clear. On the second or third day the copaiba capsules may be dispensed with, and the patient may commence a course of tonics with gymnastic exercises, sponging, etc. Violent exercise should not be indulged in for the first few days after the operation, but a moderate walk need not be interdicted. In from four to ten days the patient may take a little claret, and subsequently resume his usual mode of life, observing, however, abstinence from tobacco or strong coffee.—*Acton.*

239. This urethral irritation is sometimes relieved by external counter-irritation from a perpetual blister, irritating plaster, issue, or seton. In some cases we find it necessary to keep the penis sore in order to prevent erections, or in some exceptional cases to insure against self-pollution.

240. When lying on the back causes erection and nocturnal emission, we employ counter-irritation over the spine to prevent this, and also to relieve the spinal erythism which exists. The irritating plaster of our Dispensatory is the agent I prefer, and to the extent of two by six inches; in the majority of cases it is applied over the sacro-vertebral articulation.

241. Where there is marked enfeeblement of the perineal structure, a well adjusted elastic perineal supporter is sometimes of marked advantage, until by the use of electricity and passive movement and kneading we can stimulate normal nutrition of these structures.

242. Pendulous scrotum and dragging testes, with or without varicocele, calls for a well adjusted suspensory bandage; and sometimes the local use of Pond's Hamamelis.

243. The truss worn for hernia may not only prove a cause of impotence, but also of spermatorrhœa. It should always be examined, and the pressure so arranged as to remove the irritation as far as possible. In some cases it will not do to have any pressure upon the back, and then the simple strap with leaden ball will prove the best form. In others it is the inguinal pressure that causes the irritation, and we will employ the large soft pad for retention only.

244. Whilst in some cases we order the drinking of large quantities of water, to dilute the urine, render it less acrid, and thereby remove irritation, in others we prohibit fluids, especially in the evening. In many cases the full bladder is the cause of sexual excitation, erection and nocturnal emission. In one case under my care, the emission would occur in the day-time, under any circumstances, if the bladder was allowed to become largely distended. The patient is therefore charged to drink but little in the evening, pass water before going to

bed, form a habit of waking and passing water after midnight, and of getting up, when first awaking in the morning. Not unfrequently this will give material aid in the arrest of nocturnal emissions.

245. I need hardly say in conclusion that the patient must break off from all vicious habits and associates. Contact with the impure in thought and action is sometimes sufficient to continue the disease, despite the influence of medicine. A vicious literature is as bad as vicious associates, and our country is flooded with it. It not only includes such vile sheets as the police journals, but the more popular weeklies filled with exciting love stories, mixed with blood and thunder. The parent who allows such stuff to come into his house, is morally responsible for the debauchment of his children. If the habit of self-abuse is not given up, we insist that it shall be, and if the sufferer lacks moral power, we make use of escharotics over the course of the urethra, to make handling the organ an impossibility. It is more difficult to manage the married than the single, and sometimes it is impossible to control them without single beds.

SPERMATORRHŒA IN WOMEN.

246. Admitting that this is a misnomer, and that women can not have the disease according to our present nosology, any more than they can have prostatorrhœa, yet when we study spermatorrhœa as but a symptom of a lesion of the reproductive function, we can readily see how women may suffer similar lesions without this symptom. I am satisfied from a considerable experience that there are more cases in women than in men, and that the suffering and danger to mind and life is full as great in one as in the other.

247. The reproductive functions in man and woman are alike, though the organs differ. There is the same sexual

feeling, the same relationship with the emotions and the mind, the same connection with the spinal cord, and the same relations with all the vegetative functions through the sympathetic nervous system.

248. If we study the causes of the lesion we find that women are quite as much exposed to them as men. We have already seen that they suffer from self-abuse, not so frequently it is true, but quite as severely. And in the marital relation they suffer more frequently from excitation of the sexual organs without gratification. Let this be repeated for years, and the wonder is, not that we meet with such cases, but that they are not of more frequent occurrence.

249. Many of the nervous ills of woman, cloaked under the name *nervousness*, or hysteria, are due to this lesion of the reproductive function. Thousands of women have *enjoyed* ill health, and living a few years of a sickly wasted life, have died, without the nature of the lesion and its cause having been suspected. It is not always child-bearing and the common household cares, that bring premature age and death. These are rarely the cause, as may be seen in the improved health of women when pregnant. Pregnancy, child-birth and nursing, are physiological functions, and nature responds to the call with alacrity. Perpetual gratification of the lust of a *rutting* man is unphysiological, and is the cause of the multitude of maladies attributed to natural function.

250. It is well to think and talk in plain English on this subject, for the lesions are so serious and destructive, and the cause so gross, that they should be brought fairly to view. It may be impossible to rectify the wrong in many cases, but it is possible in a large number, and we illy do our duty as physicians if we do not use our influence in a right direction.

251. Though the lesions we propose studying here are principally nervous, it will do no harm to call attention to the fact that every form of local disease of the uterine organs may be grown from this cause. And, to the more important fact that this abuse must be stopped if we are to have successful

results from treatment. Indeed I have seen severe cases of ulceration of the cervix, that had resisted topical treatment, cured by continence and cleanliness alone.

252. The disease of the reproductive function we are studying in women may be divided into two classes—one of hyperæmia and increased sensibility of the nervous system and the sexual organs, the other of anæmia, and impaired sensibility. It is well to make this classification of cases, even though the majority may show neither the one nor the other condition as a marked feature. When they do, however, the treatment will differ very materially.

253. In the one class of cases, the general expression of the body is of contraction—pinched. The features are sharp, the muscles of the face distinctly outlined, the orbicularis orum and palpebrarum contracted, mouth retracted, eyelids do not close, alæ nasi drawn in, eyes dry, pupils immobile, hair harsh and dry, tongue contracted and incurved, etc. The appetite is variable, digestion poor, bowels inclined to constipation, or constipation alternated with irritative diarrhœa, nutrition impaired, skin parchment-like and dark, etc.

You do not have to ask the patient if she suffers, the entire expression is one of suffering. You get a history of pain in back, intense pain in head, pain in every part of the body upon slight lesion, of broken rest, unpleasant sensation of dizziness, præcordial oppression, and uneasiness in the pelvic region. But above all there is the impairment of conscious life alternating between undue excitation and the apathy of despair, which causes the most intense suffering, though it bears but little relationship to pain.

254. You make a vaginal exploration, and the touch sends an electric thrill over the person, and up the spine to the head, which is recognized at once as unpleasant. The examination will frequently show the character of the lesion in the change of the structures and their increased sensibility.

255. In the opposite cases, the body is expressionless, the movements languid, and the face apathetic. The eyelids are

full, dark lines around them, eyes dull, pupils dilated. The tongue is full, pale and slimy, the breath a peculiar sweetish fetor, bowels constipated, digestion and blood-making impaired. She suffers from a sense of fullness and weight in the pelvis, dragging sensations, difficult urination and defecation, is easily exhausted, especially when obliged to be on the feet. This patient sometimes suffers intense pain, but it is the pain of exhaustion, as if nature, wearied with the struggle for life, was about to succumb.

In this class we find atony of the sexual organs. The vulva has lost the fatty tissue, and is soft and relaxed, the vagina dilated, the uterus low, the cervix full, the os dilated and patulous, and from all the mucous surfaces there is an increased secretion.

256. We have a larger number of cases, in which the symptoms are the same as described in the lesion of the male. There is marked impairment of the general health, but overshadowing this is the *nervousness*, the desire for seclusion and rest, the downcast look, unsteady eye, languid movement, with the fear of impending danger intensified by sensations of dizziness and præcordial oppression.

257. These symptoms should excite attention, and a careful examination will lead to a correct diagnosis. It is sometimes difficult to learn the facts, from the natural diffidence of woman, and her dislike to think of, much less talk upon these subjects. This is not mitigated by the common reputation of many physicians, who more from indiscreet conversation, than from impure lives, are looked upon with distrust—a fact which should lead physicians to be chaste in speech and in their professional relations, whatever they may be outside of this.

258. The prognosis is favorable when we can control the habits of the patient, and avoid sexual excitement. In some cases absolute continence and avoidance of all exciting causes are necessary. In others the cure progresses better with very moderate indulgence.

259. TREATMENT.—In the first class of cases I usually commence the treatment with: ℞ Tincture Pulsatilla, Tincture Macrotys, aa. ʒss.; Water, ℥iv.; a teaspoonful four times a day. If the circulation shows fullness, I alternate with this: ℞ Tincture Veratrum, gtts. x. to xx.; Water, ℥iv. If it is small and shows hardness, Aconite is taken in preference. Not unfrequently there is a marked indication for the use of Acids, and we prescribe them internally and use Acid baths. Bromide of Potassium may be used where there is intense sexual excitement, and when the rest is broken. If the patient complains of persistent headache, we think of Iodide of Ammonium; if there is an epileptic tendency shown by muscular twitchings, or periodic excitement with rigidity of muscles, we give Bromide of Ammonium.

In some cases we use Veratrum and Fowler's Solution of Arsenic, alternately or together, and sometimes associated with Cod Oil. Quinine inunction is frequently an excellent means, and gives the necessary stimulation to the nerve centers.

260. Demulcent vaginal enemata are sometimes of advantage, and warm Flaxseed infusion may be taken as the type. Some cases are benefited by the wet-pack around the pelvis, others by the acid-pack, and still others by suppurative counter-irritation. The electric sponge-bath is also an efficient means. It may be used with the positive pole applied to the cervical spine, and the negative passed over the hips, perineum, back, and with a vaginal and uterine electrode through the reproductive organs.

261. The second class of cases will be benefited by the use of restoratives, good food, out-door exercise and sunshine. We prescribe here Pulsatilla and Macrotys, but alternate it with Nux Vomica and Iodine—the pill heretofore named is a good form. If there is excitement with free mucoid secretion, especially the glairy secretion from the cervix uteri, we prescribe: ℞ Tincture Staphysagria, ʒj.; Water, ʒiv.; a teaspoonful four times a day. As an alternate we may use Tinct.

Phosphorus in the same proportion. Hamamelis is the remedy where there is a tumid and doughy cervix, and full, protruding perineum, Collinsonia being reserved for the acute venous congestion.

Coca may be employed in these cases where there is involuntary excitement of the sexual organs, especially at night; Phosphate of Soda where the tissues are full, pallid, and lack elasticity. Belladonna and Ergot are occasionally useful where there is dullness, hebetude, and a disposition to sleep. Zincum will be found an excellent remedy where there is a disposition to diarrhœa, and impediments to chylous absorption—the sixth decimal trituration is recommended, or small doses of Oxide of Zinc.

Salt water frictions to spine, abdomen and perineum, with brisk rubbing with dry flannel will be found a good means in some cases. In others the dry flannel or silk friction is preferable. And in still others we use electricity for its stimulant action—superficial faradization being the best.

262. The local applications, if any are used, should be stimulant as well as calculated to arrest the increased secretion. There are cases in which Nitrate of Silver, grs. v. to grs. x. to the ounce, makes the best injection. Sulphate of Zinc, ʒss.; Chlorate of Potash, ʒij., to the pint of water, is a good injection. The Tincture of Hamamelis, one part to two or three of water, is also a good remedy where an astringent action is desired.

263. There is sometimes marked spinal irritation in these cases, which must be recognized and relieved. It will be recollected that we divide this lesion into two classes—hyperæmia and anæmia of the cord, the nervous lesion being quite the same in both. The first is met by suppurative counter-irritation, the second by salt water frictions, rubefacient frictions, faradization, or the hot iron—firing.

DISEASES OF WOMAN INCIDENT TO PROSTITUTION.

264. Some public women seem to suffer but very little from their mode of living, but these are usually persons of peculiarly strong nervous systems, well developed bodies, and good digestive organs. They are also very careful in the care of the person, cleanly, regular in their habits, and the sexual excesses are thus counter-balanced by right living in other respects. But the larger number do suffer from acute diseases of the sexual organs, and finally from confirmed chronic disease.

VULVITIS.

265. Inflammation of the vulva may be deep-seated or superficial, the last being by far the most common.

In deep seated inflammation the parts are much swollen, red and painful. The patient suffers considerable constitutional disturbance, the pulse increased in frequency, the skin dry, bowels constipated, urine scanty, tongue coated, and the nervous system excited. In some cases the inflammation is very extensive, and involves the ischio-rectal fossæ, and the patient suffers intensely. It may be days before suppuration is so far advanced, that the pus points to the surface, and sometimes it is inclined to burrow deeply, instead of coming to the surface.

266. Superficial vulvitis is analogous to balanitis in the male, and is frequently the result of want of cleanliness, the secretion of the too frequently excited organs being acrid and irritating. In some cases there is an eczematous or herpetic eruption, and an intolerable pruritus, which induces scratching or rubbing the parts, only to make the trouble worse. Continuing for some time, we have an eruption of small phlegmons, very painful, and which sometimes repeat themselves for weeks or months.

267. TREATMENT.—In the deep-seated inflammation the patient is put upon the use of Veratrum or Aconite, as indicated, alternated with Phytolacca. The patient has a hot sitz-bath, a local application of Tincture of Veratrum to the inflamed part, followed by an emollient application, cold or warm, as may give the greatest relief. The bowels are kept gently open with a saline cathartic, if necessary, and if the urine remains scant, a weak solution of Acetate of Potash is given as a drink.

Though this is an outline of the treatment in ordinary cases, we do not forget that the successful administration of remedies is based upon special indications, and we follow them here as in other diseases.

268. If called in the early stage, we may expect resolution, and if suppuration results we want to restrict it as much as possible. But when pus has formed, no advantage comes from giving it time to burrow and break down sound tissue, and the abscess is opened early. If a proper general treatment has been pursued, and the secretions restored, the process of healing is rapid and good. But should it show tardiness in healing we may fear the formation of fistulæ, and we adopt the following course.

269. Giving the patient a careful examination to determine the general treatment—and this is a very important matter—we inject the abscess with such stimulant as may serve to restore the reparative process, and granulation from the bottom. I prefer our old-fashioned Sesqui-Carbonate of Potash, though sometimes the Sulphate of Zinc will do as well or better. The general means will be Cod-Oil, Lime water, Arsenic, Iron, the Hypophosphites, Phytolacca, Rhus, Iodide of Ammonium, or other special remedies as may be indicated.

270. In superficial vulvitis with excoriation, we sometimes find Colgate's best Glycerine Soap, well applied, an effectual remedy. The "Juniper Tar Soap" is also an excellent agent where there is a constant disposition to this irritation. When

it is associated with pruritis, I prescribe Glycerole of Tar. In some cases, a solution of Permanganate of Potash, grs. v. to x. to Water, ℥iv., is a good local application, as is Carbolic Acid, grs. x. to Glycerine, ℥ij.; Rose Water, ℥iv. The old remedy: ℞ Morphia Sul., grs. x.; Sodæ Bi-Boras, ℥j.; Aquæ Rosæ, ℥vj. M.

271. In some cases the difficulty is dependent upon the irritant secretion of the parts alone, in some upon irritation of the rectum, from ascarides, constipation or hemorrhoids. When very persistent, we will always find some general lesion, and even in acute cases, a single remedy, prescribed for a special indication, will give speedy relief. Then we use Rhus, when the vulva presents a shining, bright-red appearance, dry, with the characteristic pustular eruption. Apis, if the surface is mottled red and white, like the eruption of "hive," with some burning, or burning with itching. Phytolacca, if associated with fullness and sense of weight and dragging. When the irritation becomes chronic, we think of Arsenic and Cod Oil.

272. Chronic, deep-seated vulvitis is a very troublesome affection. There is a deposit of low albuminoid material, sometimes to a very considerable extent, and as the finger is passed over the surfaces the nodulated deposits resemble cystic or fibroid growths. These break down occasionally from local irritation or impairment of the general health, and suppuration occurring, sinuses form, burrowing in the cellular tissue of the part. After a time the formation of pus ceases, and the nodules of cacoplastic material are re-formed.

In some of these cases, Lime-water is the remedy, associated with general restoratives, but in the majority permanent relief will only come from Cod-Oil, and Arsenic in small doses.

URETHRITIS.

273. In public women we are apt to regard inflammation of the urethra as specific, yet many cases of simple urethritis will be met with. It is usually associated with vaginal or vesical irritation, and sometimes with vaginitis or cystitis.

274. The patient complains of a frequent desire to pass water, and after a time the calls are every few minutes and can not be resisted. The urine is scanty, high colored and acrid, and is passed with tenesmus and burning. The skin is dry, the pulse increased in frequency and hard, and the face shows suffering.

275. TREATMENT.—In the early stage of the disease the patient may be put upon the use of Veratrum and Gelseminum, with warm demulcent vaginal enemata. If indicated, a saline laxative may be administered, but frequently they will get along better without it. Frequently the patient is markedly relieved in a few hours, and put upon the use of Aconite and Macrotys, makes a speedy recovery. In other cases it is tedious, and we follow with Cannabis Indica, Pulsatilla, Staphysagria, as may be indicated. Persistent burning pain in the urethra is sometimes speedily relieved by Rhus and Aconite alternated.

276. In some cases local medication is of advantage, especially if the disease is persistent. A bougie conveying a small portion of Carbolic Acid in Olive Oil, is good, so is an injection of Sulphate of Zinc and Morphia, but I prefer in most cases the solution of Sulphate of Hydrastia.

IRRITABLE URETHRA.

277. In the last few years we have had many cases of irritable urethra. It is not confined to public women, but is usually a result of sexual excesses.

The patient complains of burning or scalding along the course of the urethra, frequent desire to pass water, and tenesmus. In some cases it is paroxysmal, the patient suffering severely for a time, and then for some hours having relief. In some cases it is only felt during the day, and especially if she is much on her feet, but in others the patient has to pass water several times during the night and suffers constantly. Pretty soon you will see it wearing upon the general health, and as weeks go by, the patient has a worn and haggard appearance, and complains of various functional lesions.

278. TREATMENT. — I have obtained the best results in these cases from the use of Rhus, Apis and Eryngium, according to the special indications heretofore named. I select the remedy, and use it in alternation with Aconite. Prof. King's prescription of Elaterium will be found a specific in those cases in which there is inflammation of the base of the bladder with deep pain and tenesmus. Of a Tincture of Elaterium, we would give twenty drops three times a day, until it acted upon the bowels—then in doses of five drops.

279. If there is frequent micturition with pain and great tenesmus, extending to the bladder, I would recommend Stramonium as follows: ℞ Tincture Stramonium, ʒss.; Comp. Tincture Cardamom, ℥iijss.; from half to one teaspooful every two or three hours. If the patient has been in the habit of using Opium, the dose will be larger.

280. When the disease is persistent, and resists the action of remedies, forcible dilatation of the urethra may be proposed as a radical cure. Usually the patient will have to be placed under the influence of Chloroform, when a large bougie or catheter may be passed, followed by one as large as the forefinger, or the finger well oiled may be passed quite as well. The patient is kept in a recumbent position, and full doses of Veratrum are given. The operation is repeated in two or three days, usually without the Chloroform.

VAGINITIS.

281. Acute vaginitis is not of unfrequent occurrence, and is sometimes a source of great suffering and annoyance. It is usually rapid in its development. Commencing with a sense of scalding in the canal, the parts soon become swollen, hot and painful. In some cases the natural secretion is arrested and the parts are dry, but in others the secretions are thin and acrid. Not unfrequently there is an unpleasant

tenesmus and bearing down, and despite the care of the patient her sufferings are increased by involuntary contraction of the abdominal muscles. The constitutional disturbance is frequently marked. The skin is harsh and dry, urine scanty and acrid, bowels constipated, pain in head and back, temperature elevated, 102° to 104°, and the circulation excited.

282. It is impossible to diagnose the simple from the specific vaginitis further than this: that the simple comes up quicker, the symptoms are more active at first, and not nearly so severe in the second stage. The acute inflammation in simple vaginitis is sometimes followed by increased secretion of mucus or muco-pus, but the pain and uneasiness are relieved by the discharge, whilst in the specific disease it is increased by it.

283. TREATMENT.—I have treated these cases as I would an acute inflammation in other parts of the body. The patient has a hot sitz-bath followed by hot fomentations, or a cold-pack, as may be deemed best, and is put upon full doses of Veratrum, with Gelseminum in some cases. If the bowels are locked up they are gently moved with a saline cathartic after the action of the sedative has been manifest. Now continuing the sedative we add Acetate of Potash with abundance of water, until the urinary secretion is free, and follow with Cannabis Indica, Pulsatilla, Macrotys, or Stayphysagria, as indicated.

284. In some cases, warm demulcent vaginal injections will be grateful at first, but sometimes they are not well borne. But after two or three days, a weak solution of Chlorate of Potash to keep the parts thoroughly clean will be found important. If secretion becomes too free, use an infusion of Hydrastis, or better, a solution of Sulphate of Hydrastia.

CHRONIC VAGINITIS.

285. Sporting women do not suffer from vaginal leucorrhœa as frequently as one would suppose. The strict atten-

tion to cleanliness, necessitated by their position, freeing the vagina from all secretions and discharges which might undergo decomposition, is a safeguard. There is no doubt but that want of cleanliness and care is a very common cause of this trouble with most women. In prostitutes, the vagina does not suffer from irritation like the vulvæ and cervix uteri, and if not exposed to the specific disease, and free from disease above, there is little tendency to abnormal discharges from this surface. Following a badly treated gonorrhœa, or disease of the cervix uteri, we sometimes have a very unpleasant form of the disease, and one which at times will cause urethritis and balanitis in the male.

286. The symptoms are clear. There is an abundant muco-purulent discharge, varying in character, from a thin ichor to a thick, flocculent yellow or greenish fluid. The woman complains of aching in the hips and back, sense of fullness and dragging in the pelvis, some difficulty in micturition, tires easily, and suffers from menstrual irregularity.

An examination discloses the increased secretion, and determines its chatacter. When the discharges are removed and the mucous membrane exposed, it is found thickened and discolored. In some cases it is unnaturally rugose, and every fold seems like a sponge furnishing the peculiar secretion. In others all the rugæ seem to be effaced, and the mucous surface is unnaturally smooth, the vagina being very much dilated, especially in its upper portion.

287. This disease is not unfrequently associated with diseases of the rectum and bladder. There is constipation and difficult defecation, a hemorrhoidal condition, ulceration or fissure. And of the bladder, chronic inflammation, increased mucous secretion, deposits of the triple-phosphates, with occasionally prolapse.

288. TREATMENT.—In my experience a good general treatment is absolutely indispensable to success. A careful examination determines the special remedies indicated, or if there

are no such indications we then institute means to increase waste and improve nutrition with the expectation of getting a better renewal of life, and with better tissues we may anticipate an improved condition of the diseased structures.

289. The remedies which exert a special influence upon these structures will be thought of. Macrotys, if there is pain in hips, pelvis and legs. Hamamelis, if there is venous fullness, tendency to varix, and relaxation of perineum. Staphysagria, if associated with involuntary sexual excitement. Pulsatilla, if the patient is nervous and depressed. Eryngium, if there is difficult micturition. Tincture Phosphorus, if increased mucous secretion from bladder. Even Copaiba and Cubebs may find a place in our therapeutics.

290. In old and stubborn cases, with depraved nutrition, I would always think of Cod Oil as an important remedy. And if the skin showed the peculiar dusky hue, with want of elasticity, Fowler's Solution of Arsenic.

291. The local remedies will necessarily vary very greatly. Take the thickened spongy vagina, seemingly secreting from every pore, and I would use an injection of Tincture of Iodine, Solution of Nitrate of Silver, Solution of Sulphate of Zinc, or of Permanganate of Potash, the strength of the solution proportioned to the change of tissue. This treatment necessitates confinement for a few days, and the free use of sedatives, but it is sometimes the only one that will reach the difficulty.

292. In less severe cases I frequently prescribe: ℞ Chlorate of Potash, ℥ss.; Sulphate of Zinc, ʒj.; Water, Oj. ℞ Tincture Hamamelis, ℥iv.; Water, Oj. ℞ Permanganate of Potash, ʒj.; Water, Oj. ℞ Solution of Carbolic Acid in Glycerine, (℥j. to ℥iv.) ℥ss.; Water, Oj. ℞ Infusion of aa. Alnus and Quercus Rubra. ℞ Tannic Acid, ʒj.; Glycerine, ℥iv.; Water, Oj. I need hardly say, that we get along better when we study our cases well, and prescribe according to the condition of the case in hand, and not empirically.

ACUTE METRITIS.

293. Inflammation of the uterus is of more frequent occurrence than vaginitis, the lower segment suffering especially. Whilst we may have a specific (gonorrhœal) inflammation of the cervical canal, the diagnosis is generally easily made because it involves the parts below.

294. Whilst the symptoms are pretty clear if we look for them, the disease of the uterus is sometimes overlooked, because the general symptoms are so pronounced. The patient complains of the general *malaise* preceding severe disease, has pain in the back, limbs and head, a chill, followed by febrile reaction. When we are called, she feels so sick, that she finds it difficult to locate the disease. She has unpleasant sensations in the stomach with frequent nausea and vomiting, sometimes most persistent. The bowels are constipated, and she has an uneasiness and desire to go to stool, which is ineffectual, but painful. The skin is dry, urine scanty, and its passage frequent, the temperature is elevated, and the pulse small, hard and frequent. With such symptoms the disease may run on for days, like an ordinary fever, or it may be greatly intensified by bad medication, and develop peritoneal inflammation with typhoid symptoms. I recollect a case of this kind, which ran a course of ten days, without being suspected by the attendant physician, yet post-mortem examination showed suppurative inflammation of the uterine wall, and recent peritoneal adhesions.

295. TREATMENT.—The treatment here is nearly a repetition of that given for acute inflammation of other parts, yet there is no harm in repeating it. The patient must have entire rest, even from the tenesmus which is sometimes so annoying. Following a hot sitz-bath, with sometimes Chloroform applications to lower spine and over the hypogastrium, we use a rectal enema of starch-water and Tincture Opium, if necessary. Selecting the appropriate sedative, Veratrum when the pulse is full, Aconite when it is small, we give it in

the usual doses, every hour until convalescence. If the nervous system is excited, the eyes bright, pupils contracted, we add to it Gelseminum. If the patient is dull and somnolent, Belladonna. If there is muscular pain, pain in the hips, and seemingly in the pelvic bones, or deep-seated in the pelvis, Macrotys or Caulophyllum. The sharp, burning pain in pelvis, with erythematous flush of face, or surface elsewhere, Rhus. In some cases the indication for the alkalies is marked, and a Salt of Soda is curative; in the latter part of the disease Acids are occasionally required.

296. If the inflammation has come on during or immediately following the menstrual flow, or the result of abortion, (which is always to be looked to), the antiseptics become important remedies. We are accustomed to say that Chlorate of Potash is *the* antiseptic in the diseases of the uterus, when absorption of putrescent material has occurred. Though this is the general rule, it will not do to take it for granted, and we select our remedy as we would in other cases.

297. If at the time of the menstrual flow, the discharge has been prematurely arrested, we follow the sedatives with: ℞ Tincture Pulsatilla, Tincture Macrotys, aa. ʒss.; Water, ℥iv.; a teaspoonful every two hours. To be effectual, sedatives must precede their administration. We never give the stimulant emmenagogues in such cases.

298. In the majority of cases the hot sitz-bath, followed by fomentations and Chloroform counter-irritation, will give the most relief, especially if near the menstrual period. But in some cases, not at this time, the cold pack to the pelvis and perineum will do better. Occasionally benefit is had from warm enemata, of Chlorate of Potash, a weak salt water, or a demulcent; but in many cases the exertion and vaginal irritation does more harm than the injection does good.

CHRONIC METRITIS.

299. Chronic inflammation is not an uncommon disease in the advanced life of the sporting woman, as in her sisters who

have suffered sexual abuse under the marital cloak. The long continued excitement, frequent excesses, derangement of the menstrual function, and attacks of the acute disease, eventually lead to it, and when these causes persist, the patient is with difficulty cured.

300. The previous history shows repeated attacks of uterine irritation, with attending unpleasant sensations. The patient may have had gonorrhœa, which is a not uncommon cause. She has suffered from back-ache, weak back, fullness and dragging in the pelvis, pain in the limbs, and leucorrhœa. Her general health is impaired, appetite variable, bowels irregular, some urinary trouble, and general malaise. Sexual intercourse may or may not be painful, but she is nearly always worse afterwards.

301. Examination by the touch shows an enlarged uterus, sometimes to double its usual size. Elevating the organ upon the finger may not be painful, but when pressure is made through the abdominal wall above, it is always productive of pain. The lower segment alone, or the entire organ may be involved. The tumid tissue, tense yet yielding to the touch, with a sense of impaired elasticity, is characteristic. The os may be patulous and open, or tightly closed and rigid. In the first case the finger will readily dilate it and pass in to the first articulation.

302. If the disease is of the cervix principally, we will sometimes find an abundant secretion from the cervical canal of a glairy, tough mucus; or there may be erosion of the outer surface with abundant muco-purulent secretion ; or well defined ulceration within or without, or both.

303. In some cases where the disease is of long duration, the cervix is very much enlarged, sometimes full, doughy, inelastic, at others nodulated, as if suffering from malignant disease. In other cases, and especially when the result of old gonorrhœal inflammation, the surface shows a granular surface, which bleeds on being touched.

304. Almost always there is displacement of the uterus

if the disease is of long duration. Most commonly there is prolapse, the cervix resting upon the recto-vaginal septum; and here the sense of weight and dragging is greatly increased, and all the symptoms intensified. In some there is anteversion or retroversion, and the pressure upon the bladder and rectum is the cause of very unpleasant symptoms.

305. TREATMENT.—It might seem unnecessary to study these diseases here, as they are studied in detail in the common treatises on diseases of women. But there are two reasons why I think it best: The first, that they may be associated in the mind with wrongs of the sexual function. The second, that a simpler treatment may be presented. It really makes no difference whether this inflammation and its results are met with in the married or the prostitute, the causes are very similar, and the treatment will not differ materially.

306. Rest to the reproductive organs is an essential of a successful treatment. Absolute continence is not necessary in some cases, but it will be found the best in nearly all. Too much exercise upon the feet is to be avoided, and sometimes the recumbent position for a few days facilitates the cure. When there is much dragging and weight in the pelvis, the *perineal supporter* is an excellent aid, and will give marked relief. Any wrong of bowels or bladder causing tenesmus, must be relieved, as this seems to perpetuate the disease.

307. The general treatment is of great importance. In some cases there are *marked* indications for some *one* remedy, and we will find it curative. Thus I have cured cases with Macrotys, Rhus, Hamamelis, Nitric Acid, Thuja, Copper, Arsenic, alone, or as the internal treatment. The indications for a remedy not being distinct, we use those which influence the part, and in the direction opposite to the disease. In other cases, the general treatment will be directed to a *renewal of life*—such means as will increase waste and excretion, and such as will improve the appetite, blood-making, and nutrition.

308. When we come to particular remedies, we may be guided by the following: If menstruation is painful, and there is deep pelvic pain, or muscular pain, Macrotys and Pulsatilla. If there is fullness and relaxation of perineal tissues, with or without hemorrhoids, feebleness and want of elasticity of cervix uteri, Hamamelis; nodulated hardness of cervix, Iodide of Ammonium; with full leaden pallor of tongue, Iodide of Potassium; violet coloration of tongue, same color of cervix, Nitric Acid; burning pain in upper vagina, or rectum, or bright erythematous redness of cervix, Rhus; contracted os, or tense, resisting cervix, with brownish coloration of mucous membranes, Arsenic; dilated os, and free, cervical secretion, Staphysagria, Tincture Phosphorus.

309. In some cases vaginal injections are used for cleanliness alone, in others for the topical action of the remedy upon the cervix. In the main we may be guided in their selection as in chronic vaginitis. There are cases in which a topical application of a saturated solution of Tannic Acid, or Persulphate of Iron will be beneficial in strengthening the blood-vessels, and diminishing the hypertrophied cervix. Others in which there is abundant secretion from the eroded mucous membrane, in which Permanganate of Potash or Carbolic Acid will be useful.

310. In the more common condition of localized ulceration I prefer the Nitric Acid to all other remedies. Let the part be freely exposed with the speculum, using a good light reflected. Have a pine stick of sufficient length, with the extremity flattened, and adapted to reach all the ulcerated surface; dip it in strong Nitric Acid, rubbing the free acid off on paper, and apply it thoroughly to the parts. For the canal of the cervix, round the end of the stick, giving an ovoid ball termination, and the acid can be well applied to the cervical canal. No application will be found so effectual in checking profuse secretion, or arresting the progress of ulceration, and promoting rapid healing as this, but it requires to be thoroughly used.

311. If the acid is applied to a large surface, or to a cervical canal greatly diseased, or the structures are very irritable, the patient should be kept in a recumbent position, and the sedatives given every hour. If there is much pain from the application, which is very rare, a sufficient dose of Morphine may be administered.

OVARITIS.

312. Inflammation of the ovaries of a sub-acute character is frequently met with, acute inflammation more rarely.. In some cases we find an unnatural irritability of these organs, and the patient suffers from local pain and sympathetic disease of other parts, whenever she has been tempted to excess in eating, drinking, or sexual indulgence.

313. In acute inflammation the general symptoms are very similar to metritis. She suffers from general *malaise*, has pain in back and limbs, headache, loss of appetite, and following a chill, considerable febrile action. In some cases she is not able to locate the pain, the entire lower abdomen and pelvis suffering with wandering pain. But eventually it localizes itself in one or other of the iliac regions, and deep pressure elicits tenderness. In some cases the peritoneum becomes very sensitive, especially when the attack comes on during or immediately following the menstrual discharge.

314. It may continue for but a short time, or run a course of days. In rare cases it is followed by pelvic cellulitis, and the formation of deep abscesses, which are especially unpleasant where the blood contains cacoplastic material or the patient suffers from constitutional syphilis.

315. In sub-acute inflammation there is little febrile action, yet the secretions are arrested, and the tongue is furred, and the appetite impaired. The patient suffers from pelvic pain, pointing in the iliac region, and less frequently a sense of weight and dragging, with back-ache and pain in the limbs.

316. TREATMENT.—The patient requires rest in either case, and we usually order a hot sitz-bath, followed by Chloroform

counter-irritation over the ovaries, and this by a hot fomentation. Hot applications, as a rule, are much more grateful than the cold pack, yet once in a while this will prove the best. If the bowels are irritated, either from the disease or the injudicious use of cathartics, great relief will follow from the use of an Opium suppository, or an enema of starch water and Tincture of Opium. There is no treatment so bad as the injudicious use of cathartics.

317. In the majority of cases Aconite will be the sedative, and when there is a sense of fullness and weight with the pain, as is frequent, we add Belladonna. Our prescription is: ℞ Tincture Aconite, gtts. x.; Tincture Belladonna, gtts. xx.; Water, ℥iv.; a teaspoonful every hour. The Belladonna may be advantageously replaced by the Macrotys the second day, or in some cases we will see cause to use it from the first. If, as the disease progresses, the patient suffers from "nervousness," we add Pulsatilla to the treatment, using it and Macrotys associated, alternated with the Aconite.

318. We control the rectal tenesmus with Opium and keep the bowels quiet, but sometimes we have difficult micturition with tenesmus. In most cases Eryngium will be the remedy, though in some it will be Gelseminum. The usual means are employed to establish secretion from skin and kidneys, as soon as the sedative action is obtained. The internal administration of Opium, and especially of Chloral, to relieve pain, is to be deprecated.

NEURALGIA.

319. Neuralgia is sometimes met with in its most stubborn form. The pain may be localized in the diseased part, as in ovaralgia, but most frequently it points at some distance from the part specially affected. Any undue irritation of ovaries, uterus, vagina, bladder or external parts, or of the sexual function in its entirety, may determine neuralgia.

320. When one suffers pain, he is apt to think it would be more easily borne in any other part than the one affected. If it was a toothache they would rather it would be a colic,

or in the toes, but if in the toes, they would rather have it any where else. Patients may not suffer more from neuralgia of the reproductive organs, in so far as the intensity of the pain is concerned, but there is no doubt but it exerts a much greater influence in impairing the vegetative functions.

321. A very common place for this neuralgia to point, is in or near the anus. Sometimes she can cover the spot with her finger, but again, though located in this region, it is shifting. In one case of this kind dependent upon ulceration of the cervix, the pain was most intolerable, the contraction of the sphincter from irritation producing convulsions. The patient was chloroformed to relieve the suffering, a small hypodermic injection of Morphia used near the rectum, and the next day the ulcer was thoroughly cauterized with Nitric Acid, and there was no further return of the neuralgia. She had suffered from these attacks for some months. In a second case the pain seemed to point under the clitoris in the arch of the pubis, and was evidently the result of venereal excesses. The same treatment, followed by Pulsatilla and Macrotys, gave relief.

322. TREATMENT.—After what has been said, I need hardly call the reader's attention to the necessity of a careful examition to determine the cause. In the majority of cases, pointing at a distance, the location of the pain is calculated to mislead. A singular case may serve as an example: Mrs. C—— has suffered for some ten years with coccygeal pain, to such an extent that she has been forced to maintain a recumbent position for weeks at a time. In addition to various internal remedies, and local applications, she has had the sphincter ani divided, and an incision made thence to the coccyx, and a small portion removed. I came to the conclusion that the wrong was of the sexual function, and associated with a dysmenorrhœa, from which the patient had suffered for years. Whether the diagnosis was correct or not, she recovered by

the use of Pulsatilla and Macrotys, followed by minute doses of Arsenic.

323. The relationship between local disease and neuralgia is best seen in cases of ulceration. Hence the cure of the ulcer stops the neuralgia.

324. But in addition to determining the cause, we find it advantageous to recognize the ordinary classification—with predominant affection of the part where the pain is found; with predominant affection of the brain, which receives the impression—and secondly, with hyperæmia; with anæmia.

325. In some cases the treatment will be almost entirely local, and when the disease of the part is removed, the neuralgia is permanently cured. In others the treatment will be general, and especially directed to the nerve centers, and as the increased susceptibility to impressions is gotten rid of, the neuralgia is cured.

326. In the condition of hyperæmia, whether of the part or brain, we put the patient upon the use of the sedatives with Gelseminum, and follow them with saline laxatives and diuretics. In the condition of anæmia we employ small doses of Aconite and Belladonna, Quinine, Iron, and the restoratives.

The hypodermic injection of Morphia becomes an important means of temporary relief, and many times of a radical cure. As a rule I prefer to use it as near the place where the pain points as possible. The quantity will vary, usually ¼ to ½ grain is sufficient; the strength of the solution being grs. x. to water, ℥j.; the dose would be ten to thirty drops. In some cases the influence of Atropia with Morphia is better than the Morphia alone—Atropia, gr. ½ to gr. j.; Morphia, grs. x.; Water, ℥j. Sometimes we use the agent endermically. Take a thimble closed at the top, put a lock of cotton in it, and drop in a few drops of strong Aqua Ammonia, and apply quickly to the part. In about one minute the epithelium is loosened, and may be rubbed off with the finger. Dress the part with a paste of Morphia, and the influence is the same as from the hypodermic injection.

GONORRHŒA.

327. It will be advantageous to study venereal diseases of women separately from those of men, at least so far as the primary or local lesion is concerned. The parts affected are different, the diseases present different symptoms, and the methods of treatment vary to a certain extent. Especially is this the case with gonorrhœa, which in the male is confined to the urethra, but in the female may involve vulva, urethra, vagina, the canal of the cervix, and even the cavity of the uterus.

328. We will study the specific character of the venereal poisons, when we come to a full consideration of the subject, and will find good evidence to believe that they are three in number—gonorrhœal, multiple or soft chancre, and syphilis proper. We will probably reach the conclusion that each is distinct, always reproducing itself in kind, never producing the others, and so far as we know, at this day never arising *de novo*. It may be that we will find the differential diagnosis difficult in some cases, but in the majority it will be readily made, if sufficient care is used.

329. Contact with the gonorrhœal virus gives rise to a peculiarly malignant inflammation of mucous membranes; not necessarily of the urethra alone, for one mucous membrane is as susceptible as another. In the extensive mucous lining of the female reproductive organs, the part first suffers, which has received the virus. It may be confined to this part, or extend itself by continuity of structure, or the secretion of gonorrhœal virus which is brought in contact with the surface.

330. Thus we will sometimes find the disease confined almost wholly to the vulva, or the urethra, lower part of vagina, or the upper portion of vagina and cervix uteri. It is singular, in some cases, how the disease can remain localized in a small portion of this mucous surface; as it is sin-

gular in others how rapidly it will spread, until the entire mucous lining is involved in disease.

331. There is also very great difference in the intensity of the disease. Whilst in some it is so mild that they are hardly aware there is anything wrong, in others the inflammation is extensive and extremely intense, with considerable constitutional disturbance. I have known cases where the woman was diseased for weeks, and only became aware of it by inoculating her male associates.

332. There is also very great difference in its persistence. In some cases it will get well of itself in a few weeks, or is readily cured by simple means, and not a trace of trouble is left. In others it seems almost impossible to effect a cure, the contagion lurking in the folds of the vulvæ, urethra, rugæ of vagina, around the cervix uteri, or in the cervical canal.

333. In the severer cases the symptoms are very distinct. From two to six days after connection, she feels a sense of heat in the vulvæ or vagina, and if the urethra is affected, scalding on passing urine. In twelve to twenty-four hours, this sense of burning has become very unpleasant, and is associated with swelling and dryness of the parts, pelvic pain, scanty urine, desire to evacuate the bowels, and some febrile action. By the second or third day secretion is established, and soon becomes abundant, a yellowish or general muco-pus, very unlike the secretion in any other acute disease of the parts.

334. In the less severe cases there is some burning, the parts being somewhat swollen. The discharge is not so free, and there is less irritation in adjacent organs, and no febrile action.

335. The progress of the disease is very variable. In some the local inflammatory symptoms are lessened as the discharge increases, but in the majority they remain quite as severe, or are intensified for some days. Usually the acute symptoms are lessened by the end of the first week, have nearly disap-

peared by the fourteenth day, and by the the twenty-first the discharge has almost or quite stopped.

336. Mention has already been made of the rectal and vesical tenesmus, which is sometimes the cause of the severest suffering. The uterus may sympathize in the inflammation, and if a menstrual period should occur during the progress of the gonorrhœa, the sufferings may be greatly intensified. In some cases the ovaries are involved as well, and rarely there is pelvic cellulitis or even peritonitis.

337. The symptoms pointing to disease of the sexual organs will cause an examination even in the mild cases. The touch shows parts swollen and hot, smooth and elastic in the first hours, bathed in secretion after the second day. If we use the speculum we will have ocular evidence of the inflammatory process. Frequently we have no occasion for the speculum, in fact could not use it without very great suffering, the parts being so swollen and painful. The woman being exposed, the vulva is shown tense, swollen and red, and as it is pressed open by the finger, the condition may be seen upwards as far as the commencement of the vagina. The nymphæ are sometimes so swollen as to project beyond the labia, and the entrance of the vagina shows like a red ring of swollen tissue inside. When the urethra is involved, the meatus is prominent, reddened and tender to the touch, and the swollen urethra is prominent in the anterior vaginal wall.

338. Whilst the majority of women recover readily from a gonorrhœa, some never get well; the specific character of the disease may be lost, after some months, so that they can not transmit the contagion, but they suffer for life from the results of the inflammation. In some the mucous membrane of the vagina is thickened and spongy, secreting muco-pus. In others there is chronic disease of the cervix uteri, especially of the cervical canal; in others chronic cystitis, with occasional attacks of urethritis; in others diseases of the rectum; and in still others, and more intractable than any, a tendency to inflammation of the pelvic connective tissue, with a low

grade of deposits which frequently break down, and sometimes from fistulæ in various parts of the perineum.

339. TREATMENT.—In the ordinary cases of gonorrhœa in women, the treatment is quite easy if they are so situated that they can follow directions. Rest and cleanliness are two essential elements. Rest means the recumbent position and quiet until the active inflammation has passed off, if this is possible. To relieve the inflammation and for cleanliness, we order a warm sitz-bath, (sometimes a cold sitz-bath is more grateful), the diseased parts being thoroughly washed with glycerine soap whilst taking the bath. This bath may be repeated two, three, or four times a day, at first, and when there is no further occasion for the bath, a large bowl of water is so placed that the patient sitting over it can wash thoroughly. Sometimes a weak salt-water is less irritant than simple water; sometimes it is a weak solution of Chlorate of Potash, Borax, or Acetate of Lead. If the upper vagina is involved, an injection pipe will be required, but when the disease is principally at the outlet, simple washing will answer.

340. If there is tenesmus, we order an Opium suppository. Moving the bowels every second day with a saline laxative—Prof. Howe's Crab Orchard Salts and Sulphur does very well, with a small portion of Cubebs after the first week.

341. Put the patient upon the use of: ℞ Tincture Veratrum, gtts. xx.; Tincture Gelseminum, ʒss. to ʒij.; Water, ℥iv.; a teaspoonful every hour. With this give a simple diuretic as Althæa, Hair Cap Moss, an infusion of Melon Seed, until the urine becomes moderately free, and then Acetate of Potash, with an abundance of diluents to maintain the action. Usually a twenty-four or forty-eight hours of this treatment gives marked relief, and we now add Canabis Indica, Macrotys, Pulsatilla or Staphysagria, as may be indicated.

342. When the disease is confined to the urethra, I would risk the abortive treatment. Nicely round the pine stick to

the size of a catheter, the end being made very smooth, dip it in the Nitric Acid, wipe dry, and after a minute, introduce it as you would a catheter. Of course it burns, though the burning does not persist as one would suppose, and is soon succeeded by a feeling of relief. The same means may be used at any part where the disease is localized and can be reached in this way. I am sure it offers the only certain cure for gonorrhœa of the cervical canal.

343. Following these sharp applications, the patient is kept quiet, put upon the use of the sedatives, and has a hot sitz-bath, or an Opium suppository if necessary.

344. When the discharge has become profuse, I have obtained more benefit from Macrotys, Cannabis, Staphysagria and Pulsatilla, then other remedies. Sometimes the old prescription of Copaiba is very good, but very offensive. Cubebs is much pleasanter, and may be used in powder when we want a stimulant action.

345. For a wash when the discharge is abundant we may prescribe Chlorate of Potash, Sulphate of Zinc, Permanganate of Potash, Carbolic Acid, or what I prefer to all, a solution of Sulphate of Hydrastia, grs. iv. to Water ℥j. It should be used after the parts are well cleansed, and held in contact with them for some time. In some cases more benefit seems to come from keeping the mucous surfaces apart than from the medicine. A piece of soft cotton cloth or lint, of proper width, folded upon itself, and wetted with Mucilage of Elm, medicated with Acetate of Lead and Morphia, carried up with the finger, a spatula or something of this kind, will be found to give very great relief. I have also employed the remedies named in this way. Or in place of this, we may use our remedies in the form of suppository, introducing them into the vagina.

346. In chronic cases where the mucous membrane is thickened and spongy, I use a local application of Nitric Acid, a strong solution of Permanganate of Potash, Sulphate of Zinc or Carbolic Acid, as may seem best adapted, but in

either case so as to change the condition of the part and the secretion. With a good general treatment and improved nutrition these patients will frequently make a good recovery.

SYPHILIS.

We might omit the study of syphilis in women, as the treatment is very nearly the same, yet there are some points connected with it that deserve attention, and they may be better studied in this connection.

347. As heretofore named, we recognize three venereal contagions—gonorrhœa, soft chancre or chancroid, and hard chancre or syphilis proper, and we will study these more fully further on. Here we want to call attention to the important fact that the soft chancre is almost always *multiple*, the hard chancre a *single* sore. In women, at least, this is the only safe guide, as the true syphilitic ulcer will frequently present but little induration, owing to the character of the tissues. As an additional means of diagnosis we recollect that in chancroid the lymphatic glands are enlarged earlier and suppuration is a very common result; in hard chancre or true syphilis there is induration of the glands, but rarely suppuration.

348. This seems plain enough—if there is but one sore, and engorgement of the inguinal or femoral lymphatic glands, without suppuration, it is true syphilis. But if there is more than one sore, especially if inclined to spread, and the glands suppurate, it is chancroid. In the first there will be constitutional symptoms, no matter what plan of treatment is adopted. In the second there are no secondary symptoms, the disease being purely local. Notwithstanding we can state the general facts thus explicitly, and the diagnostic distinctions are well defined, still errors in diagnosis are made by the most experienced. A single ulcer may be chancroid, and the

glands may not suppurate; the ulcer may also, from local inflammation, have a degree of induration. So also we will occasionally find the true syphilitic ulcer multiple, and the glands may suppurate. In the one case we congratulate ourselves on the success of a treatment which seems to have neutralized the syphilitic poison, and effected a radical cure. In the other we are surprised to find a syphilitic eruption and other symptoms following a local disease which seemed to be soft chancre. Such mistakes should not occur often, but they will happen sometimes to the best.

349. The examination for chancre must be very thorough, else the ulcer may escape our notice. I prefer to make it with reflected light, having a good lamp set by the side of the patient and using a concave hand mirror. The first inspection will be of the vulva, and every fold should be effaced and thoroughly inspected. The obscure places are the special sites of venereal ulcers, because they escape the washing that follows impure connection. The sore may be in a fold of the *nymphæ*, in the superior commissure, in the fossa navicularis, between the *carunculæ*, by the side of the clitoris, hid by a full meatus, or just within the urethra. Using the speculum, the examination must be very thorough of the outer surface of the cervix. The little ulcer may be at the junction of vaginal wall and cervix, and with an ordinary examination may not be exposed. It is still more difficult to detect it, if located on the posterior surface of the cervix. It may be just within the os, and the swelling of the part may have so closed the opening that we only suspect the part by its localized hardness, and the unyielding character of this lip of the cervix. Chancre of the vaginal wall is more rare, yet the sore will sometimes be found hid away in one of the rugæ, small indeed, but a continued fountain of infection.

350. Whilst the venereal contagion is propagated by sexual intercourse, there are very rare cases in which it may be communicated otherwise. Thus there are cases on record, in which chancre of the lip was communicated by a kiss

chancre of the breast by nursing an infected child, and I have seen one case of chancre of the nates, communicated from an infected water closet. Chancre of the hands are not uncommon, from handling dressings, or washing the clothes of the infected.

351. Thus chancre may be developed upon any part of the skin or mucous membrane, by contact with the virus. A number of cases are on record of chancre of the rectum in women, produced by attempted intercourse *post-venereal*, under the mistaken notion that the disease could only be communicated to the genital organs. Similar cases of chancre of the *mons Veneris*, and outside of labia, have been met with.

352. Sometimes the local symptoms may be so slight, that a woman will carry a venereal ulcer for months without being aware of it, until from communicating the contagion, she is forced to have an examination made. A hard chancre may thus be allowed to lapse into a chronic form, and shows so little of the character of a sore, that it may escape notice, unless the examination is very carefully conducted. The chancroid usually presents the severest local symptoms, and forces attention until cured. True syphilis may thus lurk in the genitals of a woman, in the character of an old and indurated ulcer, or what seems to be a warty growth, and be communicated for months, possibly for years.

353. Both hard and soft chancre may be present together, and what seems singular, one person may contract the one, and another person the other. Both have had connection with the same woman, no other exposure, one has chancroid without constitutional syphilis, the other has true chancre, followed by secondary symptoms in the usual time. It has been claimed that a woman might carry the three contagions, and whilst one of her friends would have gonorrhœa, a second would have chancroid, and a third true syphilis—hence the idea with some that there was but *one* syphilitic poison, producing the three forms of disease, according to the peculiar

condition of the one exposed. If true, this would have been a fair example of *idiosyncrasy*.

354. TREATMENT.—As a general rule the treatment of chancre in women is more satisfactory than in men, if one knows what to do, and how to do it. In the treatment of the venereal we want a clear knowledge of the varying conditions of the local and general disease, cultivated senses to recognize them, and a steady hand to carry out the plan deemed best.

355. In soft chancre, and in true chancre not very much indurated, I prefer cauterization with Nitric Acid. No half-way work will answer the purpose. Have the part thoroughly exposed, one or more pine-pencils, thoroughly saturated with the strong Acid, wiped dry, and apply them thoroughly to every part of the sore or sores. It is not superficial cauterization that we want—simply making the surface white; but the pencil should reach the bottom, and follow every sinuosity, especially of the borders of the ulcer. Many physicians have a very light hand when they use an escharotic, they are afraid of burning too much — it is "a lick and a promise." This kind of practice won't do, what needs to be done, needs doing at once and thoroughly. It is just as bad practice to use the pine-pencil with a drop of free acid adhering, for this only reaches the surface, and runs off on to adjacent sound tissue, and not unfrequently serves as a cause for spreading the disease. Make a note of this—*cauterization must be thorough and deep.*

356. But it don't do any good, in the majority of cases, to use Nitric Acid on an indurated chancre, still less good to use Nitrate of Silver. Indeed, many times we will see the chancre harden under the application, and a sore that might have been cured in one or two weeks, is made to last for many months. Complete destruction, rapidly effected, is the object, if we use means for the destruction of the chancre.

357. If the chancre is so situated that it can be wholly

excised, this is the quickest method of removal. Cleanse it thoroughly, grasp the tissue with serrated forceps, or the ordinary dressing forceps, lift it the length of the connective tissue, and snip it out with the scissors; slightly apply the Nitric Acid to the surface, and use a simple water dressing.

358. If we use an escharotic, it will be Potassæ Fusa or Chloride of Zinc. In using the stick of Caustic Potash, we protect adjacent parts with lint wetted in vinegar, and the pencil is carried to the complete destruction of the entire induration. The Chloride of Zinc is used in the form of a paste—℞ Chloride of Zinc, (crystals), Gum Arabic, aa.; water to form a paste; spread it upon leather the proper size, and apply until the diseased structure is entirely removed. These remedies are not selected, unless there is marked induration, and they will not always give satisfaction. You think you have used your escharotic thoroughly, and yet you find the wound left shows hardness, and presently the characteristics of chancre, and you have gained nothing. The disease is constitutional, and the local disease can not be cured, except with general treatment.

359. In very many cases, a good Mayer's ointment (made strictly according to the formula) will be the best dressing after cauterization. It is sufficiently tenacious to remain where placed, protects the part thoroughly, and gives the necessary stimulation. The sore heals by granulation, and the part needs rest and protection.

360. In some cases an astringent and stimulant application is necessary, and then we think of the old-fashioned dressing of Port Wine and Tannin—℞ Port Wine, ℥vj.; Tannic Acid, ʒij.; apply with lint. I should use this application when the part was spongy and deep colored. A solution of Permanganate of Potash will also be found a good dressing in some of these cases; and once in a while a weak solution of Carbolic Acid.

361. Sometimes we find that a dry dressing answers a better purpose; most usually in cases where there is a free and

somewhat ichorous secretion. If the part is tumid and pallid, I would use Sub-Nitrate of Bismuth; if pallid but spongy, Oxide of Zinc. Dry Calomel has been very highly recommended as a dressing for some chancres, but I doubt whether it possesses any advantages over those named. Once in a while a case will present, in which the chancre is spongy, secretes profusely, and is very irritable, when Oxide of Lead (powdered White Lead) will serve our purpose best.

362. If we conclude not to cauterize the hard chancre, we will keep steadily in view the fact that it will be best removed by suppuration, and anything that will favor free suppuration, without producing irritation and determination of blood, will serve our purpose as a dressing. The Mayer's Ointment spoken of above, is a favorite remedy of mine, and I frequently dress the sore from first to last with this alone. Where the chancre was a nodule of induration, like the half of a split pea, secreting but very little, and showing no irritability, I have dressed it with the irritating plaster until it suppurated freely, then with the Mayer's Ointment.

363. But the constitutional treatment should be closely looked after here, as sometimes the local disease will not yield until we have made an impression through the blood. It is all romance to talk of a single plan of treatment, or a single anti-syphilitic, for all cases. Just as foolish to expect that "Compound Syrup of Stillingia and Iodide of Potash" will prove a cure-all, as that Proto-Iodide of Mercury is a cure-all. The physician who has an "invariable prescription" will fail here as well as elsewhere. We find cases that need Veratrum, Quinine, remedies that increase waste and elimination, remedies that give an appetite and favor blood-making, restoratives, Alkalies, Acids, Iodide of Potassium, Iodide of Ammonium, etc. It is hardly worth while to describe the indications for these here, as we will bé obliged to take them up in detail hereafter.

DISEASES OF THE MALE ORGANS OF GENERATION.

INFLAMMATION OF THE PENIS.

364. Whilst there are rare cases of simple inflammation of the penis, the majority of cases are erysipelatous in character. It is not a common disease, but an unpleasant one to manage, as there is a constant tendency to destruction of tissue.

365. The inflammation here commences with the usual symptoms. The part is swollen, hot, red and painful, and with these local symptoms there is considerable constitutional disturbance. In the majority of cases the erysipelatous character of the disease shows itself in the erythematous redness of skin, and effusion into the cellular tissues. Sometimes, within twenty-four hours, the swelling of the subcutaneous tissue is almost sufficient to strangulate the organ. In one case the prepuce drawn back was so swollen as to cause lividity of the glans, and free incisions were required to prevent sloughing.

366. The disease runs the usual course of such inflammations. The appetite is lost, the bowels irregular, the tongue shows blood-poisoning, and the nervous system the influence of the zymotic disease. In some cases the skin vesicates, and large blebs form, which discharging gives relief. In others suppuration of the cellular tissue occurs, and when opened there is a discharge of a thin unpleasant pus. The inflammation may extend to the abdomen, perineum, scrotum, or may involve the tissues of the corpora cavernosa and spongiosum.

367. TREATMENT.—Let the patient understand at once that absolute quiet is necessary to a successful treatment. With a good bath for cleanliness, and a hot foot-bath, put the patient to bed. Select the proper sedative, and give it in the usual way. In some of these cases — where the part shows the

bright redness of arterial blood, and the pulse is full—Veratrum is specific. If the pulse is small with sharp stroke, Aconite with Rhus—as: ℞ Tinct. Aconite, gtts. x.; Tinct. Rhus, gtts. v.; Water, ℥iv.; a teaspoonful every hour. If erysipelatous in character we select the proper antiseptic by the appearance of the tongue. True, we may give Tincture of Iron empirically, and hit it in three-fourths of the cases, but I think it better to start with a correct diagnosis. Iron is the remedy where the redness is not vivid, and especially if there is a tinge of blueness. The indications for Veratrum have been noticed already. Sulphite of Soda is the remedy where the mucous membranes are pallid, and the tongue covered with a pasty-white coat. Sulphurous Acid where the mucous membranes have a normal color, but the coating is thick, pasty and dirty. Rhus Toxicodendron is the remedy if the part is tense, glistening, and vividly red.

368. The local treatment will vary in different cases. In simple inflammation the part is painted with Veratrum, and a wet dressing applied, either cold or hot, as may be most agreeable. In sthenic erythematous erysipelas we use Veratrum as the local remedy, painting the part with the strong tincture. When we give Tincture of Iron internally, we would use it as a local application, either of full strength, or diluted with Glycerine or water. In phlegmonous erysipelas, after the first day, a solution of Permanganate of Potash is usually the best remedy; the strength being from ℨss. to ℨij. to Water, Oj. Carbolic Acid is also a good remedy in some cases, especially where pus has formed and a tendency to sloughing is manifest. It should not be forgotten that if the infiltration and swelling of the cellular tissue impairs the circulation, and there is a gangrenous tendency, free incisions are necessary to ensure safety.

BALANITIS, POSTHITIS.

369. Superficial inflammation of the mucous membranes covering the glans and lining the prepuce, takes these names,

and either or both, when secretion has been profuse, has been known as *gonorrhœa spuria*, or *balanorrhœa*. In some cases it is undoubtedly caused by an impure connection, the female organs suffering from a similar disease, or from an irritant leucorrhœal discharge. In many it is a sequel of venereal diseases—the sufferer has had gonorrhœa, chancroid, or true syphilis, and ever after has tenderness of these parts, and is obliged to look after them carefully to prevent irritation. Still in the majority of cases, the inflammation is the result of a want of cleanliness, the secretion from the glands of the parts being retained become acrid and irritant.

370. The patient knows he has a sore penis and tells the story clearly. If the prepuce can be retracted, we can see the exact condition of the organ. In *balanitis* there is superficial excoriation, and the surface denuded of epithelium secretes pus freely. Sometimes the excretions are very irregular, and the surface dark red and velvety in appearance : sometimes the redness is vivid, or there are vivid red granulations showing upon the surface. In *posthitis* we frequently find an irritated mucous membrane, and a number of small superficial ulcers, almost as clearly defined as chancroid. In many cases we see them in every stage, from the minute red spot, the vesicle, the complete ulcer, and the erosion. The follicles of the *corona glandis*, are frequently enlarged, and secrete abundantly.

371. When the prepuce is long and narrow, phymosis occurs early, and the diagnosis is somewhat obscure. The extremity of the penis is swollen and painful, there is a more or less free discharge of a yellow purulent matter from the opening of the prepuce, and there may be difficulty, pain and burning in micturition. Sometimes it is almost impossible to tell where the discharge comes from, the prepuce being so contracted that we can see the meatus with difficulty. It is quite as difficult sometimes to diagnose it from soft chancre. Usually, however, the enlargement of the inguinal glands, and suppuration in the last comes in to help our diagnosis.

372. If the prepuce is short and retracted, it may become

œdematous, or a state of *paraphimosis* induced. Some of these cases are very unpleasant and persistent. The swollen prepuce interferes with the freedom of the circulation, and covering up the fossæ of the coronæ glandis, ulceration may go on there, hidden away from ordinary applications.

373. TREATMENT.—Prof. Blackman was in the habit of saying, "that no man should have a penis unless he thought enough of the organ to keep it decently clean," and so say we all. This means "soap and water" freely used. Some men will find, that they can not get along comfortably without the use of soap and water, to keep the parts free from acrid secretions. We prescribe soap and water in every case as the basis of good treatment. There is a choice in soap, and it is well to say "Colgate's *best* Glycerine Soap," with soft water. Turn the prepuce well back, and dipping the cake of soap in the water, rub it thoroughly into the part, and then wash clean.

374. If the prepuce is in a condition of phimosis, a piece of the soap may be cut so that it can be introduced through the contracted opening and brought in contact with the diseased surface. Or it may be used with a thick camel's hair pencil, or a strong soap suds may be used with a syringe. In either case the part should be thoroughly rinsed in clear water.

375. If this does not seem sufficient we use in addition: ℞ Permanganate of Potash, grs. v. to grs. x.; Water, ℥iv.; to be applied two or three times a day. If there is much pruritus, Glycerole of Tar is an excellent application. If there is an erosive eczematous eruption, resisting the means named, we would think of Citrine Ointment, one part, to simple Cerate, three to five parts; apply morning and night.

376. The only trouble with the local treatment in minor cases is, that it cures too quickly, and patients do not like to pay for "soap and water." In such cases a *placebo* always goes with the treatment—"to purify the blood," and act on

the patient's imagination. It is not worth while to give anything nasty, or any of the "Compound Syrups," at the expense of the doctor's pocket.

377. But there are cases, in which an internal treatment is necessary to a cure. Sometimes the patient will want Iodide of Ammonium for a few weeks; or a cooling purgative, as Crab Orchard Salts and Sulphur. Sometimes Sulphur alone or Sulphurous Acid, etc. When the disease has been of long duration, and is very stubborn, we frequently find an indication for Arsenic, and give Fowler's Solution in doses of two to three drops, three times a day.

VERUCCA.

378. Warts may appear upon any part of the genitalia, either of the skin or mucous membrane. They may be non-venereal, and arise from irritation of the surfaces, or from the obscure and unknown causes, that change nutrition, and give rise to these growths in other parts. They sometimes follow the irritation of balanitis and posthitis, or pruritus. Or they may be venereal, either a sequel of the disease which has run its course in the person, or contracted by intercourse with one having these vegetations.

379. Gonorrhœa is a not unfrequent cause of verruca, and what is singular, these warts are sometimes as contagious as the primary disease, and they are propagated by intercourse. They are of less frequent occurrence after chancroid, yet sometimes they will secrete a contagious pus, which will produce soft chancre in some, verruca in others. They may follow hard chancre, growing from the site of induration, and continue to secrete an inoculable virus. Or they may follow the primary disease, being induced probably by the local irritation, and possess none of the characteristics of syphilis.

Or they may follow as a secondary symptom, associated with mucous tubercle.

380. In the male, the most common seat is immediately behind, or upon the *corona glandis*, though they may appear upon the prepuce, glans, or at the meatus. Varying in size from a small point to a growth as large as a strawberry, there may be but one, or they may cover the entire extremity of the organ with their red, granulated surface. In the female, the most common situation is at the entrance of the vagina, though we may find them in every portion of the organs.

381. In both sexes, they give rise to irritation of adjacent surfaces, increasing secretion from the mucous follicles, and sometimes causing erosion and secretion of pus. It is sufficient to say they are always unpleasant companions, and should be gotten rid of.

382. TREATMENT.—A great many methods of removal have been advised, but the most of them are worthless. Powdering the surfaces with powdered Savin or Alum, don't amount to anything, unless the warts are ready to leave of their own accord. You can snip them off with the scissors, or cut them off with a scalpel, or strangulate them with a ligature, but in a few days they are back as bright and vigorous as ever, and you will be lucky if you don't find that others have come to attend the funeral, and concluded to stay. It is very much the same with the use of the common escharotics. You may burn them off, but it only serves like good cultivation—they grow more vigorously afterwards.

383. There are three methods which will give success, and one of the three I advise. If the wart is rather loose in its structure, not very flaccid, or a rapid grower, use Nitric Acid. Shape your pencils to suit the growth—always pointed; saturate them with the strong Acid, and carry them thoroughly down to the base in every interstice of tissue, and take time enough to do the work thoroughly. Superficial cauterization will not answer, and we want no free Acid upon the surface.

Chromic Acid probably stands first in destructive power. It will destroy the warts, but it is difficult to circumscribe its action, and it would quite as soon burn sound as morbid tissue. Unless used with care, it is very apt to burn where you don't want it, and not enough where you do want it. The best means of applying it is with a pointed glass rod, not using too much free Acid, but working it well down to the base of the growths. It is especially the remedy for syphilitic verruca. My favorite remedy is the irritating plaster, (Emplastrum Picis Compound of our Dispensatory). Take a piece of sufficient size to cover the wart, put it on the end of a probe, and hold it to the fire or lamp until soft, and apply to the wart; and repeat the dressing with fresh plaster every day, until the growth is gone. I hardly know how it acts, but one thing is certain, the wart goes, and goes quickly, and is so disgusted with the treatment that it never returns.

384. In some cases constitutional means are necessary. It may be the evidence of depravation of the blood, and associated with impaired nutrition in other parts, and will require means to promote waste and restoratives. When gonorrhœal, and the warts are very persistent, it is well to suspect the continuance of the gonorrhœal virus, and employ the proper remedies for it. In my early practice I saw a case cured with Copaiba and Cubebs, that had resisted ordinary means for a twelvemonth. If syphilitic, of course an anti-syphilitic treatment will be necessary to a cure.

PHIMOSIS.

385. Phimosis may be congenital or acquired. Up to the age of ten or fourteen the prepuce covers the glans, and can not be retracted. Now in the development of the organ, the foreskin is shortened in proportion to the entire length, and the opening becomes so dilated that it can be retracted. In

some cases we find that this infantile condition persists, the prepuce being long and narrow, and the glans is never exposed, or exposed with difficulty. In other cases it is narrowed, and slight irritation is sufficient to cause the contraction of phimosis.

386. In many cases of chancre, especially the multiple or soft chancre of the prepuce, it becomes so swollen that it can not be retracted, and the parts distended with the secretion, become very unpleasant. We may have phimosis from hard chancre, but it is not of such frequent occurrence. We have already seen that in balanitis and posthitis, phimosis might occur, and sometimes gives rise to considerable trouble.

387. TREATMENT.—Whilst an operation gives the speediest relief, it is not always the best plan of treatment. Indeed, in some cases it should not be resorted to if it is possible to avoid it. These are especially the cases of soft chancre, in which the disease almost always appears in the incisions, and makes the case very unpleasant.

388. In the majority, careful attention to cleanliness, using soap and water as heretofore directed, with the camel's-hair brush or syringe, will be sufficient to remove the irritation of the mucous membranes. Painting the part with Veratrum will remove acute inflammatory action, and the application of a solution of Alum, or Pond's Hamamelis, will strengthen the tissues and relieve the swelling.

389. When there is œdema of the prepuce, the administration of a hydragogue cathartic, followed by a diuretic, will frequently give speedy relief. Or in place of this we may give: ℞ Tincture Apocynum, ʒss.; Water, ℥iv.; a teaspoonful every two hours.

390. If there is necessity for operative interference the surgical procedure is very simple. Introduce a grooved director under the upper part, and cut the prepuce upon it, the entire length of the constricted portion, so that it may be freely retracted. Now apply an adhesive strap, so that

the wound is kept *open* to its full extent, and apply a water-dressing. It has been recommended to make several of these incisions to free the prepuce, but I think when more than one is required, circumcision is the better operation.

CIRCUMCISION.*

391. It is well in this place to study briefly the ordinance of circumcision, and its relation to the reproductive function. If of Divine ordination, it must have had an important use in

---

*ADVANTAGES OF CIRCUMCISION FROM A SURGICAL POINT OF VIEW.—Dr. Cadell read a paper on this subject before the Medico-Chirurgical Society of Edinburgh. He considered it in four aspects: 1. In infancy. 2. In boyhood. 3. In adult life. 4. In old age. He described:

1. The local and constitutional disturbance which may be set up by a long prepuce in infancy, and showed how these might be immediately relieved by circumcision. He read notes of a case, and also referred to those of Mr. Bryant, illustrating the effects of an adherent prepuce on the urinary organs, and the relief obtained by circumcision.

2. In boyhood, he believed that a long prepuce, by imprisoning the secretion from the glans, might be an exciting cause of masturbation; and if there was an hereditary disposition to nervous affections, epilepsy and insanity might be thereby induced.

3. In adult life, circumcision would facilitate cleanliness, diminish the secretion from the glans, so that the great cause of non-venereal excoriation would be removed, and thus render the mucous surface less susceptible to the venereal poison.

4. In old age, he cited Mr. Hey's opinion, that a congenital phimosis was an exciting cause of cancer in the penis.

In conclusion, Dr. Cadell remarked that he would strongly recommend circumcision in boys between infancy and puberty, whenever a congenital phimosis caused them the slightest inconvenience.

Prof. Lister said the cases alluded to by Dr. Cadell, of irritation caused by adherent prepuce, must be admitted to be of great interest. They knew that where adhesion existed there was often an accumulation of secretion, and they could understand that to be a cause of irritation. He should like to have it clearly brought out how far the symptoms in these cases were attributable tc

the world, and it is possible that in neglecting it, we have neglected a wise provision for health.

392. The social laws and observances of the Jews were certainly conducive to physical well being; of which we have the evidence in their existence as a people through so long a period of time, their power to endure persecution and oppression, their health as a people, and especially their exemption from the diseases we are now studying.

393. The elongated prepuce keeps the covering of the glans delicate and sensitive, and as we have already seen, this might be a cause of sexual irritation and spermatorrhœa. The extremely sensitive glans makes copulation brief, and

---

that cause, as distinguished from mere length of the prepuce. Though all would allow that cases of phimosis ought to be subjected to operation, it ought to be considered whether circumcision was the best that could be done. The object could be obtained without mutilation. Mr. Jordan, of Birmingham, has written an interesting paper on the subject, showing that a perfectly natural condition of things might be obtained by the simple means of notching the ring of skin to the requisite extent, and then dividing the mucous membrane up to the *corona glandis*, and, avoiding all use of stitches, simply have the part drawn backward and forward twice every day. As regards the question of malignant disease, he might have been unfortunate, but he had now seen a large number of cases of cancer of the penis, not one of which was associated with the phimosis.

Dr. J. Bell said his experience in regard to circumcision was in cases of long standing, and perfectly incurable nocturnal enuresis by small children who were in the habit of wetting the bed. In as many as four or five cases he had succeeded in effecting a perfect cure, by simply removing the redundant portion of the prepuce. In one case, a very bad case, a poor little fellow made his water first in the prepuce, which was like an orange at the end, and then he got rid of the water by squeezing it with his hand, the water coming out by a small aperture. That case was in George Watson's Hospital, and it became a question with the managers how to provide the necessary bedding for the boy. The operation performed was very simple, and was a complete cure. He (Dr. Bell) had very little experience of adherent prepuce; cases of adhesion of the prepuce were not so common as those of long prepuce.

Dr. Halliday Douglas said, that several years ago he was waited upon by a gentleman who had been married a few days before, and who had failed to effect connection. He was laboring under a very tight phimosis. He had

though the venereal orgasm is perfect in the man, it is more rarely experienced by the woman. This we have seen is sometimes a cause of disease. The elongated prepuce and tender structures offer a better field for the venereal disease, and we find here one element of free contagion.

394. So far as recommending circumcision, I am free to say this, that it is especially applicable where the penis is extremely sensitive; when a person from this suffers nocturnal

---

never experienced any inconvenience during his life of twenty-five or twenty-eight years. He (Dr. Douglas) transferred him to Mr. Syme's hands, and, within twelve months, there were twins born to him. Another curious fact in this gentleman's history was this: In early life his brother had been relieved of phimosis, and three of his children, nephews of the first gentleman, had required to have the operation performed.

Dr. Watson was glad that the conclusion to which Dr. Cadell had arrived was, that where an elongated prepuce was a source of annoyance, it was right to relieve the person by removing it. As regarded the question of the comparative frequency of venereal complaints among persons who had been circumcised and those who had not, he might refer Dr. Cadell to a paper which appeared in the *Medical Times and Gazette*, 1st of December, 1855, by Mr. J. Hutchinson, in which it was shown that at the Metropolitan Free Hospital, situated in the Jews' quarter, in London, in the year 1854, the proportion of Jews to Christians among the out-patients was as *one* to *three*—at the same time, the proportion of cases of syphilis in the former to the latter was only as *one* to *fifteen*. Yet, that this was not the result of any higher degree of morality on the part of the Jewish population was obvious, because fully one-half of the cases of gonorrhœa occurred in Jews. This preventive influence of circumcision, as regards chancrous infection, led to hereditary syphilis being rarer among the children of Jews than of Christians. . . . . He was surprised that Dr. Cadell did not quote that greatest of all authorities on such matters, viz., Dr. Ricord, who had said, in one of his published clinical lectures: "The prepuce is an appendix to the genital organs, the object of which I could never divine; instead of being of use, it leads to a great deal of inconvenience, and the Jews have acted kindly in circumcising their children, as it renders them free from one at least of the ills to which flesh is heir. The prepuce is, in fact, a superfluous piece of skin and mucous membrane, which serves no other purpose than as a reservoir for the collection of filth, especially when individuals are inattentive to cleanliness." This was very strongly confirmatory of Dr. Cadell's views, though it appeared to Dr Watson a little extreme.—*Edinburgh Medical Journal.*

emissions, over-sexual excitement, nervous irritation, spermatorrhœa and prostatorrhœa; or where there is continued disease from its closeness.

395. The operation of Gross is the simplest: "With this view, the redundant parts, steadied with a pair of slender forceps, applied just in front of the head of the penis, are cut off with one sweep of a long bistoury from above downwards and from behind forwards. The contracted and tightened membrane is then, if necessary, divided with the scissors. Any little arteries that may bleed are secured with fine ligatures, when the muco-cutaneous edges of the wound are approximated by four sutures, placed at equi-distant intervals. Elevation of the penis, with cold-water dressing, recumbency, light diet, and a purgative the morning after the operation, constitute the after treatment. The sutures are removed at the end of the third day."

PARAPHIMOSIS.

396. In paraphimosis we have a contracted prepuce, but it is drawn back and strangulates the glans. We sometimes find cases of this kind in boys, who having worked the prepuce over the head of the penis, find that they can not get it back. We will also see some rare cases of this in the adult. In the majority, however, the opening of the prepuce has been contracted by disease, usually *posthitis*, but sometimes soft or hard chancre, and it being retracted whilst the organ is very flaccid, it can not be returned on account of the swelling. It may also be caused by a rapidly induced inflammation of the prepuce. I saw a case of this kind, in which it followed the irritation of connection, there never having been any previous difficulty. In some rare cases it will follow erection, the glans not losing its state of turgescence.

397. The symptoms are very clear, and usually very unpleasant, if the constriction is severe. The contracted prepuce has prevented the flow of blood from, though it does not prevent the admission of blood into the head of the organ. The glans is very much swollen and discolored, and in the majority of cases there is some pain. Pain, however, is a good symptom, for where there is pain, there is life; absence of pain and want of sensibility are precursors of gangrene. If the strangulation is severe and protracted, a low grade of inflammatory action may follow, or the glans may slough in part or the whole.

398. TREATMENT.—In the minor cases, relief is speedily given by the local application of cold to the part. We may use pounded ice, or even suspending the organ in ice-water, or cold well or spring water will answer. If the case is still more serious, we use a *cold* sitz-bath, a good sized tub of water being preferable to a small quantity.

399. Should this not be sufficient, or if from the appearance of the organ, we deem there is imminent danger to the tissues we relieve the constriction with the scalpel. I do not think it is essential to work a grooved director under the contracted prepuce, though if this can be done it is well enough, and will give the ordinary practitioner confidence in the use of the knife. In the severer cases, the director can not be used. Take the head of the penis between the thumb and finger, bending it sharply downwards, have the patient or an assistant retract the prepuce as much as possible, and with a sharp scalpel sever the constricted portion from above downwards. There is but very little danger of cutting the body of the organ—none at all if the knife is held steadily.

400. Dress the part with an ordinary water-dressing, adding a small portion of Tincture of Aconite and Camphor if the constriction has been of some hours duration, or use a weak solution of Sulphate of Zinc, if there is danger of sloughing.

URETHRITIS.

401. Inflammation of the urethra in the male, may result from various causes, but in a majority of cases it follows connection with a woman suffering from vaginitis, leucorrhœa, or during the menstrual period. There are times when the secretions from the vagina become very acrid, and give rise to urethritis, balanitis, or posthitis. It is rarely the case, however, that these affections can be transmitted from the male to the female. Women suffering from secondary syphilis, and having inflammation of these organs, or leucorrhœa, will sometimes communicate local diseases of a very severe character, not, however, specific.

402. SYMPTOMS.—The symptoms of urethritis resemble to some extent those of gonorrhœa, though not usually so severe nor persistent. At first a feeling of fullness, tension, or constriction along the urethra, with frequent desire to urinate, is followed in a couple of days by burning in passing water, sense of soreness afterward, and a milky-white discharge. In the majority of cases, the ardor urinæ commences to decline by the fourth or fifth day, there is no chordee, and the discharge ceases, or becomes yellowish and creamy.

403. There is no possible means of determining between a specific and non-specific urethritis, other than that the symptoms of the last are much milder, as would appear by the description. It usually runs its course in a week or ten days, though it may be protracted for months, or give a great amount of trouble by continually recurring upon slight exciting causes.

404. We occasionally see cases in which the inflammation runs higher than in gonorrhœa, but these are quite rare. In gonorrhœa the favorite seat of the disease is the lacunæ of the navicular fossa; in simple urethritis the disease involves the entire urethra, and is severest when it principally affects

the membranous and prostatic portions, and especially when it extends to the bas-fond of the bladder. In the latter case, there is deep-seated, burning pain, with an almost constant desire to pass urine, and great tenesmus—so much so at times that the patient passes blood with each discharge.

405. TREATMENT.—In the majority of cases a very simple treatment gives excellent results. Put the patient upon the use of Veratrum and Gelseminum, in the proportion of—℞ Tinct. Veratrum, gtts. xx.; Tinct. Gelseminum, ʒij.; Water, ℥iv.; a teaspoonful every hour. If the bowels are constipated use a saline laxative, as a Seidlitz powder, Bitartrate of Potash, or Crab Orchard Salts and Sulphur. Give diluents freely, sometimes an infusion of the milder diuretics, usually a weak solution of Acetate of Potash.

406. This treatment gives relief in twenty-four hours, and it may be all that is necessary. Usually, when the acute symptoms pass off, we follow with: ℞ Tinct. Cannabis Indica, gtts. x.; Water, ℥iv.; or with small doses of Pulsatilla, Staphysagria or Macrotys.

407. When the upper portion of the urethra is principally involved, we have the patient use a hot sitz-bath, until the tenesmus is relieved, go to bed, and have an enema of starch and Laudanum, or Tinctures of Opium and Lobelia, or an Opium suppository. The bowels may be relieved before these are used, as named above, but afterwards should be kept confined. The sedatives should be given as in the less severe cases, and the after treatment will be the same.

HEMORRHAGE FROM THE URETHRA.

408. Hemorrhage from the urethra may occur as the result of injury to the parts, especially when the penis is in a state of erection. It may also result from over-excitation

during sexual intercourse, or in some rare cases of chordee. I recollect a case of hemorrhage in a man aged some forty-five years, which was caused by great venereal excitement and connection with a woman under the influence of liquor. The flow of blood was profuse, and the sufferer was almost exsanguined before it was arrested; in this case it was from the bulb of the urethra. In another case the hemorrhage was caused by a kick from a prostitute, and it was months before the sufferer could have an erection without some bleeding.

409. The diagnosis is easy, a stream of bright blood wells out of the meatus, and if an attempt is made to arrest it by compressing the head of the penis, the urethra becomes distended, and presently involuntary contraction ensues, and the blood is forcibly expelled. The locality of the ruptured vessels may sometimes be determined by the uneasiness in the part.

410. TREATMENT.—Suspending the penis in ice-cold water, or the application of pounded ice will suffice in a majority of cases. But if the locality of the ruptured vessels can be determined, compression can be made to the urethra over the part, and the patient kept still until the vessels are closed. When the hemorrhage is persistent, I should use a large sized bougie, with moderate compression and the application of cold.

URETHRAL CALCULI.

411. Occasionally we meet cases in which small calculi formed in the bladder or in the kidneys, pass into the urethra with the stream of water, and either from their size, or from irritation then lodge there, and the sufferer can get them neither forward nor back. In some of these cases the suffering is extreme. The flow of water is suddenly stopped, and

the desire to micturate becomes very pressing, and is attended with tenesmus and forcible expulsion. The angular or sharp projections of the stone irritate the urethra, which contracts against the further advance, and as the stone progresses it tears the tissue, causing severe pain and hemorrhage. Calculi have thus remained in the urethra for many hours.

412. TREATMENT.—Surgical authorities have recommended the extraction of calculi from the urethra with forceps, which is all well enough if the stone is near enough the meatus to be readily reached and grasped. Even then its removal is attended with severe pain. But in the majority of cases, the forceps will not reach it, and the patient must suffer intensely until it has worked its way sufficiently forward. Here my treatment will be found especially applicable — Introduce a large bougie or catheter back as far as the stone, and gently press it backward so as to dislodge it; hold the parts quiet for a few moments until the involuntary contraction ceases, and then slowly withdrawing the instrument have the patient make the effort to pass urine. The stone follows immediately behind the instrument, which dilates the urethra, and it is passed without difficulty or pain.

STRICTURE OF THE URETHRA.

BY PROF. EDWIN FREEMAN, M. D.

413. A stricture of the urethra may be defined to be an organic contraction of that canal, at some particular part. This interferes with the passage of the urine, and becomes more and more serious, according to the degree and permanency of the contraction. Strictures are essentially of two kinds: *transitory* and *permanent*.

414. *Transitory* strictures consist of two well defined kinds, *spasmodic*, and *congestive* or *inflammatory*. In *spasmodic*

stricture, there is involuntary contraction of the circular muscular fibres of the urethra, in some part, or of the compressor urethræ muscle, which may be associated with some degree of irritability of the mucous membrane at that point. In *congestive* or inflammatory stricture, there is usually chronic congestion, or inflammation of the mucous membrane of large tracks of the urethra, principally the prostatic, membranous, and bulbous, which from various causes, is suddenly increased to an acute condition, with swelling or thickening of the mucous membrane and narrowing of the canal. This condition may be, and frequently is associated with a spasmodic action of the muscular fibres just referred to, the two causes acting temporarily to completely occlude the urethra.

415. The exciting causes may be, errors of diet in dyspeptic and irritable persons, or the effects of cold, suppressing the secretions of the skin, or the intemperate use of liquors, and other like causes, increasing the acidity of the urine, and as a consequence, the irritability and inflammation of the urethral canal. The congestive form is especially liable to occur in persons of a rheumatic or gouty diathesis; and the spasmodic form in those given to excesses in drinking and in venereal indulgences, or in those afflicted with piles, ascarides, fissure, stone in bladder, etc. Symptoms of spasmodic stricture are: Inability to pass the urine, resulting suddenly, and quickly passing away. It may be accompanied with some heaviness in the perineum, and as the bladder fills up there are expulsive pains in the hypogastric region, which increase in severity if the urine does not pass.

416. TREATMENT.—These attacks are usually quickly relieved by a saline cathartic; the free use of Acetate of Potassa with Gelseminum and Hyosciamus; or with Sweet Spirits of Nitre, with Opium and mild mucilaginous diuretics, as the Marsh Mallows, etc. The hot hip bath, with a Dover's powder internally, may be the only thing necessary to give relief in some cases. It may be necessary to introduce a

bougie or catheter in some cases, before relief can be obtained.

417. *Congestive Stricture.*—The symptoms are: Inability to pass the urine, with great heaviness and pain in the perineum, occurring as the result of cold or dissipation, etc., in persons having a persisting inflammation or congestion of the urethra. There is also extreme sensation of burning if a few drops of urine escape; pain in hypogastrium extending frequently to back and hips; eversion and redness, with sometimes gleety discharge at the meatus, with other indications of acute urethritis. On testing the urine, the blue litmus paper will usually turn a bright red if the urine be highly acid.

418. TREATMENT.—Subdue the inflammation by the use of Aconite, Sweet Spirits of Nitre, Hyosciamus and Gelseminum internally. Use fomentations of Hops and Stramonium to the perineum and hypogastric region, covering the external genitals. Give freely of Acetate of Potassa or Bicarbonate of Soda if the urine be found to be acid. Administer freely infusions of Marsh Mallows and Flax Seed, and by injections and mild cathartics get the bowels into a soluble condition. It may be necessary to introduce a bougie or catheter, if the urine can not be made to pass otherwise, but it should be done with great care, lest the inflamed and swollen urethra be injured and increase the difficulty. In the after treatment it may be necessary to pass a bougie occasionally, of as full size as possible, and also to use mild injections of infusion of Hydrastis Canadensis, in which a little Borax has been dissolved, or the infusion alone will be sometimes most grateful. Sometimes Iodide of Potassium in large doses, alone or combined with other antilithics, have the best results, while in other cases in persons suffering from malarial influences, antiperiodics, such as Quinine, etc., must be given before much relief can be obtained.

419. *Permanent or Organic Stricture.*—In this form, the contraction remains permanently, and is only removed by instrumental interference. It may be the result of chronic in-

flammation, leading to plastic deposits in the mucous membrane at some part of the urethra, or in the sub-mucous tissues, or else ultimately extending to them and the corpus spongiosum. In the initiatory stages, it is probable that there is some muscular contraction resulting from the frequent passing of the urine over an inflamed and slightly thickened mucous membrane, and this occurring at the time that the plastic deposit is becoming organized, results in the formation of a more or less wide circular band around the urethra, narrowing its canal. The persistence of the cause, and the additional cause resulting from the narrowing of the passage, the extension of the inflammation and deposit into the submucous tissues, and possibly the effects of careless instrumental interference, ultimately result in so close a contraction of this band, and such an indurated condition of it and adjacent tissues, that urine can no longer be expelled, excepting after long waiting, much effort, and then only in a very small twisted or divided stream, or in very bad cases only in a few drops at a time.

420. Another definition of the causes of stricture is, that it is the result of a proliferation of the elements of the submucous cellular tissue. According to Rokitansky, there is sometimes found at the site of the stricture, and deposited upon the walls of the urethra, a copious secretion of pasty mucus, the result of chronic inflammation. It "may or may not be attended with an exuberant formation of epithelium, and in which accordingly the epithelium is either rapidly thrown off from an almost bare, and, as it seems, excoriated mucous membrane, or accumulates over the whole or parts of the surface, and thus forms a complete laminated covering for it, or patches of various thickness here and there upon it." He also describes a croupy deposit upon the mucous membrane without any external contraction—the result of acute inflammation. Sir Henry Thompson has only found three cases in a large number of examinations, and two of these he thinks owe their appearance to dilated lacunæ.

421. *Age.*—Stricture of the urethra seldom occurs before puberty. It usually takes its origin between the ages of twenty-five and forty, and may continue for an indefinite period. It has, according to Mr. Erichsen, been known to occur as early as fourteen years of age, and a case of traumatic stricture at eleven years of age is reported by Dr. Chas. C. Lea, in the American Journal of Medical Sciences, July, 1862.

422. *Seat.*—On this subject much might be written, as eminent surgeons have remarkably differed. But examinations on the living subjects are, from various causes, liable to be inaccurate, while post-mortem examinations, carefully and honestly made, must necessarily be determined to be decisive. Sir Henry Thompson has made a careful examination of more than three hundred preparations of stricture, in the museums of Paris, London and Edinburgh. His statement is this: That part of the urethra which is most frequently affected with stricture, is the portion comprised in the niche anterior to the junction," (of the membranous and spongy portions), "that is, the posterior or bulbous part of the spongy portion. The liability of this part to stricture appears to diminish as it approaches the junction, where it is less common; while behind it is very rare. Most rarely is a stricture found so far back as the posterior part of the membranous portion." The strictures occurring in all this region just mentioned amount to sixty-seven per cent. of the entire number. The next most frequent seat of stricture is that part of the urethra included between the meatus urinarius and two and a half inches within that orifice, the number being seventeen per cent. The central portion, including the part between the two portions above mentioned, has a ratio of sixteen per cent. Examinations by other surgeons fully sustain these decisions. Mr. Thompson, however, has not seen a case of stricture in the prostatic portion of the urethra. Yet Mr. Walsh describes a preparation in the Museum of the Royal College of Surgeons in Dublin. Other surgeons have also described other cases.

423. *Number and Character.*—In the largest number of cases there is only one stricture, but often there are more. Mr. Thompson never met with more than three or four in one person, while Mr. Hunter has met with six; and Colot with eight. Sometimes the stricture is a simple fold of the lining membrane containing the constricting fibres, a narrow annular stricture, called by Mr. Thompson the "linear stricture," the "pack-thread" or "bridle" or "valvular" stricture of other writers. This fold is sometimes oblique, or may extend only part of the way around the urethra. It has sometimes been perforated by instruments, and forms bridles or frona, stretching from one side to another. The "elongated annular" stricture may occupy a considerable part of the urethra, being closely contracted at the beginning and ending and less in the centre. When the course of the passage through an elongated stricture differs from its normal direction, it is called "irregular or tortuous."

424. *Degree of Contraction.*—Cases present themselves of all degrees of closeness of constriction. Many are rigid, others are readily dilatable, but as quickly contract. These are usually situated in the bulbous and spongy portion of the urethra, and are called by Mr. Syme the "resilient strictures." In some the walls are indurated and firm like cartilage, allowing the urine to escape only drop by drop, in many cases allowing the passage of only the finest instrument after long and tedious effort, and sometimes entirely preventing the passage of any instrument through them. A stricture that is strictly impermeable to urine probably does not occur, excepting as a "traumatic" stricture, the result of injury and possibly sloughing of the urethra, in which a urinary fistula would be present, through which all the urine passed.

425. *Results of Stricture.*—The principal changes in the genito-urinary track are found posterior to the seat of stricture. The urethra may be largely dilated, even forming a true pouch, which may present itself in the perineum as a fluctuating tumor. The walls of the bladder, from the effort

to expel the urine, may become thickened and fasciculated. The ureters may become dilated, and even the kidneys irritated and congested and structurally changed, and their functions materially interfered with. The ejaculatory ducts may be dilated, and the testicle may become irritable and inflamed. The patient, in severe cases, may become hypochondriacal from the remote effects upon the nervous system of incomplete depuration of the blood through kidneys. He may also become dyspeptic and be subject to chilliness and wandering pains in back, limbs and thighs.

426. SYMPTOMS.—These are a greater or less delay in the evacuation of the urine or waiting for it to appear, and after it has passed, the retention of a few drops which afterward escape. The stream of urine is small, often twisted or forked, scattered, fan-like or passing in two currents, one forward and the other directly downwards. There is often a sensation of pain or aching in the perineum in passing the urine. This becomes almost constant and severe in bad cases. Often in such cases there is over-distension of the bladder and a constant dribbling of decomposed urine, loaded with mucus and triple-phosphates. The severe straining to expel it sometimes gives rise to hernia, hemorrhoids, prolapsus ani, or severe irritation about the rectum. There is often also a gleety discharge from the meatus, often quite profuse, which arises from the mucous surface around the stricture, and is the result of chronic inflammation. It is especially so when the stricture is the sequel of gonorrhœa. One of the effects of straining in a severe stricture is a slight rupture of the mucous membrane behind the stricture, the insinuation of a little urine through the fissure, which gives rise to inflammation and the formation of abscess and fistula. Blood sometimes appears in the urine, but it is not common.

427. CAUSES.—In two hundred and twenty cases, according to Mr. Thompson, twenty-eight strictures were from "injury

to perineum," eight were true "inflammatory," seven were true "spasmodic," six were from "congenital" causes, seven from various other causes, as phagedœna, cicatrization of chancre or chancroids, lithotrity, masturbation, etc., and one hundred and sixty-four were from gonorrhœal inflammation. Of these latter, ninety were from chronic inflammation or gleet.

428. DIAGNOSIS.—As many of the symptoms of stricture are found in other diseases, as sub-acute inflammation of the prostate gland, and urethral neuralgia and hyperæsthesia, it is necessary to make a careful exploration of the urethral canal. This may be performed with steel sounds, solid or flexible catheters or with certain bougies. The instrument should always be large enough to well fill the urethra, and should be passed in with a firm and careful hand, until the obstruction is reached, and fairly recognized. Smaller sizes may then be passed until one passes through to the bladder. In this manner the seat and degree of the stricture may be pretty accurately determined. In certain slight strictures where there is doubt, it is best to pass a bougie of sufficient size with an acorn point, "bougie a boule." This may be readily passed through, but being withdrawn, the shoulders of the point are restricted by the fold of the stricture and thus determine it.

429. TREATMENT.—There are four principal methods of treatment, viz.: Dilatation, Rupture, Incision, Caustics.

430. Dilatation may be performed in three ways: gradual, continuous, over-distension or rapid dilatation.

431. Gradual dilatation is the usual method and a very successful one of treating ordinary strictures. In this method instruments that can be closely crowded through the stricture are used daily, or every two or three days, always increasing the size, and the pressure from within, besides enlarging the canal, causes an activity of the absorbents that soon results in the lessening and removal of the indurated material of which

the stricture is composed. The instruments by which this may be accomplished are: 1st. Steel sounds well polished in oil or nickel plated. The curve should, according to Thompson, be made to correspond to the sub-pubic curvature of the urethra, which is an arc of a circle three and a quarter inches in diameter. 2d. Silver or gum elastic catheters of similar size and shape may also be used, and sometimes it is an advantage to use them, where there is accumulation of urine in the bladder. A bell wire may be bent upon itself, and then given the proper curve and used as a catheter in case of emergency. 3d. Bougies of lead, wax, elastic, catgut or whalebone, may be used, and they are made of various sizes and shapes. The English mahogany colored, and the French black bougies are most used. The latter are the most preferable, on account of their flexibility and adaptability to the canal. They are also furnished with olive shaped points which prevent their being caught in the lacunæ of the mucous membrane, or catching in and penetrating the folds of the stricture, which is possible with the sharp pointed ones. They readily engage themselves in the opening through the stricture, and are more easily insinuated through it. The English bougies are stiff, and in those furnished with an olive point, the neck beyond the point is so slender and brittle, as to be easily broken on slight pressure.

Filliform bougies, either of gum elastic or whalebone, are indispensable in the treatment of very tight and close strictures. These are made with the acorn point, or with variously twisted points to suit the various conditions. The large extremity of the gum elastic filliform bougie may have a metallic cap securely fastened to it, by which it may be screwed on to an instrument for over-distension, rupture, or internal urethral incision. The finest whalebone filliform bougies are of great use in first passing an almost impermeable stricture, even where the gum elastic filliform can not be made to pass. When at last the latter can be got through, if there is to be forcible enlargement or incision, the instrument may be at once attached and passed in, the bougie acting as a guide through the stricture, and coiling up in the bladder, whence it is withdrawn after the operation is completed. It is safe to attach a fine strand of strong silk to the bougie, near the metal cap, previous to passing it into the bladder, lest by accident it become detached from the cap, and left in the bladder when the instrument is withdrawn. In such a case the silk will guide the end of the bougie into the urethra, and draw it out of the bladder, thus saving much trouble and danger.

432. *Introduction of the Instrument.*—This may be accomplished with the patient either standing or lying down. If standing, the surgeon stoops or sits in front; if reclining on his back, he places himself on his left side. The instrument being well oiled, he grasps the penis near the head, between the ring and middle fingers of the left hand, the thumb and forefinger being left free to retract the prepuce and open the meatus. The instrument is seized with the right, and by the thumb and fore and middle fingers, lightly like a pen. If it be a bougie it passes in with slight manipulation and pressure. If a sound or catheter, etc., with a fixed curve, it must enter the meatus, with the shaft parallel to the surface of the abdomen or left groin. The penis should be well drawn up, so as to put the mucous membrane on the stretch, and the point of the instrument should be made to follow the course of the upper wall of the urethra, as it passes under the pubes to the bladder. In this operation the handle of the instrument is, at first, raised to a perpendicular, and then depressed between the thighs, the instrument being pressed firmly in the direction towards the point if there be much resistance. In some cases where there is difficulty in the introduction of an instrument, besides oiling it well, the injection of oil into the urethra opens and lubricates the canal, and facilitates the passage of the instrument. When it has passed into the bladder it should be retained from one to three or five minutes, or it may be immediately withdrawn. In one or two days a larger one may be attempted, and this course should be persevered

in until a No. 26 to 30 French scale, or 16 to 19 English scale, is passed. This large instrument should then be passed once a week, once a month, or once in three months, and persevered in for a long time, to prevent further contraction. During this course proper attention should be paid to the general condition of the system and the urine, and such measures taken to allay any irritation produced by the instruments. The urine should be rendered as bland as possible; and the general condition improved by proper tonics, etc. Sometimes a stricture can not be dilated by this method beyond a certain size, and resists further efforts. For these cases and all others in which we wish to hasten the cure, the following methods are adapted:

433. *Continuous Dilatation.*—In this method the catheter is retained for several days in succession, producing ulceration at the point of stricture, and a free discharge. The urethra becoming enlarged, a larger catheter is inserted, and so on. Care should be taken not to allow it to remain so long that incrustations form around it. This method is allowable when there are false passages, or when, the catheter being inserted, if withdrawn it would be very difficult to again pass it in. The disadvantages and dangers attending this mode of treatment, and the more frequent recurrence of contraction, prevent its being often resorted to.

434. *Over-Distension or Rapid Dilatation.*—This operation is performed by an instrument of two blades, united at their points, and separable in the curve, by the working of a screw between them. It allows of distension at the stricture, greater than an instrument of the size of the meatus could produce. The distension proceeds slowly, requiring from seven to ten minutes to complete it. A full sized gum catheter is then passed, and allowed to remain twenty-four hours, and then withdrawn, and on the third day a large sound may be passed and occasionally afterward repeated.

435. *Rupture.*—This method has come much into use, chiefly through the exertions of Mr. Holt of the Westminster

Hospital, London. An instrument invented by him, "Holt's dilator," consists of two blades with a handle, and united at the point, which is somewhat tapering. A wire passes through the handle and to the point between the blades. Upon the wire, cylinders of various sizes are made to slide, the rod guiding them while they separate the blades. The point of the instrument may be removable, so that the metallic cap attached to the filliform bougie may be screwed upon it. In very close strictures the filliform-bougie should be introduced first, and then the instrument being attached it will follow the bougie through the stricture, until its widest part becomes engaged in it. In an open stricture, the instrument may be used without the bougie. The proper slide is then placed in position, and firmly pushed down to its place. The rupture of the stricture is sudden and complete, yet the mucous membrane may not be injured much, excepting the stricture was very close, or the slide a very large one. If there be some hemorrhage, it is readily arrested by the application of cold cloths, and the internal use of Hamamelis or other astringents. Fomentations may be used for several days, and such other treatment as may be necessary to reduce the inflammation. At the end of three or five days, a No. 8 or 10 English, 14 or 18 French bougie may be passed, and rapidly increased daily to the largest size. This should then be introduced occasionally for several months or a year. Voillemier's rupture instrument is on the same principle, excepting that in that the central slide is grooved and the blades are made to slide in them. In Thebaud's instrument, the blades are made to separate at the end, which when they are closed is blunt, and can only be used on a stricture which is quite open. The blades are separated by a screw working in the handle.

436. *Incision.*—There are two methods of incision: Internal urethrotomy and external urethrotomy. Internal urethrotomy is performed from before backwards; or from behind forwards. In the former method a grooved staff is in-

serted, guided by a filliform-bougie through the urethra, and a triangular blade sharpened at the edges before and behind, but blunt at the apex, is pushed down the groove of the staff. The blunt apex protects the urethra, while the stricture is encountered and cut through by the sharp edge of the blade. This is Maisoneuve's instrument, which has been modified by Voillemier, by furnishing the blade with a sheath until it reaches the stricture, and then withdrawing it. The stricture is incised from behind forwards, by an instrument (Civiale's) in which the blade is concealed in a terminal bulb, of the size of No. 7 or 8 of the English scale, and can only be used when a stricture is dilated to that size. It is passed through the stricture, the blades are projected during its withdrawal, and it cuts its way through. The blades are sheathed and the instrument is withdrawn. The after treatment in either case is essentially the same as in rupture. In stricture of the spongy portion of the urethra, nearest the meatus, the lanceted catheter may be used, or when close to the meatus, Civiale's concealed bistoury or a probe-pointed bistoury.

437. External urethrotomy may be performed in certain forms of stricture, in which the cure is not possible by either of the other methods. This operation may be performed in certain forms of permeable strictures, and in the impermeable ones. Permeable strictures accompanied with extreme sensibility of the urethra, preventing the use of instruments, and resilient strictures under similar conditions, may require external urethrotomy, although in most cases it will be possible to use the urethrotome or to rupture, the sensitiveness being overcome by the use of an anæsthetic. Slightly permeable and impermeable strictures with fistulæ, may need external urethrotomy. If the stricture exist in the spongy urethra near the meatus it may be incised upon a grooved director. If, however, it be situated more deeply in the perineum, the operation is more severe. If a guide can be passed through it, to be cut upon, it is called "Syme's operation," or perineal division. If no instrument can be passed through

it, the operation is called especially "perineal section," and "external urethrotomy," or "external perineal urethrotomy." In the first case the operation is performed upon a Syme's staff. This is a steel staff of proper size, terminating at the extremity in a grooved probe of smaller size, and joined to the staff by a distinct shoulder. This is passed into the urethra, the probe passing through the stricture and the shoulder engaging against it. The patient is secured as in the operation for lithotomy, and an incision an inch in length is made in the median line, behind the scrotum and in front of the anus. Penetrating carefully, so as to avoid the rectum, and keeping well in the median line, the grooved probe is felt in the urethra within the stricture, the knife is made to enter the groove behind the stricture, and it is opened from behind forward, the edge of the knife being kept forward, so as to avoid opening the deep perineal fascia. After making certain that the stricture is entirely relieved, a catheter may be inserted, and guided into the bladder. It is then withdrawn, the patient placed in a natural position, with the bed well protected, and the urine is allowed to pass out of the wound, which it will for a time, until the perineal orifice closes, when it will pass out of the urethra. In impermeable stricture the incision is made upon a staff, or catheter, which is passed as far as the stricture. It may then be possible to pass a fine probe or even a bristle through the incision and stricture, as guide for the urethra. If so, it will not be very difficult to find that canal behind the stricture. But if the canal is entirely obliterated, as it sometimes is, the difficulty becomes vastly increased. It is then necessary to work carefully backwards, in the median line, from the point of the staff, until the healthy urethra is reached. It will sometimes be dilated, and present itself in the incision as a fluctuating tumor, and must be opened, and from this point to that of starting, the urethra can be traced. The catheter will then be guided into the bladder and withdrawn, and the after treatment pursued as before.

438. *Caustics.*—This method is so entirely superseded by those already described, being so harsh and dangerous, and liable to produce fresh and greater complications, that but little need be said of it. The exact distance of the stricture behind the meatus is ascertained, and marked upon a bougie. A depression is made in the extremity of it, and a piece of lunar caustic or caustic potassa is firmly fitted into it. It is then passed down rapidly to the stricture, and pressed firmly against it, and withdrawn. A gleety discharge is the result, but the application must be renewed every two or three days, until a bougie of the proper size can be passed, and the dilatation will then be continued with the bougies.

439. *Consequences of Operations upon Stricture.*—Frequently, in sensitive patients, rigors will follow the insertion of an instrument, which soon pass off. In more severe cases, the patient is suddenly seized with a chill, vomiting, acceleration of the pulse, and often with delirium and great prostration, seemingly the result of a partial shock to the nervous system. This must be met with the administration of stimulants and opiates, and Quinine if necessary, also with sinapisms to the back, abdomen and extremities, and hot foot-baths and bottles of hot water to the feet and sides, and such other measures as will restore the equilibrium.

440. *Retention of Urine.*—A person suffering from a tight stricture may, from cold or some imprudence, have superadded a spasmodic condition, which will suddenly and completely close the urethra. The bladder fills up, rises above the pubes, and expulsive efforts become serious, with no resulting discharge of urine. Eventually the urethra behind the stricture will give way, and extravasation of urine occur, if by some means relief be not obtained. Care should be exercised by the surgeon not to wait too long, before giving relief, lest permanent injury be sustained by the kidneys from the pressure upon the delicate glandular structure, through the pressure of the urine through the ureters.

441. TREATMENT.—In most cases by placing the system thoroughly under the influence of opiates and relaxants, the hot bath, fomentations, etc., and effecting an evacuation of the bowels if necessary, the urine may pass or a catheter of small size, or Thompson's probe-pointed catheter, may be passed. If not, the patient should be placed under the influence of an anæsthetic, and the attempt made, with care and perseverance, to pass the instrument. It is sometimes the case that a small acorn-pointed French bougie or an acorn-pointed filliform whalebone bougie may be made to pass through the stricture, after injecting oil, and the effect of the withdrawal may sometimes be a partial or complete evacuation of the bladder. What is called forcible catheterism should not be resorted to, for in the attempt to reach the bladder at all hazards, the urethra may be punctured, and the instrument pursue an uncertain course between the rectum and bladder. If, however, it should find its way into the bladder, it would be by making a false passage, which would very materially complicate the treatment of the case.

442. If relief can not be obtained by such methods, and if the condition of the patient and the surroundings warrant it, the operation of external perineal urethrotomy should be performed, which will at once remove the stricture, as well as give relief to the patient's more immediate symptoms. This operation, called opening the urethra beyond the stricture, may be performed in the manner already described, by cutting down upon a catheter in the urethra; or by plunging a bistoury into the perineum, just in front of the anus, the cutting edge forward, and with the finger in the rectum guiding it, cutting forward one or two inches. The bulging urethra can soon be felt in the wound and opened, giving relief to the urine, which would escape with some force. The stricture can then be severed upon a director. A director should follow the knife into the bladder, to facilitate the passage of a catheter afterwards.

443. Puncture of the bladder through the rectum is another method of relief in an extreme case. In this method the bowel being evacuated, the finger, well oiled, is passed into the rectum, and guides the trochar and canula to a point beyond the posterior border of the prostate gland, directly in the median line, to a triangular portion of the bladder not covered by the peritoneum, and bounded laterally by the vesiculæ seminales. In its passage the trochar is slightly withdrawn into the canula, and at the point named, firm pressure is made toward the interior of the bladder, counter pressure being made from the hypogastric region. The trochar is withdrawn, and the urine escapes through the canula, which is then fastened in with tapes for several days, until relief of the stricture can be obtained.

444. Puncture above the pubes is a simple operation, in lean persons, when the bladder is fully distended, but not under other circumstances, and is especially dangerous if the peritoneum be wounded, or if infiltration of urine occur. This operation is especially applicable in those cases in which there co-exists an enlarged prostate-gland, rendering perineal section dangerous, and puncture of the rectum impossible, from the finger not being long enough to reach beyond it. An incision is made in the median line above the pubes, about two inches in length, and the bladder felt for between the recti and pyramidales muscles. Its position being ascertained, the trochar and canula should be passed into it, in a direction downwards and backwards, the trochar withdrawn, and the urine evacuated. The canula should be fastened in for several days until the wound closes around it, and care should be taken to guard against urinary infiltration. The stricture to be treated as in the other methods.

445. Puncture through the symphysis is another method of relief, in which the trochar is forced by a rotatory motion, with or without a previous incision, between the pubic bones and into the bladder. A flexible catheter is inserted through the canula.

446. *Extravasation of Urine* is a very serious consequence of retention of urine from stricture. After great distension of the bladder and severe expulsive pains, there comes a sense of relief, after a feeling of something giving way in the perineum, followed after a time, by throbbing and pain, and a sensation of swelling and fullness in the same region. This usually extends forward to scrotum, thighs and penis, and is soon followed by a dingy red coloring of the skin, increased to a dusky red and purple color. The parts become often enormously distended, with a crackling feel, œdematous and emphysematous. It is confined to this region by the deep perineal fascia, which also prevents the extravasation extending backwards and into the pelvis. If relief be not early obtained, they quickly become gangrenous, and the testes and cords become denuded, the sloughing involving all the parts affected by the infiltration, until the patient sinks from exhaustion.

447. TREATMENT.—If not much urine has escaped, and the bladder be still distended, make a deep incision in the median line and enter the urethra at the point of rupture, in the manner described for entering it behind the stricture. In all cases free incisions should be made, wherever the appearances indicate the presence of urine in the areolar tissues, to allow its escape. The patient should be put on sustaining treatment, using lotions and injections as much as possible, of solutions of Sulphate of Zinc or Carbolic Acid, Labarrague's solution, with charcoal and yeast poultices to the parts.

448. *Urinary Abscess* may occur in the perineum, external to the urethra, and not communicating with it primarily, being the result of irritation produced by passing of instruments or from other causes. Pus is formed, becomes circumscribed by a dense wall of plastic deposit, and ultimately opens into the urethra. Or a few drops of urine may escape from the urethra, as the result of stricture and severe strain-

ing in urinating, and an abscess be formed, communicating primarily with the urethra.

449. SYMPTOMS.—The appearance in the perineum, under such circumstances, of a hard, somewhat circumscribed and painful tumor, with a sensation of weight and throbbing. There may be fluctuation if in the neighborhood of the scrotum.

450. TREATMENT.—It should be laid open by deep incision, and treated according to the indications.

451. *Urinary Fistulæ* form in the perineum and scrotum, commonly as the result of abscess. They may appear in the groin, thighs or anterior abdominal wall, and usually communicate with the bulbous or membranous portions of the urethra. Their external orifices may be quite numerous and some of them may be quite small, while others are large. They may sometimes communicate with large cloacæ or cavities beneath the surface. The tissues, in which they have burrowed, become indurated almost like cartilage. Frequently nearly all the urine passes through them, but little passing through the meatus. Fistula may occur in the anterior portion of the urethra, and is usually single.

452. TREATMENT.—If there be stricture, the relief of that once accomplished, the fistulæ will usually close themselves. Either of the methods, by rupture or urethrotomy, may be resorted to. Where there are many external openings and much induration, perineal section will produce the best results. The patient should be instructed how to draw off the urine himself with the catheter, or the catheter may be fastened in and a rubber tube attached to the external extremity, so that the urine may be continuously passed off without distending the bladder, thus keeping it out of the fistulæ. If they do not entirely close up, a fine wooden probe may be dipped in Nitric Acid, or some caustic solution, and passed into them, cauterizing their sides. This repeated occasionally

will usually cause them to close. Sometimes scrotal fistulæ require to be laid open to the bottom of cavities with which they communicate, and to be healed from the bottom. Sometimes the edges may be pared, and brought together by the quilled suture, with free lateral incisions.

453. *Penile Fistulæ*, situated in the anterior part of the urethra, often require the operation of urethroplasty for their cure. De Gros Clark's method is essentially this: Pare the edges of the fistula, after introducing a catheter into the bladder, and securing it. Make a transverse cut through the integuments of the penis, about an inch in length, above and below the fistula. Dissect up the skin subcutaneously. Unite the edges of the skin at the borders of the fistula by means of clamps or the quilled suture. By this operation a wide, raw surface from each side is brought into contact, with consequently a greater chance of a successful union resulting. The rubber tube should be attached to the catheter, so that, by keeping the bladder emptied, the danger will be avoided, of a drop or two of urine being forced by the side of the catheter, and through the fistula, which might be the result of an effort to evacuate the bladder.

ACUTE PROSTATITIS.

454. The prostate gland is but a small organ, and seems to serve an unimportant function, yet its diseases are among the most severe and stubborn that we are called to treat. This is to be attributed in great part to its situation and relation to the bladder and urethra. As the neck of the bladder terminates in it, and the urethra is excavated through it, any cause producing enlargement will alter the position of the bladder so as to cause retention and difficult expulsion of urine; and diminishing the size of urethra and changing its

course, will cause difficulty in its passage. It seems also to be freely supplied with nerves from the hypogastric plexus, and also from the spermatic, hence all the pelvic viscera sympathize in a marked degree.

455. Acute inflammation of the prostate may arise from the ordinary causes of inflammation, being excited by a blow or other injury of the part, but more frequently by sitting on something wet or cold—the perineal structures being thoroughly chilled. It may also be caused by an extension of gonorrhœa, by the use of irritant injections, and occasionally by the use of irritant diuretics.

456. SYMPTOMS.—The patient complains of a sense of weight and tension in the perineum, with deep, tensive pain. There is a frequent desire to pass water, difficulty in its passage, and an increase of pain at the time and afterwards. Movement increases the suffering so much sometimes, that the patient is confined to his bed, and can hardly change his position. Deep pressure also produces pain.

457. There is usually considerable constitutional disturbance. In some cases there is marked febrile action for two or three days; in all there is more than usual irritation of the nervous system.

458. When the disease is very serious, the difficulty in passing urine becomes very great, and the patient suffers intolerably at these times. Indeed, I have seen cases in which it could only be passed after an injection of Opium per rectum, and in a hot sitz bath.

459. The duration of the disease is variable. Terminating in resolution, the inflammation may subside in two or three days, or it may continue a week or more. It is very rare for it to terminate in suppuration. Occasionally a case will present, in which the inflammation extends to the cellular tissues adjacent, and an abscess forms in this, finally opening in the perineum, and inclined to terminate in fistula.

460. DIAGNOSIS.—The location of the symptoms will call our attention to the organs situated at the outlet of the pelvis, and an examination will readily determine the character of the lesion. The pain points just below the scrotum, and an examination at the point elicits deep tenderness. If a catheter or bougie were passed up to the prostatic portion of the urethra, it would meet with obstruction and cause great pain. (I do not advise this method of examination). If not satisfied, a finger passed into the rectum will determine the enlarged prostate very tender to the touch.

461. PROGNOSIS.—We can generally procure relief within forty-eight hours, and an entire removal of the disease. If the person has suffered from previous attacks, we will be governed by the history of the disease.

462. TREATMENT.—It is a rule in the practice of medicine, that no matter how small the structure involved in inflammation, the treatment will be just as active as if a larger part or organ was affected. Especially is this the case with the specific means we use.

463. We put the patient upon the use of Veratrum and Gelseminum in full doses, and continue it until the hardness and frequency of pulse has passed away, and the secretions established; then in smaller doses. Cathartics are always injurious, indeed we are careful that the bowels shall not be opened until the acute inflammation has passed by. After the influence of the sedative, the patient should take the Citrate or Acetate of Potash to the extent of two or three drachms daily, largely diluted with water.

464. To relieve the local suffering, we may employ the hypodermic injection of Morphia over the gland. Or in place of this, we may use an injection into the rectum of: ℞ Tincture of Opium, ʒss.; Tincture of Lobelia, ʒj.; Warm Water, ℥ij. M. The hot sitz-bath may be used for thirty minutes to an hour at a time, if the pain is severe; or a hot fomenta-

tion may be employed in its place. I prefer a hot brick wrapped in flannel with Tincture of Opium and Lobelia in water, and placed between the thighs near the perineum, to either the bath or fomentation.

465. In sub-acute cases, we will occasionally succeed well, with the use of Hamamelis alternated with Staphysagria. Of the distilled Extract of Hamamelis, I give twenty drops every three hours; of the Tincture of Staphysagria, ʒj. to Water, ℥iv.; a teaspoonful every four hours. These may be also given during convalescence. It will rarely, if ever, be necessary to attempt to draw the urine with a catheter. The injections of Opium and Lobelia, the hot sitz-bath, and the internal administration of Gelseminum being sufficient.

CHRONIC PROSTATITIS.

466. Chronic prostatitis is a disease of advanced life, very rarely occurring before the age of forty, and from that to sixty years. Whilst it is more frequently found in good livers, persons who have indulged freely in the pleasures of life, we will occasionally see cases where the person has lived a very regular and temperate life.

467. It is difficult to determine the cause in many cases. It may result from an acute attack, or from a badly managed or frequently repeated gonorrhœa. But in the majority, it is developed slowly, and comes on like hæmorrhoids, or other slowly progressing diseases.

468. SYMPTOMS.—The disease pursues a very irregular course. There is all the time an unpleasant sense of fullness and weight in the perineum, and more or less difficulty in micturition. When the patient has been on his feet for some time, or undergoes unusual exertion, these symptoms are increased.

469. Then there are violent outbreaks in the disease, arising from over-exertion, from injury, or from cold. The prostate increases in size, becomes very tender, the seat of a deep, tensive, aching pain, with occasional lancinating pain, like a toothache. There is a feeling of tenesmus, with desire to go to stool and pass water frequently. But the passage of urine is tardy, very difficult, and attended with much suffering. In some cases it is almost impossible for the patient to void urine, and for many hours none is passed. In some cases, the bladder being dilated to its greatest extent, the urine dribbles away involuntarily. Such a paroxysm may continue but one or two days, or it may last for as many weeks. The sufferer slowly recovers his usual health, and continues to suffer in moderate degree until the next paroxysm.

470. DIAGNOSIS.—The symptoms point to the urinary apparatus, as the seat of disease. On examination, we find tenderness on deep pressure just below the scrotum, and in persons thin in flesh, we can detect the enlargement through the perineum. An examination per rectum is necessary, however, to determine the extent of the disease. The finger can be passed over the entire gland, determining its size, position, and degree of tenderness.

471. PROGNOSIS.—Chronic prostatitis has been deemed incurable by most writers, and treatment was confined to palliatives. I think, however, we may succeed in curing the disdisease in quite a number of cases, and giving very marked relief in nearly all.

472. TREATMENT.—If called during such paroxysm as described, we would adopt the treatment named for the acute disease. The difficulty in passing urine and its retention will be overcome by the administration of Veratrum and Gelseminum, the enema of Opium and Lobelia, and the hot application. In some of the severe cases I would use the hypodermic injection of Morphia.

473. In the general treatment, if the health was impaired, such means should be employed as would restore it. In the majority of cases we will find it of advantage to stimulate the skin, kidneys and bowels, so as to get increased waste. Then by the use of bitter tonics and restoratives, and a nutritious diet, get an active nutrition and renewal of tissue. We will sometimes find, as in other forms of chronic disease, that this is the most important part of the treatment; indeed, that it will accomplish the object without specific means.

474. The special remedies that I have relied on in these cases are, the Hamamelis, Staphysagria, Collinsonia and Phosphorus. Of the first I use the distilled extract (Pond's), in doses of twenty to thirty drops, four times a day. Of the Tincture of Staphysagria, ʒj. to Water, ℥iv.; a teaspoonful four times a day. Of the Fluid Extract of Collinsonia, ʒij.; Water, ℥iv.; a teaspoonful four times a day. Of the Tincture of Phosphorus, ʒij.; Water, ℥iv.; a teaspoonful four times a day. These may be given singly, or may be alternated; and changed sufficiently often to continue the good effect. As a local application, I prefer a small seton, as being less annoyance than any other means of counter-irritation.

475. When there is considerable urethral irritation, the prostate offering an obstruction to the passage of a bougie, we will sometimes find advantage from injections. The solution of Sulphate of Hydrastia acts very kindly, as does a weak solution of Carbolic Acid. The injection is used with an Acton's long-tube syringe.

PROSTATORRHŒA.

476. Associated with spermatorrhœa we not unfrequently find an excitation of the prostatic and Cowper's glands, and possibly of the vesiculæ seminales. These glandular structures furnish an increased secretion, having a mucoid appear-

ance, and slightly resembling seminal fluid, which is passed with the urine, on going to stool, on lifting or straining, and in some cases, when profuse, there is an almost constant oozing. The patient's mind having been excited by what he has been told by designing persons, calling themselves physicians, or the private circulars he has received from the same source, he is constantly on the look-out for the discharge, and is excessively troubled by it, so much so that he is not unfrequently on the verge of insanity.

477. Not only do we find this discharge in those who truly have spermatorrhœa, but quite as frequently where that disease does not exist, the prostatorrhœa being the only trouble. The sufferer has, however, been told that he is suffering from the former affection, and religiously believes it, the influence on the mind being such as to frequently impair the general health. It is useless in these cases to attempt to persuade them of the mistake in the nature of the disease, and when we arrest the discharge we invariably get credit for curing a case of spermatorrhœa.

478. In rare cases the bladder is the principal seat of the disease, giving rise to irritation of adjacent parts. Generally, the chronic inflammation is confined to the trigone vesicæ, giving rise to but few of the common symptoms of cystitis, though there is an increased secretion of mucus, and frequently copious deposits of the triple phosphates.

479. TREATMENT.—What treatment can we adopt in these cases, that will relieve this irritation, and arrest this discharge? Upon this will frequently depend the success of our treatment for spermatorrhœa. If we are to successfully manage this affection we must gain the confidence of our patient, and cause him to believe that we can cure him. If this prostatic discharge continues, we can not attain this end; if we arrest it, he has visible assurance of the efficacy of our medicines. Spermatorrhœa is, to a considerable extent, a

mental disease, and unless the mind can be favorably influenced, there is but little prospect of a favorable result.

480. Those who have had much to do with these affections will bear me out in saying that nothing favorable may be expected from injections into the urethra, no matter what their character, and in many cases most serious results have followed their use. Where there is irritation of the prostatic portion of the urethra, marked by burning or pain on passing water, Lallemand's porte caustique may sometimes be used with advantage, otherwise all irritant local applications are useless. If there is much excitement of the genital organs, with frequent erections, nocturnal emissions or masturbation, this *must* be controlled, and may be very readily by any irritant material applied to the penis, that will make it so sore that erection is impossible. I usually use the Spanish-fly plaster, sometimes Croton Oil, at others Potassa Fusa. There should be no hesitation in the use of these means, and to such an extent as to accomplish the object.

481. As to internal measures, I have used all that have been recommended, but have not attained the success with the common means that I was led to expect. Agrimonia, Hydrangea and Collinsonia seem to have some influence, but not sufficient for a cure. Buchu and Uva Ursi are inferior to the first named. Pareira Brava has, in some cases, a decided influence, as has also Cubebs, Hydrastis and Carbonate of Iron, aa. The remedies upon which I depend now are three in number, and their use is empirical. I am inclined to believe the first one is almost or quite a specific. They are, the Staphysagria, Apis Mellifica, and Phosphorus. I use the Tincture of each, ʒj. to ℥iv. of water, a teaspoonful four times a day. I place more dependence on the first one named, which, by the way, is worth studying, as it possesses marked medicinal properties.

CHRONIC CYSTITIS.

482. Chronic inflammation of the bladder is of more frequent occurrence than the acute. It is almost always confined to the mucous coat, giving rise to the various changes of structure noticed during chronic inflammation, as thickening of the mucous membrane, enlargement of the follicles, ulceration, etc. Its causes are various; it may arise from cold, injuries, irritating diuretics or injections, the presence of calculi, irritation from disease of the kidneys, extension of disease from the urethra, as in gonorrhœa, and from extension of disease from adjacent organs.

483. Persons suffering from chronic cystitis usually complain of a sense of weight in the hypogastrium and perineum, with a dull, dragging pain. There is also tenderness on deep pressure over the hypogastrium. More or less difficulty is experienced in passing urine, sometimes on account of the increased mucous secretion, and at others, from the seeming acridity of the urine. The patient frequently complains of pain in the neck of the bladder, extending the entire length of the urethra, and sometimes of a sensation of scalding or burning referred to the region of the bladder. In severer cases, when complicated with disease of the prostate, or when ulceration has occurred, the pain and heat in the bladder is very severe, the call to urinate urgent, and attended by violent tenesmus and straining.

484. The general health becomes markedly affected when the disease is severe; the bowels are constipated; the appetite impaired; the skin dry, harsh and sallow; and considerable loss of flesh and strength. The urine varies greatly; in the milder cases it seems nearly natural, but in the more severe cases, it contains mucus, pus, and the phosphates. Sometimes it is so thick by the presence of these materials that it is voided with difficulty.

485. In some cases, when of long duration, we find the symptoms very severe. The urine is passed frequently both night and day, and with great tenesmus. There is no resisting the inclination to its passage, and if resisted, the tenesmus only becomes greater. In some cases it starts with difficulty, and the patient suffers intense agony for some minutes before the stream starts. In other cases, it starts freely, but is suddenly arrested, either by the contraction of the circular fibres, or by a forcing down of the mucous membrane from undue contraction of the *detrusor urinæ*, and in still others from the passage of mucus. In some cases, the tenesmus is such that prolapse of the bowel occurs during micturition.

486. Chronic cystitis is determined by the location of the pains and tenderness, and its association with difficulty in passing water, and alteration in the urine dependent upon the changed secretions of the bladder. Mucus in urine may be determined by its action on litmus paper, by its particles coagulating into a thin, semi-opaque membrane, on the addition of Nitric Acid, and by its soon undergoing putrefactive decomposition, becoming ammoniacal. Pus in urine generally falls to the bottom when allowed to stand; Acetic Acid has no effect on it, but if agitated with Liquor Potassæ it forms a dense, translucent, gelatinous mass. If the urine contains phosphatic deposits it is often very fœtid, sometimes pale, at others greenish, and viscid from abundance of mucus. On placing some of the mucus beneath the microscope, abundant crystals of the triple phosphate are found entangled in it. Dr. Bird remarks that: "One point must be borne in mind in forming a prognosis from the state of the urine, viz., not to regard it as ammoniacal because the odor is offensive, and not to consider the deposit as purulent because it looks so. A piece of litmus paper will often show it to be neutral, and even sometimes acid, while microscopic inspection often proves the puriform appearance of the urine to be an admixture of the phosphates with mucus. For want of these precautions, I have seen some cases regarded as almost hopeless which

afterward yielded to judicious treatment. It is quite certain that the mucous membrane of the bladder may, under the influence of chronic inflammation, secrete so much of the earthy phosphates and unhealthy mucus, as to render the urine puriform and offensive without having necessarily undergone any structural change."

487. POST-MORTEM EXAMINATION.—In the milder forms of this affection, we find the mucous membrane thickened, injected and discolored, and its follicles enlarged. It is frequently softened so as to separate from the muscular coat with considerable readiness. In a still more advanced stage the entire coats are thickened and contracted, the mucous follicles enlarged; and more or less ulceration, sometimes regular and well defined, and at others irregular and sloughy. According to Copland, "When the ulceration is extensive, the hypertrophied muscular fibres appear, and resemble the columnæ carnea of the heart, presenting a purplish-red color, the mucous coat between the columns thus formed being pale, soft and swollen. Pouches or sacks generally co-exist, with dilated ureters, between these muscular columns, and are formed by the contraction of the bladder and of the abdominal muscles in expelling the urine, forcing the mucous coat in places between the muscular fibres. These pouches are lined with a diseased mucous coat, which secretes an alkaline mucus, and are sometimes the receptacles of a mortar-like matter, and finally of calculi, consisting generally of Phosphate of Lime. As the disease progresses, it frequently extends to the ureters, pelvis of the kidney, and at last so involves its structure as to occasion death."

488. TREATMENT.—The treatment of these cases will vary greatly, and here as elsewhere, we will find that success comes from a careful study of our cases, and the employment of "specific" remedies so far as possible. I do not know that there is greater variation in these cases, than in disease of other organs, but very surely the variation is more marked.

489. It will be well to study the special means seriatim, pointing out so far as possible, the special indication for each remedy. Of course these are not peculiar to a disease of the bladder and its therapeutics, but are quite as applicable in any other form of disease.

490. Where there is an irritable bladder, with burning pain, and scalding in passing water, a tendency to erysipelatous inflammation of the skin, or simple erythema with burning, I would prescribe Rhus.

491. If there was irritation of bladder, frequent micturition, and a severe burning with pruritus, acute formication of surface, Apis.

492. If there was difficult micturition, with sense of fullness and weight at the neck of the bladder and perineum, Eryngium.

493. Where there was difficulty in starting the flow of urine, and tendency to retention, Santonine.

494. If with the disease of the bladder, there was undue nervousness, and unpleasant forebodings with regard to the termination of the disease, the tissues being somewhat tense and contracted, Pulsatilla.

495. If associated with deep pelvic and perineal pain, lumbago, muscular pain in every portion of the body, deep sense of soreness in the bladder, especially when called into contraction, Macrotys.

496. Frequent desire to urinate, but a very small stream, passed with difficulty, and great excitation of the nervous system, Gelseminum.

497. Increased mucous secretion, with sense of fullness and weight, Staphysagria, Phosphorus.

498. Impaired venous circulation, feebleness and relaxation of pelvic tissues, protrusion of perineum, atonic hemorrhoids, varix, Pond's Hamamelis.

499. Frequent desire to urinate, with pain if the urine is retained for a short time after the desire is manifested, and a

severe, cramp-like, aching pain in the region of the neck of the bladder, Elaterium.*

**Specific for Chronic Inflammation of the Neck of the Bladder.*—PROF. J. M. SCUDDER—*Dear Sir:* As you are at this time engaged in preparing a list of specific remedies for the readers of your Journal, I now present you with one, from which I have derived success in every instance where it has been employed. I will state in advance that as far as I have been able to learn, the agent, to which I here refer, Elaterium, has never been employed for this purpose. All the writers who have written upon this article, view it merely as a drastic purgative, from Pliny to the present time. In a Dispensatory I have, which is 111 years of age, it is spoken of as a dangerous drastic purgative. Nor have I been any more successful with Homœopathic writers, whose provings have never led them to view it as a remedy in the disease under consideration, or for its symptoms. Though, I have no doubt, since I now mention it, that they will soon solve the matter, as they did with the honey-bee, after I had first made its value in urinary difficulties known to the classes to whom I lectured. I, therefore, claim the right to the discovery of Elaterium as a specific in chronic inflammation of the neck of the bladder, until some other party can show a distinct and definite priority.

I have used this remedy since 1849, and during that time have treated about 45 cases, (some of whom were patients of other physicians), and with invariable success. The symptoms among these patients were more or less severe, and nearly of a similar character; they may be summed up as follows: frequent desire to urinate, with pain if the urine was retained for a short time after the desire manifested itself; one or more urinations during the night; urine frequently voided with pain and difficulty; with some, during urinations, "it seemed as though the urine was poured into the urethra;" a constant sense of weight or pain in the region of the neck of the bladder, frequently increased upon standing, or walking; with some, standing occasioned a paralytic sensation and uneasiness in one or both thighs. In the worst cases, a "severe indescribable, cramp-like, aching pain" in the region of the neck of the bladder, and in the perineum, was experienced immediately after urinating, which sensation frequently extended, with more or less violence, over the whole of the lower region of the pelvis, and low down into the thigh; the region of the neck of the bladder was distended, and painful to the touch as well as on standing or sitting. With a few, in whom the disease had been of long standing there were also present, cold feet, swollen feet, hectic fever, colliquative perspiration, cough, etc.

In the more severe cases, I have usually commenced by giving half a fluid drachm of the Tincture of Elaterium, one, two, or three times a day, until it acted upon the bowels; and afterward continue its use in doses of from 5 to 10

500. If there is some tenesmus, with spasmodic contraction of the pelvic and perineal muscles, with expulsive pain, Stramonium is the remedy. It may be given in doses sufficient to give relief, the usual proportion being: ℞ Tincture of Stramonium, ℥j.; Compound Tincture of Cardamom, ℥ij.; Syrup, ℥j.; a teaspoonful every three hours.

501. If there is a tendency to emission without the evidence of vesical contraction, Belladonna would be suggested.

502. If the bladder is emptied with difficulty, and the perineum has to be elevated with the hand, that the last portion may be passed, Ergot or Strychnia would be suggested.

503. If the tongue has a violet coloration, the urine being strongly ammoniacal, we would give Nitric Acid.

---

drops, gradually increasing it as it could be borne. Great relief has always followed in these cases, as soon as the purgative effect came on from the first large doses, and that too, in cases where other purgatives had been frequently taken without any relief whatever. In less severe cases I commence with 6 or 8 drops three times a day, gradually increasing it as could be borne, and being very careful to avoid giving it in doses to act upon the bowels. This action I have only deemed necessary at the commencement of treatment in the more severe and obstinate cases.

A great difference will be found among different persons as to the doses they can bear; while some can take from 6 to [illegible] drops three times daily for weeks without any unpleasantness arising therefrom, others will be found who can not bear more than 1 or 2 drops for a dose, on which account, some care and attention is required on commencing the treatment.

As the agent is apt to excite nausea and vomiting, I have generally administered each dose of it in a teaspoonful or two of syrup, Sarsaparilla syrup, or Compound Yellow Dock syrup, etc. In cases of cold feet, general sensation of cold or chilliness, Tincture of Prickly Ash Bark may be added to each dose; if the liver is torpid, Tincture of Apocynum Androsæmifolium, etc., etc. Gastric acidity, constipation, nervous irritability, anæmia, etc., when present, require the usual treatment for their relief or removal. I prepare the Tincture by adding one drachm of pulverized Elaterium to one pint of Alcohol, 95 per cent.; allowing it to stand two or three weeks, with frequent agitation. I will here remark, that I have likewise found this remedy very beneficial in chronic gastritis, and other chronic inflammations of mucous tissues. In procuring the Elaterium, be very careful that it is good, as there is much in the market that is worthless.—*Prof. John King in E. M. Journal*, 1870.

504. If the urine is markedly acid, we would use Alkalies; if markedly alkaline, Acids.

505. These are special agents, and in addition we have the large class of tonic diuretics, Uva Ursi, Buchu, Chimaphilla, Agrimonia, etc., which may be occasionally employed, though the common treatment with these agents has not been very successful.

506. A general restorative treatment is sometimes necessary to a cure. Take a patient who has suffered long from these urinary troubles, and has had his vital power impaired, and waste and nutrition enfeebled, and a cure will only follow improvement of the general health. Relieve the local irritation and give rest to the parts, and we find by the use of the usual means there is a rapid improvement in the general health.

507. The measures above named answer very well in the milder cases, and though we use them in the severer forms of the disease, we do not depend upon them. In such cases we resort to injections to remove morbid accumulations, and for their topical action. It is surprising to see the benefit that will result from simply washing out the bladder with tepid water, in cases of phosphatic urine with increased mucous secretion; the distressing tenesmus and burning pain and difficulty of passing water, all disappear, but return when this material again accumulates. In some cases the use of simple tepid water is all that is necessary, but in others we medicate the injection. If there is much irritability of the bladder, we might employ equal parts of Glycerine and Rose-water after the tepid injection; or: ℞ Chlorate of Potash, ʒss.; Glycerine, Rose Water, aa. ℥ij. M. Use one ounce as an injection; or: ℞ Zinci Sulphas, grs. x.; Morphia Sulphas, grs. iij.; Glycerine, Aqua Rosæ, aa. ℥ij. M. One ounce to be used as an injection, after washing the bladder out with tepid water, and if it produces too much burning, to be followed by the injection of more water to wash it out. Chloride of Zinc may be used as an injection in the proportion of one, or

at farthest two grains to the ounce of water. A decoction of Hydrastis or Cornus Florida have been used with success in many cases.

508. Formerly I employed counter-irritation extensively, and would not think of treating a case without the irritating plaster over the hypogastrium, or sacrum, or an issue in the perineum. Now I use the acid pack at night with a thorough washing with water in the morning. Usually a flannel ten inches in width, wrung out of good vinegar, passed around the pelvis, and a dry towel over all will answer; but if the case is a serious one, I would use water acidulated with Muriatic Acid.

ORCHITIS.

509. Inflammation of the testicle may be produced by any of the ordinary causes of inflammation, and we occasionally meet with cases, in which there has been no special cause. Usually, however, it will have been excited by an injury of some kind in the simple form of the disease, or by the venereal poison in gonorrhœa and syphilis.

510. The symptoms of orchitis do not differ materially, whether it has arisen from ordinary causes, or from gonorrhœa. The patient first complains of a sensation of weight and dragging in the scrotum, and pain on any sudden movement or jar. In a few hours these symptoms have become more marked, and the patient finds that all movement is painful; and at last has to assume the recumbent position, and keep the part supported.

511. As these symptoms develop, the testicle increases in size, until finally it attains a diameter of a couple of inches, and a length of three, or sometimes four inches. It is quite sensitive to the touch, and when allowed to drag upon the cord, is very painful. Sometimes there is considerable heat

of the part, and the scrotum is reddened. The pain in the organ is of a tensive character, with occasional lancinating pains; sometimes they are of a throbbing character, and are very severe.

512. The disease runs a variable course; sometimes coming up rapidly, the organ attaining its greatest size in one or two days, at others slowly increasing for a week. It will sometimes pass away, under appropriate treatment, in forty-eight hours, but in others may last for days.

513. Gonorrhœal orchitis is usually developed coetaneous with the suppression of the discharge from the urethra. Many have thought that such arrest was the cause of the inflammation—that the orchitis was a metastasis. This opinion is strengthened by the fact, that with the subsidence of the disease of the testes the discharge reappears—or, as others would state it, with the re-appearance of the clap, the orchitis abates. There is no doubt but there is an intimate relation between the two, and a treatment that looks to the sudden suppression of a gonorrhœal discharge will frequently be followed by the inflamed testes. The constitutional disturbance varies in different cases. In some there is marked febrile action and arrest of secretion, in others but little disturbance.

514. The diagnosis of orchitis is readily made. No one making a careful examination would fail to determine the solidity of the testicle in inflammation, from a distension of the scrotum from serum, blood, or the pressure of the intestine in hernia.

515. It has been deemed more difficult to determine whether it was simple or specific. An examination of the penis will give the necessary information. In simple inflammation there is no evidence of recent disease of the prepuce and glans, or of the urethra. In gonorrhœal orchitis, though the discharge has usually ceased, the mucous membrane is tumid, dusky or livid, and irritable. If syphilitic, the disease has developed slowly, there are evidences of previous

chancre, and almost invariably a cutaneous eruption of the syphilidæ.

516. With proper treatment, we may safely promise speedy relief, in a large majority of cases. Once in a while, we will meet with a very stubborn case, continuing until both patient and physician are discouraged. Gonorrhœal orchitis, as a general rule, is most readily managed; and syphilitic orchitis the most stubborn.

517. TREATMENT.—If the inflammation is of an acute character, I usually prescribe: ℞ Tincture of Veratrum, ʒss.; Tincture of Gelseminum, ʒij.; Water, ℥iv. M. A teaspoonful every hour. If, however, there is a sluggish circulation, I prefer Aconite and Belladonna in the usual doses. The patient's bowels are moved with a Seidlitz Powder, or some mild cathartic.

518. If it has arisen from gonorrhœa, the use of means to check the discharge should be stopped, and nothing used but a mild lead wash or a solution of Sulphate of Hydrastia, as an injection.

519. Rather than use local applications, I prefer supporting the testicle by means of adhesive straps. Let the patient lie down, and cut the hair from the pubes and perineum, where it is necessary to attach the straps. Cut the adhesive plaster in strips over an inch broad, the width of the roll. Have the person support the testicle on the abdomen, and with the straps well heated, apply them from the perineum upward on the abdomen, and from side to side around the testicle crosswise. The object is to bind it firmly to the abdominal wall, giving it uniform support and compression.

520. Prof. Howe employs the adhesive straps in a different way. The testicle being suspended in its natural position, he applies the straps spirally, so as to give uniform compression, and finally attaches them to the abdomen so as to take the weight off the cord.

521. If we do not employ the adhesive straps, the testicle should be supported in a suspensory bandage, or by a sling, which may be easily continued. As a local application, I prefer painting the part with Tincture of Veratrum, or Aconite and cold water, or occasionally Belladonna. A hypodermic injection will give speedy relief to the suffering, and will sometimes effect a cure. I prefer to use it at the affected part, raising the skin of the scrotum.

CHRONIC ORCHITIS.

522. Chronic inflammation of the testicle is occasionally developed from the ordinary causes, but in the majority of cases it will be found to be the result of gonorrhœa or syphilis. Occurring in persons who have lived *fast*, we have no hesitation in asking such questions as will determine this fact. True, it will make little difference in the treatment, whether it has been produced by repeated attacks of gonorrhœa, but it would make a difference if it could be traced to syphilis.

523. The patient describes having an enlarged testicle, which is a source of annoyance from its size, its weight, and unpleasant sensations of fullness, dragging, and occasionally aching. The enlarged organ is in the way, and is constantly getting hurt.

When we examine it, we find the testicle three or four times its natural size, sometimes as large as a goose egg, hard, and sensitive to pressure. In some cases the enlargement will be almost wholly of the body of the testicle; in others it will be in part of the epididymis.

Occasionally it is associated with hemorrhoids, at other times with an irritable bladder or urethra. I have seen cases in which the general health was markedly affected, but usually there is nothing of this to attract attention.

If syphilitic, we will have the evidence of the lesion in some other form. Whilst we may have acute orchitis with the syphilidæ, the chronic inflammation is usually one of the last of the secondary symptoms, and is associated with maculæ, ulceration and nodes

524. Though it is easy to determine the enlarged testes, it is not always so easy to say that it is simple inflammation. The diagnosis between an orchitis and enlargement from fluid in the tunica vaginalis is readily determined, as it is from scrotal hernia. Cystic disease may frequently be determined by the uneasiness and variable degree of hardness. Malignant disease may be determined by the irregular form, unequal consistence, and nodulated character of the growth. The diagnosis is confirmed by the cancerous cachexia, which is always soon developed in cancerous testes.

525. In the majority of cases we may promise a cure, though in most of these cases it will require time and patience. Of course there are some cases that can not be cured. Old syphilitic orchitis has been deemed peculiarly intractable, but even this can be cured.

526. TREATMENT.—If the general health is good, our treatment wiil be confined to such special remedies as influence the testicle, and to local applications. If it is impaired, we will adopt the appropriate means to restore health, waste and excretion, and good nutrition.

527. In some cases, where there has been considerable deposit, good results will occasionally follow the use of the vegetable alteratives and the saline diuretics to stimulate absorption.

528. I have used the Hamamelis with excellent effect; the distilled extract is preferred. This is alternated with small doses of Veratrum, Tincture of Phosphorus, and small doses of Collinsonia.

529. In *irritable* testes Bromide of Potassium will sometimes exert a good influence. It may be given in doses of ten

grains, three or four times a day. I have also used the Staphysagria and Pulsatilla in the same cases.

530. The local application will vary in different cases. When the scrotum is dense, and will bear it, I prefer a solution of Iodide of Ammonium, used in this way: ℞ Tincture of Iodine (strong), Aqua Ammonia, aa. Let them stand until decolorized, and apply with a camel's hair brush.

531. Occasionally a dressing of Mayer's Ointment, Black Salve, or Ointment of Stramonium, will serve a good purpose. A lotion of Iodide of Potash has also been employed with advantage, as has the Belladonna.

532. Whatever application we may use in this way, the testicle should be well supported with a suspensory bandage. In some cases the continued use of a water dressing, with such support, will answer the purpose. In some cases, compression by means of the adhesive straps, as advised in the acute form, will give the speediest cure.

533. If the cause is syphilitic, the patient should also receive the appropriate treatment for this. It is true, that a general antisyphilitic treatment will not cure the testes, but it is equally true that they will not get well without this. (See Syphilitic Orchitis.)

STRUCTURAL DISEASE OF THE TESTES AND SCROTUM.

534. We may briefly notice a number of structural lesions of the testes and scrotum, more especially to point out their differential diagnosis. They are not of very common occurrence, and yet the testes suffer more frequently than some other portions of the body.

STRUMOUS DISEASE OF THE TESTES.

535. When irritation of the testes, from injury or other causes, is set up in a person who has a low grade of albumi-

noid material in the blood, it will be deposited in these organs, as it would be elsewhere under similar circumstances. Two conditions are represented in tuberculosis—the presence of a low grade of albuminoid material in the blood, and a local irritation with determination of blood to a part. In this case these organs may suffer without any fault of the patient, but many times the irritation that causes the deposit has been induced by sexual excesses and abuse.

536. The disease announces itself with a sense of uneasiness and weight in the scrotum, especially on prolonged exercise, and the patient gets relief by supporting them with the hand or the clothing. At a further stage, he notices that they are really enlarged, and that the increase in size is continuous; there is also greater weight and uneasiness, with sometimes dragging pains in the scrotum. In this way it may go on for months or even years, before the tubercular material loses its life and breaks down.

537. On examination we find the body of the testes irregular in form, and many times the tubercular nodules can be distinctly felt, especially in the epididymis. At a later stage, the enlarged organ forms attachments to the scrotum, which assumes a livid hue, ulceration occurs, and the matter is discharged with but little inflammatory action. In this case unpleasant fistulæ are formed, which discharge a thin serous pus, and continue for a long time.

538. In other cases, acute inflammation results from the deposit, presenting the usual symptoms of orchitis, but running on to suppuration, and the formation of an abscess, discharging through the scrotum. Abscess of the scrotum is very rare, except from strumous disease, or severe injury.

539. TREATMENT.—Two indications of cure are here prominently presented. The one looks to the removal of irritation of the affected organ, and its proper support and rest, to remove the tendency to local deposit; the other, to getting rid

of the imperfect material in the blood, and its replacement by a well elaborated albumen.

540. If there is considerable irritation when the case is severe, we order rest, a well adjusted suspensory bandage, and the local use of Veratrum, or Aconite. If the irritation is not so acute, we may prescribe Hamamelis, Belladonna, a solution of Iodide of Ammonium, or an infusion of Alnus and Quercus Rubra. If the testes are irritable with neuralgic pain, Camphor Chloral will be a good remedy.

541. The general treatment will be varied to suit the particular case in hand. We determine carefully what needs be done to facilitate retrograde metamorphosis, and increase secretion from skin, kidneys and bowels, bearing in mind that great over-activity can not be maintained, and will be followed by corresponding depression. This is but one-half of the treatment for a "renewal of a better life." The digestive organs must be put in good condition to receive food and make it into blood, and the necessary restoratives must be given. Sometimes the one half, sometimes the other half, of this treatment will preponderate, but neither must be forgotten.

DEGENERATION OF THE TESTES.

542. Degeneration of the testes is a rare form of disease, but still it is met with in all of its variations, *fibrous*, *cartilaginous*, *osseous*, *fatty* and *granular*. The causes which give rise to it are obscure, but probably there is always the general tendency to degeneration, and the local manifestation is due to causes which debilitate these organs. I think in all degenerations we find these two factors. There is an impairment of the blood, and a want of formative power, and locally the organ or part has been over-worked, and its power of renewal impaired.

543. In all cases of degeneration, the size of the organ is increased. It will frequently affect but one testicle at first, and involves the other only after some months or years. In some cases there is deep pain at times, but in the majority,

there is simply a feeling of discomfort from the enlargement, and the dragging upon the cord. At first it may increase sexual excitement, but gradually as the structure of the testes is lost, especially if both are involved, venereal passion and power are lost.

544. TREATMENT.—Though treatment has not proven very successful, we would adopt the rational plan in this as in other cases. The organ affected needs rest, and gentle stimulation; especially does it need support. Whilst the general treatment should look to a better renewal of life. In the early stage of the disease, I would think it possible to arrest its progress; of course, the tissues lost would never be replaced, yet if but one testicle was saved, it would well repay the necessary care.

545. As degeneration, like other chronic structural diseases, involves but one of the testicles at first, and commences in the second when the first is destroyed, we may well consider whether the removal of the diseased organ may not be necessary to the preservation of the sound one. Here, as in structural disease of the eye, I am satisfied that the disease of one affects the other sympathetically, as well as by their close relationship and arterial and nervous supply. In other words, that the presence of the diseased organ will frequently prove a cause of disease in the other. Hence the importance of removing the affected testicle when it is a source of irritation, and if the disease in it can not be controlled.

CYSTIC DISEASE OF THE TESTICLE.

546. Cysts may form in the testicle, and eventually destroy its structure. They may be large or small, from the size of a pin's head to a pigeon's-egg, and number from one or two, to many hundred. Cystic disease usually occurs in early life, from the age of sixteen to thirty.

547. As a rule, the patient suffers little pain or uneasiness, except possibly a sense of fullness and weight as the organ

enlarges, until sometimes attaining a very large size, it becomes very inconvenient from its bulk.

548. The only remedy is excision, which should be performed sufficiently early to save the other organ, when but one has suffered from the disease at first.

CANCER OF THE TESTICLE.

549. The testes suffer from malignant degeneration, though not so frequently as might be expected from their structure and exposed situation. Encephaloid is the most common form of the disease, and it usually occurs in young persons, and runs its course rapidly. Scirrhus is less common and occurs in advanced life, running its course slowly.

550. If we find that the testicle has enlarged rapidly, with little suffering at first, but afterwards with deep tensive pain, in addition to sharp pains radiating from a centre, and passing up the spermatic cords, to the groins, back and thighs, we will suspect encephaloid. The diagnosis will be confirmed by finding an irregular and nodulated growth, of unequal elasticity, enlargement of the blood-vessels in the vicinity, and eventually attachment to and discoloration of the skin. The evidence of a cancerous cachexia is soon shown in the general appearance.

551. Scirrhus progresses very slowly. The testicle is enlarged, hard, nodulated, and is the seat of a severe, tense, burning pain, with the occasional radiating, lancinating pain spoken of above. The patient bears in his general appearance the evidence of severe suffering, and impairment of nutrition.

552. In both cases the attachment of the skin is the precursor of ulceration, and the symptom of open cancer. Encephaloid now runs its course quickly, the patient being exhausted by severe hemorrhages. Scirrhus runs its course still slowly, and may involve much of the perineal tissue before death results.

553. TREATMENT.—The treatment of cancer is not yet very successful. and though the testes seem favorably located for

removal, operative means have not been followed by the good results expected. One reason for this is found in the tenacity with which a man clings to his testicles. He can not bear the thought of losing them, and postpones the time until attachment is formed to the skin, or the lymphatic glands have become diseased. There is but one chance of success here, and that is in early excision. If the diseased structure is extirpated before the lymphatics suffer, and the patient is then put upon a treatment which will improve waste and nutrition, he may be cured, or it will be many years before the disease returns.

VARICOCELE.

554. Varix of the spermatic veins is a disease frequently met with. In many cases it is slight and increases slowly, or not at all, giving rise to but very little disturbance. In others the vessels become much enlarged from causes which disturb the organs, and then shrink away when they are at rest. And in still others, the enlargement of the veins continually increases, until from their size they become a source of constant annoyance.

555. Any cause that unduly excites, or debilitates the sexual apparatus may be a cause of varicocele. Thus it is induced by onanism, by sexual excess, or by injury of the organs by much horseback riding. But it only occurs in those who have an enfeebled venous system, and a tendency to varicose veins, and is thus frequently associated with varix of the legs, or hemorrhoids, or as it occurs in early life, it may be the precursor of these.

556. It is usually slow in its progress, and at first gives rise to but little disturbance, except a feeling of weight and dragging in the groin. As the veins enlarge, however, the patient suffers aching and dragging pains in the parts, much

increased by being upon the feet, by walking, or riding. In some rare cases it causes venereal excitement, but in the majority it lessens it, and may finally prove a cause of impotence.

557. An examination shows a marked enlargement of the spermatic cord, forming an elongated conical tumor, the enlarged veins giving a sensation very much like a bundle of earth worms.

558. Treatment.—In the early stage of the disease, the patient may be very much relieved, sometimes cured, without an operation. We order a well fitted suspensory bandage for the day time, a linen band to retain a compress at night. The scrotum is wetted with Pond's Hamamelis, morning and night, and for a time a compress wetted with the same, may be used at night. If there are acute attacks, with determination of blood, and venous enlargement from this, I should prescribe: ℞ Tincture of Collinsonia, ʒss.; Water, ℥iv.; a teaspoonful every two or three hours. But if it was purely from venous atony, the prescription would be Pond's Hamamelis, gtts. x. to gtts. xx.; three times a day.

559. Prof. Howe has permitted me to extract from his surgical papers what he says in reference to operative means for the radical cure of varicocele:

"Surgical treatises usually contain descriptions of several operative methods for the radical cure of varicocele, yet none of them are devoid of danger from erysipelas, phlebitis, tetanus, or pyæmia—accidents which generally arise from the puncture-nature of the wounds inflicted, and from the subcutaneous strangulation of the veins. A ligature—even if it be made of virgin silver—twisted tightly around vessels beneath the skin, will produce irritation enough to call out fluids which have no means of escape except through the opening in the integument occupied by the ligature. Therefore, it is my opinion that a subcutaneous strangulation of the enlarged veins is more hazardous than ligation applied through a free incision in the integument. But fatal consequences have followed all kinds of strangulation of the spermatic veins, though the degree of danger is diminished by an open incision at the point of constriction.

"To shun the risk incurred by all of the well-known operative procedures, I have excised a segment of the varicose veins, and used no ligatures or sutures. I make an incision an inch in length along the course of the cord about half way between the external abdominal ring and the bulge in the scrotum produced by the testicle. The hair is snipped off before the incision is made. A fold of the loose integument is raised by the thumb and finger along the course of the spermatic cord, and the crest of the fold is incised, including skin, dartos and whatever fascia is grasped. The wound is then spread with the fingers, and the true spermatic fascia seized and incised. The dilated veins may now be separated from the vas deferens, nerves, arteries, and other structures of the cord. After the varicose plexus has been well isolated and brought out of the incision, scissors are used to excise a segment of the veins, by dividing the vessels in two places, each a half inch from the other. The operation is not attended with excruciating pain, and the hemorrhage is never profuse. In fact, the size of the dilated veins has little influence over the amount of blood passing through them. Besides, vessels cut with scissors do not bleed so persistently as when divided with a knife.

"If the divided veins do exhibit a disposition to bleed, the bleeding ends may be compressed with the thumb and finger for a few minutes, or until the hemorrhage ceases. I can assure the most timid that there is no danger of exhausting hemorrhage.

"After the operation is performed, and the hemorrhage, if there be any, has ceased, the edges of the wound are to be laid together, and a wet compress applied. If Chloroform has been used, as it may be with irritable and apprehensive patients, the reaction from its effects may start afresh a hemorrhage which has been checked, therefore the surgeon is not to leave his patient too soon, lest he be re-called to arrest what the patient and attendants may consider a dangerous bleeding.

"The patient should keep the recumbent posture for three or four days, when, if everything be favorable, he may be dressed and take moderate exercise. Of course, the scrotum should be supported by some kind of a suspensory apparatus, when the patient assumes the upright attitude. The wound will suppurate moderately, and heal by granulation. No sutures being used, the traumatic condition is rather simple; and the wound being open there is little danger of pus burrowing in the scrotum. After the healing process is complete, a suspensory netting should be worn to afford comfort, and to prevent, as far as may be, the dilatation of other veins. It is not to be supposed that all the veins in the spermatic cord become varicose, therefore when one set is obliterated or occluded, enough are left to convey the blood, and even to reproduce the original difficulty. Occasionally a patient *radically cured*, may, some years after, need a second operation.

"I have operated four times in the manner described, each case proving a satisfactory success, and no untoward circumstance interfered with the healing process. In the rare cases of varicocele needing an operation, I feel like commending the plan described. The operation is easily performed, and there is no danger of seriously disturbing vessels or structures proximate to the varicose veins. The excision obliterates the dilated vessels as circulating media, and does not interfere with the functions of the testicle or spermatic cord. The wound is too unimportant to admit of dangerous complications; and is attended with less pain and shock, than other operative procedures designed to accomplish the same result. An anodyne may be needed the first night to ensure rest, but, after a day or two, the patient considers the operation an insignificant affair."

HYDROCELE.

560. The *tunica vaginalis* is arranged like all serous membranes lining cavities, having a visceral layer investing the testes, and a reflected layer lining the scrotum, and secretes sufficient moisture for the lubrication of these surfaces. Like other serous membranes, it may be so changed by disease that it will secrete considerable quantities of fluid, and dropsy results. The more common causes are such as cause irritation and subsequent enfeeblement of the serous membranes. The fluid is generally of a specific gravity of 1010 to 1020, but sometimes becomes quite thick and contains considerable flocculent material, or may even be purulent.

561. The swelling commences in the lower portion of the scrotum, and as the fluid increases gradually extends up to the abdominal ring, pressure does not produce pain, except it is brought to bear upon the testicle, and then there is pain with a sense of faintness. The tumor is pyriform in shape, and gives the sensation of a bladder filled with water, with sometimes distinct, sometimes obscure fluctuation. If there is doubt in the diagnosis, the room may be darkened, and a light placed behind the scrotum will show a degree of translucence and determine its character.

562. TREATMENT.—In the early stage of the disease we may sometimes effect a radical cure without an operation, but when of considerable duration we would not attempt it. Keep the patient's bowels moderately open with a saline cathartic and Sulphur, and apply a compress, wetted with a solution of Hydrochlorate of Ammonia, or Pond's Extract of Hamamelis. A fine elastic suspensory bandage is necessary to success. In some cases, firm strapping to the abdomen with adhesive strips, as recommended in orchitis, is an excellent means, and will sometimes effect a cure alone.

563. The operation is a very simple one. The scrotum is punctured with a trocar, and the perforator being withdrawn,

the canula is pushed into the sac and all the fluid drawn off. It is necessary to be careful about this, and the position of the canula will sometimes need changing, and the scrotum pressed in order to remove the last portion of fluid. Now a stimulating injection is thrown into the sac through the canula, in order to set up adhesive inflammation. The injection commonly used is Tincture of Iodine, one part to two, three, or four of Alcohol, bringing it in contact with the entire surface by movements of the scrotum, and pressing out all the free fluid. The canula is now withdrawn, and the scrotum supported by a well adjusted bandage. In old cases, or where the operation has been previously unsuccessful, the scrotum should be firmly strapped to the abdominal wall, as in cases of orchitis.

564. If acute inflammation follows the operation, we would apply a lotion of Aconite, Aconite and Camphor, or Veratrum. Keep the patient quiet in bed, and give the sedatives internally.

565. In the hydrocele of *children*, a cure can almost always be effected without an operation. The local application of the Hamamelis or a solution of Hydrochlorate of Ammonia, proper support, and the internal administration of small doses of Apocynum Canabinum, soon removes the effusion.

HEMATOCELE.

566. Hematocele, or an effusion of blood into the tunica vaginalis, is usually the result of an injury, though sometimes the patient may not be able to account for it. It usually comes up quickly, though the distension may be to the full capacity of the scrotum.

567. Not only does the swelling come up quickly, but then it has more solidity, no fluctuation, or very obscure, is dark

in color, and not translucent. The history of the case, and the fact of an injury, aid the diagnosis.

568. TREATMENT.—The object of treatment is to prevent inflammation, and promote absorption. Following an injury the part should be dressed with a lotion of: ℞ Tincture of Aconite, ʒss.; Tincture of Camphor, ℥j.; Water, Oj.; until all excitement had passed away. Then with a compress wetted with Pond's Hamamelis. The patient might have small doses of the sedatives, followed by an alkaline diuretic.

569. If inflammation should ensue, and we fail to control it by these means, and suppuration is likely to occur, an incision is made, the blood turned out, and the part healed by granulation.

TUMOR OF THE SCROTUM.

570. Occasionally fibroid tumors are developed within the *tunica vaginalis*, and may attain considerable size. They are annoying from their weight, and especially when they press upon the testicle, sometimes give rise to severe suffering. Usually the diagnosis is easy. The fingers can trace the spermatic cord and testicle, and separate them from the enlargement; the tumor may be above or below the testicle, growing from the scrotum, or may be attached to and grow from the testes, though this is rare.

571. If the growth is annoying, the operation for its removal is quite simple. Make an incision into the tunica vaginalis of sufficient size to remove the growth. Separate it with the finger nail from its attachment, and close the part with silver ligatures. Keep the patient quiet for a few days, using the sedative lotion named above.

572. Occasionally we meet with *sebaceous* tumors of the scrotum, evidently arising from disease of one or more of the

sebaceous glands. Sometimes it attains considerable size, is painful, and has been mistaken for malignant disease.

573. Most usually, when it possesses the character of a growth, it can be readily turned out with the finger after a first incision is made with the knife. But when it is associated with hypertrophy of the skin, it is the safest method to apply the Chloride of Zinc paste, establish free suppuration until the growth is removed, and then dress with some simple ointment.

EPITHELIOMA OF SCROTUM.

574. In the olden time, chimney-sweepers or "soot-cancers" of the scrotum, were among the most common of the epithelioma. There was probably nothing in the soot, further than as it and the occupation caused irritation of the scrotum, and consequent depraved nutrition. But outside of this cause I am inclined to believe that the scrotum is a favorite seat of epithelial cancer, and it will probably be met with here more frequently than in any other situation, the face excepted.

575. Paget thus describes the growth: "Among the examples of the superficial epithelial cancer, the greater part derive a peculiar character from the share which the papillæ of the skin or mucous membrane take in the disease. These being enlarged, and variously deformed and clustered, give a condylomatous appearance to the morbid structures, which has led to their being called papillary or warty cancers, and which renders it sometimes difficult to distinguish them from common warty growths. According to the changes in the papillæ, numerous varieties of external appearance may be presented; I shall here describe only the chief of them.

"In the most ordinary examples of epithelial cancer of the lower lip, or of a labium, or of the scrotum in the soot-cancers, if they be examined previous to ulceration, one can feel an outspread swelling, and an unnatural firmness or hardness of the affected skin. The width and length of the swelling are much greater than its thickness. The diseased part is enlarged; the lip, for example, pouts, and projects like one overgrown; and the swelling is slightly elevated, rising gradually or abruptly from its borders, and having a round or oval or sinuous outline. Its surface, previous to ulceration, may be nearly smooth, but more often is coarsely granulated, or tuberculated, or lowly warty, like the surface of a syphilitic condyloma, deriving this character usually from the enlarged and closely clustered papillæ. The surface is generally moist with ichorous discharge, or covered with a scab, or with a soft material formed of detached epidermal scales. The firmness or hardness of the diseased part is various in degree in different instances: it is very seldom extreme; the part, however firm, is usually flexible and pliant, and feels moderately tense and resilient on pressure. Commonly, it is morbidly sensitive, and the seat of increased afflux of blood. Its extent is, of course, various; but, before ulceration, the disease makes more progress in length and breadth than in depth; so that when, for example, it occupies the whole border of a lip or of a labium, it may not exceed the third of an inch in thickness.

"In the form of epithelial cancer just described there may be no considerable enlargement of papillæ, or it may only appear when the growth is cut through. But, in many instances (especially, I think, in the epithelial cancers of the prepuce, glands, and integuments of the extremities), the changes of the papillæ are much more evident. In some, as in the adjacent sketch, one sees a great extent of surface covered with crowds and clusters of enlarged papillæ set on a level or slightly elevated portion of the cutis. Singly (when the ichor and loose scales that fill their intervals are washed away), they appear cylindriform, flask-shaped, pyriform, or conical; clustered, they make nodulated and narrow-stemmed masses. They may be in one or in many groups; or groups of them may be scattered around some large central ulcer. They appear very vascular, and their surface, thinly covered with opaque-white cuticle, has a pink, or vermilion, or brightly florid hue.

"In other instances, or in other parts, a large mass is formed, the surface of which, when exposed by washing away the loose epidermoid cells which fill up its inequalities, is largely granulated or tuberculated, and is planned out into lobes by deeper clefts. Such growths are upraised, cauliflower-like; and, with this likeness, may be broken through the clefts, into narrow-stemmed masses, formed each of one or more close-packed groups of enlarged, tuberous, and clavate papillæ. The surface of such a growth shows, usually, its full vascularity; for if it be washed, it appears bare, and, like the surface of common granulations, has no covering layer of cuticle. It may be florid, bleeding on slight contact, but, more often, it presents a dull or rusty vermilion tint, rather than the brighter crimson or pink of common granulations, or of such warts as one commonly sees on the prepuce or glans penis.

"Occasionally, we meet with an epithelial cancer having the shape of a sharply bordered circular or oval disk, upraised from one to three lines above the level of the adjacent skin or mucous membrane, and imbedded in about the same depth below it. The surfaces of such disk-shaped cancers are usually flat, or slightly concave, granulated, spongy, or irregularly cleft; their margins are bordered by the healthy integuments, raised and often slightly everted by their growth. Such shapes are not unfrequent among the epithelial cancers of the tongue, of the lining of the prepuce, and of the scrotum. I removed such a one also from the perineum, and have seen one in the vagina."

576. It may maintain these appearances for months, before involving deep seated tissues, and during this time the patient suffers only from a superficial burning pain, which only be-

comes very troublesome when the part is irritated. But after a time the skin and cellular tissue are markedly thickened, and nodules of cacoplastic material are deposited. The ulceration becomes deeper by the softening and breaking down of this, and finally we have complete destruction of the skin and an extension of the disease to the testes, perineum, or penis, and the patient presents very much the symptoms of open scirrhus.

577. TREATMENT.—Whilst we do not profess to cure cancer in general, at least after the lymphatic glands are involved, this variety is usually amenable to treatment. In some cases, the epithelial disease is scarcely malignant, and though the ulceration is corroding, and destroys tissue after tissue, it does not cause constitutional infection.

578. In these less severe cases, the progress of the disease may be sometimes arrested by the use of Carbolic Acid dissolved in Glycerine, (℥j. to ℥iv.); or by a dressing of Tilden's "Bromo-Chloralum," or by the use of a strong Tincture of Iodine.

579. But in the majority I would prefer to use the Arsenical paste, prepared as follows: Take of the Hydrated Sesquioxide of Iron a sufficient quantity, throw it on a filter to drain off the water, until it has the consistence of a paste; add to this one part of Lard to three or four parts of Iron, thoroughly mix. In this we have the basis of the ointment, and to it we add Arsenious Acid in the proportion of ʒj. to ℥iv. to ℥iv.; usually the weaker preparation gives the best results, though it requires more time. It is spread on soft cotton cloth, and applied once or twice daily, until the malignant character of the disease is removed, and the tissues seem soft and healthy, when we use the simple Iron dressing until the parts are healed.

580. In some cases the Chloride of Zinc will be the preferable remedy, as in other forms of cancer. If deemed best, it will be used in the usual manner.

PEDICULUS PUBIS.

581. The capilli or hair covering the external organs, occasionally suffers from disease, but it is rarely of much moment. It is, however, the habitat of a parasite, the *pediculus pubis*, which is occasionally a source of great annoyance, and sometimes of quite severe disease.

582. A patient complains of persistent pruritus of the parts covered by hair, that is not relieved by scratching. It has been a source of uneasiness for some time, but they have not yet determined the cause; in such cases an inspection will frequently detect the louse. Remaining for some time, they spread to other parts of the body where there are short hairs: about the anus, the hair of breast, abdomen and axillæ, the hair of the neck, the eyebrows, etc. In some cases they give rise to severe irritation of the skin, which, increased by scratching, causes ulceration. In the female they sometimes cause severe leucorrhœa.

583. This louse will be recognized by its brownish color, and its close adherence to the skin and the hairs with its fore legs. "It has a shield shape and a much broader body in proportion to its size than either of the other forms of lice; and there does not appear to be any distinct separation between its thorax and abdomen. It does not run about like other lice, but grasps the stems of the hairs with its fore legs, and adheres so firmly that it is difficult to remove it without pulling out the hair. The *nits* or egg-capsules are attached to the hairs in the same way as on the head. Pruriginous or eczematous eruptions, which may become pustular, are the results of their existence," (Anderson.)

584. They are propagated by contact, like other lice, and though frequently *in veneris*, yet quite as commonly from male to male by sleeping in the same bed. A husband may catch them innocently by occupying a strange bed, and transmit them to the wife, and both may suffer long and severely

before they know what is the matter, and if the wife choose to be jealous, she may have grave suspicions of her husband on finding out the character of the disease, but which will be dissipated by the explanation of the physician.

585. TREATMENT.—It has been proposed to destroy these parasites with Sulphur, infusion of Tobacco, Staphysagria, and Mercury. As a general rule the Sulphur Ointment will be found insufficient as well as filthy. A solution of Potassæ Sulphuretum has been recommended, but it is not very certain. The strong decoction of Tobacco is both unpleasant and uncertain. Staphysagria is more likely to irritate the skin than kill the lice, and to the common Mercurial Ointment we have the objection that it is sometimes absorbed and causes salivation. When Mercurial Ointments are used, it is generally the "*red* or *white* precipitate."

586. I prefer Prof. King's treatment—a thorough application of a good *Cologne;* two or three applications are usually sufficient to destroy the pests. Should it fail, and Mercury become a necessity, the solution of the Bichloride, three or four grains to the ounce of water and Alcohol, will be found decidedly the best. The application should be especially to the hair, and very thorough, once or twice a day for a week, reaching every part affected.

VENEREAL DISEASES.

587. As a result of venereal excesses men suffer from certain infectious diseases of the reproductive organs. They are propagated by contact of the virus with a mucous or sometimes cutaneous surface, and so far as we know, at the present time, are never produced *de nova*. As we have already seen in the brief discussion of prostitution, the origin of these diseases dates back to very early periods in man's history, as we have evidence of it in the earliest preserved writings. How the diseases were originated we know not, but have reason to believe that they were the result of intense animalism in the early periods of the race.

588. We have already noticed the fact that there are epidemic cycles, in which contagious diseases are greatly intensified, as there are periods when the contagious virus loses a portion of its virulence. This we find to be the case in all diseases produced by a specific contagion, as has been noticed and described in such common affections as variola, rubeola, and scarlatina. We do not know what peculiar conditions intensify these diseases at regular intervals of some years, but the fact is well established.

589. This is also true of the venereal virus, and one need but to read its history to be satisfied of this. It will account for the sudden outbreak and spread of the venereal at certain periods, as at the siege of Naples, as it will also account to some extent for the discrepancies between authors.

590. This variation of the disease in epidemic cycles is not only in its intensity, but also to some extent in its character, and will account for the differences in treatment. I am quite

sure that these, like other affections, do not present such uniform lesions, that a stereotyped treatment can be successfully employed in all cases. Even the diseases of a single year will show a diversity of pathological peculiarities, and demand skilled diagnosis and therapeutics.

591. It is hardly worth while at this day to discuss the *unity*, *duality*, or *triality* of the venereal poison, and adduce the arguments *pro* and *con*, for the best observers have determined that there are three distinct venereal diseases—*gonorrhœa*, *chancroid* and *syphilis*. This view agrees with all we have seen of the disease, and is the only one that will explain its phenomena, and offers a classification that will be intelligible to the student.

592. Each of these has its peculiar virus, is propagated by direct contact, and produces its own specific poison. The gonorrhœal virus always produces gonorrhœa, and never chancre or chancroid; chancroid produces chancroid and never gonorrhœa or true chancre; and true chancre reproduces itself, and never either of the other diseases.

593. It is true, as already noticed, that a person, the woman especially, may have two, or even three of these diseases, at the one time, and that free connection may inoculate one with chancre, another with chancroid, and a third with syphilis. These cases are rare, but they have been relied upon to prove the unity of the venereal poison. As a general rule the three diseases are distinct, and their history very clear.

594. We will find that whilst this is a true classification, there are cases in which our diagnosis may be at fault. We can not always tell from the appearance of the local disease whether we have chancre or chancroid, and we are obliged to make the diagnosis by the appearance, or non-appearance of constitutional symptoms. Just as in some cases we can not distinguish between a specific urethritis—gonorrhœa, and a simple inflammation of the urethra. So there are cases of concealed chancre—of the urethra for instance, which, causing

a free muco-purulent secretion, simulates gonorrhœa. Or a concealed true chancre, with outer chancroid, and secondary symptoms result, though the physician has only the evidence of the disease which produces no constitutional infection.

595. Here as elsewhere we must learn not to give credence to exceptional phenomena, at least not to form theories from isolated cases. The habit of superficial observation is so ingrained in the majority of physicians, that the wonder is not that they make mistakes in diagnosis, but that they are not more frequent. Theories are very frequently formed from the superficial observation of a few cases, possibly from a single one, and then all facts are bent to its support.

596. These three specific contagions are very much alike in their origin and propagation. They are each produced in the course of the disease in the form of a specific pus, that does not materially differ from ordinary pus formation, whether we examine it chemically or under the microscope. They are each propagated by contact—the specific virus, whatever it may be, possessing the power to change the life of the tissues, and produce the characteristic local disease. If we wanted a theory to account for this, we could probably find it in Beale's bioplasm, the secretion of thediseased surface or ulcer containing a peculiarly diseased material of this character, possessing the power of reproducing itself in a protoplasm.

597. In diseases produced by contact with a contagious material, the only absolute safety is in avoidance of the danger; in the case of the venereal it is, "touch not." These contagions may be and are found outside of prostitution, but outside of prostitution there is very little danger. It is illicit intercourse with unknown persons that usually transmits the disease, for even the confirmed prostitute will be careful not to endanger her personal friends, if she is aware of the disease. I am sorry to say that the male prostitute has not so much honor, and will sometimes out of pure maliciousness disease those with whom he has been friendly. The woman,

as a rule, degraded though she may be by these associations, is far more honorable than the man.

598. When one risks infection by intercourse with persons known to live such lives that they may contract these diseases, they take a well known risk, for which there is no protection except cleanliness. Some men might and do have intercourse with diseased women and not be infected. It may depend upon a well developed epithelial tissue, the immunity being natural, or upon thorough washing with soap and water immediately after the act. The public woman always protects herself by free ablution, especially of the external genitals, which are more likely to suffer than the internal organs.

599. In this description of the venereal virus, we have only studied the propagation of the primary or local disease. True syphilis, as we will see hereafter, may be produced in other ways. Very certainly certain forms of secondary syphilis may be inoculated. The lesion is hereditary to a certain extent, and both mother and child may be diseased from the male germ, the one from its inception, the other through the placental circulation.

600. It might be asked how one suffering from these local diseases could be induced to have sexual intercourse? Looking at the fully developed disease, we would think a man or woman suffering from gonorrhœa, chancroid or chancre, would find it a source of discomfort and pain rather than pleasure. So they may from the fully developed disease as frequently seen, but we find it in an obscure form in a large number of cases, and its only influence may be to increase sexual excitement. One thing is very certain, that the infectious material is produced in all these before there is much local disturbance, and a slight secretion may retain its infectious character when the patient seems to have recovered. A man will frequently disease his wife with gonorrhœa before he has felt the first symptom of urethral irritation, or feel it first or immediately after such intercourse. He may transmit a soft chancre from a sore not noticed, or that seems little

more than an erosion; and true syphilis from the secretion of the diseased membrane before the chancre has formed. In woman, these unconscious sources of disease are far more common, for it may lurk in her genitalia, without producing sensible irritation, the secretion being but little if any changed. She may convey the contagion in this way for months, without being aware that there is anything wrong.

601. As a rule, when a person has venereal disease, we may conclude that they have contracted it in the *natural* way. Modest persons are frequently very much surprised when they learn the character of the disease, and feel inclined to blame water-closets or privy-seats. It is all well enough, and makes no difference in the therapeutics, and we have charity in such cases.

GONORRHŒA.

602. As we have already seen, gonorrhœa is a specific inflammation of mucous membranes, produced by contact with gonorrhœal virus. Whilst confined to the urethra in the male, and the external and internal organs of generation in the female, in the majority of instances, it may affect any mucous surface in the body. Whilst the disease is caused by contact with gonorrhœal virus, in its progress it reproduces the same, which may serve as a center for further infection.

603. As regards the gonorrhœal virus itself we know but little, further than it is a muco-pus, produced during the gonorrhœal inflammation. In its physical properties, it does not differ materially from the products of simple inflammation, further than it is usually in large quantity.

604. As the disease is dependent upon a specific virus, contact with this is essential to its production. This usually occurs during sexual congress with a person diseased; and we may take it for granted, in a large majority of cases, that the

disease is thus contracted. Of course there are exceptions: in one out of a thousand cases a man may contract a gonorrhœa from sitting on a privy-seat used by a person having the disease, sleeping in a bed occupied by such person, or occasionally by using clothing, cloths, towels, etc., contaminated by the virus. The eyes are diseased by carrying the virus to them with the hands or cloths. The nose in the same manner, the rectum by want of cleanliness, and the bladder by a gradual extension of the inflammation from the urethra.

605. A period of *incubation*, of longer or shorter duration, ensues after exposure. The closest observers claim that this is from thirty-four hours to three days; but we find many patients who contend that a week, ten days, or even two or three weeks have elapsed before they experienced any symptoms. While I am of the opinion that the disease manifests itself before the fourth day, in a majority of cases, I must still believe there are cases in which the virus remains dormant for a considerable time.

606. Sexual intercourse with one suffering from gonorrhœa is said to produce peculiar sensations, by which danger may be suspected. Among these is a sense of pungent heat and burning, sometimes associated with an intense erotic excitement. These sensations are somewhat persistent, and the organs may not lose them until the disease is fully announced.

607. In the male, the first symptoms of gonorrhœa are—a feeling of pricking and itching in the urethra and at the meatus, which soon becomes so intense as to be very unpleasant; the patient, also, feels a sensation of fullness, and as if there was something foreign there, and a desire to urinate and evacuate it. By the end of the second day these symptoms have become real pain, the urethra is dry, with frequent desire to urinate, and a scalding sensation when the urine passes the urethra. The discharge now commences having a milky-white appearance.

608. By the fourth or fifth day the disease is fully developed. The desire to urinate is very frequent, with sharp,

pricking pains previous to the passage of water, and scalding while it is passing. The pain is usually more severe after the bladder is emptied, and toward the last the urine passes in drops with much tenesmus. There is a constant sensation of fullness, tension, and soreness, which is very unpleasant. The discharge has now become free, and is a yellowish, somewhat creamy muco-pus, its fluidity varying in different cases; sometimes it possesses a peculiar unpleasant odor.

609. If the penis is now examined the meatus will be found red, slightly everted or pouting, and on separating it the mucous membrane will be observed red and swollen. The part of the urethra diseased is swollen and hard, and pressure produces pain. In a majority of cases the disease is located, at first, about an inch and a half from the meatus, where there are numerous large lacunæ, but as time passes it gradually extends to other portions.

610. Painful erection, or chordee, makes its appearance now in many cases. These erections occur when the patient gets warm in bed—sometimes several times in a night—and prove a source of very great annoyance. In consequence of the inflammation, complete distension of the corpus spongiosum is impossible, or the urethra fails to attain the length necessary in erection, hence the downward curvature of the penis, the pain being consequent upon traction upon the inflamed structure.

611. When the case is left to itself the discharge usually increases for a week or ten days, remains stationary for the same length of time, and then decreases until nothing remains but a slight gleet. During the first period the suffering is greatest, but the pain and scalding in passing water, gradually diminish during the second, and at last become so mitigated as to give but little trouble.

612. In some cases the prepuce becomes much swollen from serous exudation, and phymosis is the result. These are usually troublesome cases, and sometimes complicated with balanitis, or posthitis.

613. Though from the symptoms enumerated we might suppose there would be little difficulty in diagnosis, and in a majority of cases a simple inspection of the penis tells the story, there are cases which require a very careful examination, and even then we are sometimes left in the dark. I have already described simple urethritis, having no relation to the gonorrhœal virus, as a disease so similar that the best observers might be mistaken. Numerous cases are on record in which the husband was informed by the surgeon that he had gonorrhœa, and he well knowing that he could have contracted it from but one source accused his wife of unchastity. But an examination of the wife revealed no disease. These facts should cause us to be very careful in giving an opinion, when there is any doubt.

614. Chancre of the urethra sometimes simulates a gonorrhœa in all its symptoms, though there is not usually near so great a discharge. I have, myself, been deceived in this case, though I use much care in examination. One case came to my notice in which the patient was said to have an intractable gonorrhœa, having lasted for months; careful examination detected an indurated chancre about half an inch within the meatus.

615. TREATMENT.—Persons suffering from gonorrhœa are extremely anxious for a speedy cure, and with very good reason, for the disease is not only painful but extremely filthy, and thus annoying to a person accustomed to cleanliness. In many cases the mental suffering is more intense than the bodily, and the chagrin and loss of self-respect is sometimes sufficient to impair the general health. Some persons, of course, get used to it, and some are so constituted as to bear it stoically as a boy would a whipping, but in all the first question is, as to a speedy cure.

616. Speedy cures do not come from internal remedies, and in the *abortive* plan that we are about to study the treatment is often wholly local. It is a mooted question whether

the risk in the abortive treatment does not more than balance the prospect of speedy cure, and this will require consideration in each individual case, and the answer will depend somewhat upon the peculiarities of the patient, and the character of the disease.

617. It is well to understand that the disease is self-limited, and will run its course in a majority of cases in from three to six weeks. Still there are some in which the gonorrhœal virus is reproduced for a long period, though the local symptoms are but slight. This is the case even where the disease is treated with the ordinary remedies.*

---

*For the satisfaction of the reader, I append my treatment, as found in Hill's Surgery: "The treatment of gonorrhœa is almost entirely empirical, and hence we have an abundance of means recommended, and such marked difference in its management by different practitioners. It might properly be divided into two parts, the *abortive* and *symptomatic;* in the first remedies being used for the immediate arrest of the disease, and in the second the symptoms met as they arise.

"In the first stage of gonorrhœa, the disease being still confined to the fossa navicularis, the inflammation not being too acute, the abortive plan may be employed with success. This consists in substituting a common inflammation for the specific one, by the use of caustic injections. I might premise the description of the means employed by saying that in order to prove successful, the injection should come in contact with the entire surface affected, for if but the smallest portion escapes, the gonorrhœa again extends.

"The injections employed should be used by the physician in most cases, the syringe working accurately, a rubber one being the best. Have the patient place his finger upon the urethra above the disease, then insert the pipe of the syringe well up, pressing the glans with the fingers to prevent the escape of the fluid, and completely fill the urethra. The injection should be used soon after urinating, and retained for from two to five minutes. After using it, the penis may be held in a vessel of water as hot as can be borne, which relieves the pain to a very considerable extent.

"Nitrate of Silver has been most extensively employed as an abortive, and when used with the precautions above named, rarely produces any unpleasant consequences. The strength of the solution used varies in different cases, from fifteen to forty grains of the crystallized nitrate to the ounce of water, being the usual quantity. I have employed it of a strength of from twenty to thirty grains. It is sometimes necessary to repeat the injection the ensuing

15

618. LOCAL TREATMENT. — Cleanliness is essential in all plans of treatment, not only for the patient's comfort, but to facilitate the cure. Frequent penis baths of cold water, the parts being thoroughly cleansed, give very marked relief. In some cases the warm bath is preferable, and we have it used frequently, and for twenty or thirty minutes at a time.

619. Three objects may be had in view for local treatment. The first looks to the speedy destruction of the gonorrhœal virus, and the production of a simple acute urethritis to replace the specific inflammation. The second looks to the destruction of the specific character of the virus, without causing inflammation. Whilst the third looks simply to the topical action of remedies opposing the inflammatory process.

620. In the first, Nitrate of Silver, Nitric Acid, Sulphate of Zinc, Carbolic Acid, Chloride of Zinc, and Permanganate

---

day, but usually one is sufficient. Sulphate of Zinc is an excellent remedy, and I have used it in the following proportion: R. Sulphate of Zinc, ten to fifteen grains; Sulphate of Morphia, three grains; Water, one ounce. M. It does not produce as much pain as the Nitrate of Silver, or cause such intense inflammation. Chloride of Zinc has been employed by some in the proportion of three to five grains to the ounce of water, with Morphine. Tincture of Iodine, Tincture of Muriate of Iron, Solution of Persulphate of Iron, have been used for the same purpose, but with what success I am unable to say. In using the injection of Sulphate of Zinc, it is frequently employed of twice the strength named, and then diluted each day until the disease is arrested.

"In a few hours after using the injection, the discharge becomes free; by the end of the first day it commences to diminish, and soon ceases. I usually give a brisk cathartic at the time, and direct the use of some simple diuretic infusion, as Althæa, with small doses of Tincture of Gelseminum.

"Sometimes an intense inflammation follows the use of these injections, and after the use of Nitrate of Silver more or less blood is passed. This should be combated by frequent use of the hot water, the bowels kept open, mucilaginous diuretics, and the special sedatives and Gelseminum. If not successful, the gonorrhœal discharge reappears in three or four days. The objections urged to the treatment is the occasional production of stricture, and rarely a chronic contracted condition of the corpus spongiosum. These objections have been considered so grave by some surgeons that they discountenance the abortive treatment."

of Potash are in most common use. This plan may properly be called the *abortive*.

621. It may be employed in any case before acute inflammation has been set up, when the inflammation runs high, but there is but little contraction of the urethra, and after the acuteness of the inflammation has subsided. It should *not* be used when the gonorrhœa has extended back to the membranous or prostatic portion; when the stream of urine is small, and its passage is accompanied by lacerative or tearing pains; or when there is severe and painful chordee. In such cases as these, even the careful use may cause stricture.

622. A solution of Nitrate of Silver, grs. x. to grs. xx., to the ounce of water, was the abortive in the olden time. If used, the strong solution is preferable, for the object should be accomplished with a single injection. A good, well-fitted syringe is necessary, and the physician should apply it himself in most cases. Let the urethra be well washed out with an injection of a weak solution of common salt, and then, having the patient hold his finger firmly upon the urethra about midway, fill the anterior portion with the injection, retaining it as long as possible, (which will not be very long.) Have the patient go home and lie down, using a warm penis bath frequently, and take internally Veratrum in usual doses, and a solution of Acetate of Potash with an abundance of diluents. The pain following this injection is most intense for some minutes, and the parts feel very unpleasant for some hours. The tendency to micturition should be restrained, using the hot penis or sitz bath when the desire becomes strong. Usually first micturition is very painful, and not unfrequently attended with slight hemorrhage, but in twenty-four hours the parts are quite comfortable.

623. A very great deal depends upon how the injection is used, whatever remedy is employed, the first washing of the urethra to fully expose the diseased surface for the action of the remedy, and not less the thorough filling of the canal, bringing the injection in contact with every portion of it, and

especially with the lacunæ, which are the favorite seat of the disease. The directions are—catch the head of the penis between the finger and the thumb, so that the meatus can be compressed upon the nozzle of the syringe, which is *gently* introduced to avoid irritation and tenesmus. The syringe should never be introduced more than one-half inch, if the ordinary instrument is employed—just so that the fingers can hold the meatus well to it. In some cases the long-tube Acton syringe is preferable, carrying it back beyond the seat of the disease and gradually discharging its contents as withdrawn.

624. Nitric Acid is used in the proportion of gtts. x. to gtts. xl., to Water ℥j.; and the same precautions are observed. Probably the stronger injection is preferable, as in the case of Nitrate of Silver.

625. Sulphate of Zinc is the favorite injection of many physicians who treat large numbers of these cases. The proportion is usually: ℞ Sulphate of Zinc, grs. x.; Sulphate of Morphia, grs. iij.; Water, ℥j. The canal of the urethra may be freed by a first injection of this, which is allowed to escape at once, and then a second injection is thrown in to distend the canal, and is retained for three to five minutes. In some cases it is best to repeat it once or twice the same day, and rarely the second day, after which it is diluted with from four to nine parts of water, and used on until the disease is entirely removed.

The Sulphate of Zinc does not produce the severe pain of the preceding injections, nor the acute inflammation which was so likely to follow them, and is not near so likely to cause stricture—indeed some claim that stricture never follows its judicious use.

626. Chloride of Zinc is preferred by some to the Sulphate, being thought to exert a more direct influence in destroying the specific character of the secretion. If it was as manageable it would be the preferable agent. But whilst some can bear an injection of grs. x. to the ounce, others will suffer acutely from grs. iij. to the ounce: the latter strength is the

one I should recommend. The Dublin solution of Chloride of Zinc was employed in the Irish metropolis, and a similar, but stronger solution by French surgeons, though it had no advantage over the solution prepared from the crystals.

627. Permanganate of Potash has not been employed as much as either of those named, excepting Nitric Acid, yet it will be found an excellent remedy in some cases. To obtain the action we are studying I would recommend a solution of the strength of grs. v. to the ounce of water, employing it in the same way as the Sulphate of Zinc until the specific character of the disease was destroyed.

628. In using these stronger injections for the abortion of the disease, we must insist on comparative, or sometimes absolute rest for twenty-four or forty-eight hours, and be ready to apply means to relieve the inflammatory action if it runs high. It is always safe, and I think advantageous to prescribe the following sedative: ℞ Tincture of Veratrum, gtts. x. to gtts. xx.; Tincture of Gelseminum, ʒj.; Water, ℥iv.; a teaspoonful every one or two hours. If the urethra becomes very much swollen and painful, pencil it on the outside with the Tincture of Veratrum and Aconite. If the urine becomes scant and irritant, the free use of diluents with a small portion of Spirits of Nitre, or some mild vegetable diuretic, will be found advantageous.

629. The second use of local remedies looks to the destruction of the specific virus, without inducing inflammation. It is doubtful whether this can be done, at least whether it can be done quickly, and yet the treatment in some cases is very successful. The same remedies are employed, but of very much less strength.

630. Probably Chloride of Zinc in the proportion of grs. ij. to Water, ℥iij.; used every four to six hours, would hold the first place in this list. Dr. Lloyd of London employed it and gave it a very strong recommendation. I have used it with advantage. In this strength the burning is not unpleasant, and is usually followed by very decided relief.

631. Permanganate of Potash, gr. j. to grs. ij. to Water, ℥j. would probably take the next place, and will sometimes be found an excellent remedy, especially when the characteristic fetor is strong. This is the only class of cases in which I would recommend it, as in others it sometimes proves very irritating, and increases the discharge.

632. Carbolic Acid, grs. v. to Water, ℥ij., has been employed with advantage. It is better to use the officinal solution in Glycerine, the strength being the same. Probably in the larger number of cases the addition of Tannic Acid improves the injection, and our prescription would read: ℞ So-Solution of Carbolic Acid, gtts. xx.; Tannic Acid, grs. v.; Water, ℥ij.

Mr. Ashmead's formula for a Carbolic Acid injection was: ℞ Carbolic Acid, grs. viij.: Tannic Acid, grs. viij.; Glycerine, ℥ss; Water to ℥j.

633. In some rare cases Chlorate of Potash, grs. x. to Water, ℥iv., will be found the best injection. In these the discharge is very free—a greenish, muco-pus, having a peculiar cadaveric odor. It is not only used freely as an injection, but the parts are thoroughly washed with it, and the cloths kept wetted.

634. Solution of Chlorinated Soda, diluted with ten to twenty parts of water, may be used in similar cases to the above. It is a powerful disinfectant, and will remove the unpleasant odor in a few hours. Probably it will be found most useful where the secretion is very profuse, and the parts enfeebled.

635. Baptisia in infusion (strained), affords an excellent injection where the parts are full and tumid, with dark, purplish discoloration, the discharge being abundant, dark, and fetid. It should be given internally, as well as used locally.

636. In the third use of local remedies, the object is to relieve the local inflammatory action, without reference to the specific character of the disease. The treatment could hardly

be termed *abortive*, though it is sometimes relied upon to the exclusion of internal remedies.

637. Cold water (iced) may occupy the first place in this list, and it has been claimed that it would be found preferable to any other, even as an abortive. I have employed it in but one case, and the result was not satisfactory. Iced water was ordered as an injection, to be used four times a day, and retained each time for five minutes. The symptoms were quite acute, but the inflammatory action had entirely passed away by the morning of the fourth day, and the discharge was but slight, of a thin glairy mucus, not gonorrhœal. But the patient did not get well of this, and suffered for months from the gleet, and probably may suffer for years. But the case was not well selected, the young man being spare, anæmic, and of relaxed tissue; it would be better adapted to the full blooded, with sthenic inflammation.

638. Cold applications externally are a very common means, and will sometimes give marked relief. The water may be used in the form of a penis bath, or wet dressings may be applied, especially at night. But as we have already seen, hot applications are to be preferred in other cases, and I have no doubt that warm water injectious will sometimes be found preferable to those which are medicated.

639. Glycerine, one part, Rose Water, three to five parts, sometimes forms a pleasant injection, and gives marked relief.

640. Sulphate of Zinc, grs. v.; Acetate of Lead, grs. v.; Water, ℥iv.; is a very common injection, and was a favorite of Ricord. In some cases the strength may be decreased with advantage.

641. A solution of Tannin in Claret Wine makes a most excellent injection, and was a favorite remedy of Niemeyer. The solution may be of the strength of ʒss. to ℥vj., and should be repeated two or three times a day.*

---

*The best therapeutic results are to be obtained in a perfectly recent gonorrhœa before the symptoms have become severe, as it then generally can be

642. My preference in ordinary cases, after the acute symptoms have been relieved is: ℞ Sulphate of Hydrastia, grs. iv.; Warm Water, ℥j. Use it two or three times a day, and continue once a day for a week after the discharge is checked.

643. Within the past four years it has been claimed, that the use of remedies in the form of a suppository, would give better results than their use as an injection. The great diffi-

---

cured in a few days. In order that the number of tractable cases of this kind may be increased—for it is only now and then that we see one—we should make all our patients aware that the disease is continually increasing in extent and violence, so that each day of delay only makes it worse. Such opinions, delivered by physicians who have the confidence of that portion of the public among whom gonorrhœa is most common, have marked effect. It is scarcely credible how coolly and with what cynicism these people talk of their debaucheries and their consequences, what an extensive knowledge of the subject is shown by some of the laity, and how much one can learn from them. For instance, in Magdeburg, where the innumerable commercial travelers of the various mercantile houses meet annually at the hotels, report is always made as to whose pox has relapsed, and who remained cured, and what injections have answered the best for gonorrhœa, etc. Only a short time after I had begun to prescribe injections of Tannin in recent claps, where the symptoms were still trifling (and I had been very successful with this treatment), the number of recent gonorrhœas which sought my aid multiplied considerably. I usually ordered three powders, each of which contained half a drachm of Tannin. One of these was to be dissolved in a half pint of red wine, and the solution was to be used as an injection. If the result was unsatisfactory, the two other powders were to be put into the same quantity of wine, and the injection to be continued with this doubly-strong solution. It has repeatedly happened to me that a patient has pulled one of these very powders out of his pocket which I was about to prescribe for him, and which he had obtained from a friend, and has asked whether he might try that first. In order that these injections may be of service, we must give them once or twice ourselves, or let a skilled assistant give them. If we neglect this precaution, it often happens that the liquid does not enter the urethra at all, or perhaps is merely thrown under the prepuce, and flows back past the syringe. Gonorrhœa syringes must be so small that they will not hold more liquid than the urethra is capable of containing. It is then unnecessary to compress the posterior end of the canal. The best plan is to have a supply of suitable syringes at some particular instrument maker's, and to give them some unobjectionable

culty with an injection is to bring it in contact with the diseased surface, and to maintain the contact long enough to be of advantage. This is claimed to be accomplished by the introduction of a suppository, which distending the parts brings the remedy in contact with the entire affected surface, and maintains it for a sufficient length of time.

644. "Dr. Schuster, of Aix-la-Chapelle, describes a method of treating gonorrhœa and gleet, to which he was led by observing the results of a similar plan in uterine catarrh. Tannin, when mixed wiih Glycerine, forms a waxy mass, which soon becomes smooth, hard, and brown, but readily dissolves under a gentle heat. He makes rods, three or four inches long, consisting of Tannic Acid, two parts, powdered Opium, 0.12 part, with a sufficiency of Glycerine. These are soft in Summer, but very brittle in the Winter. The rod, moistened with hot water, is introduced into the urethra, and a piece about an inch and a half long is left in: it melts down and forms a whitish mass with the mucus of the canal. The rod may, after remaining from five to ten minutes, either be removed by the finger, or be expelled by the stream of urine. The remedy is applied twice or thrice daily."

645. In this case, the remedy gives a consistent supposi-

---

name, since many patients, feeling too much embarrassed to ask for a "penis syringe," get an "ear-syringe," or other unsuitable article instead. I have cut short a large number of recent virulent gonorrhœas in two or three days by injection of Tannin. Even where the disease is not quite recent, but where the inflammation is not very violent, I have often used the Tannin, and obtained excellent results, although the cure was less rapid. I have no idea of claiming especial qualities and merits for Tannin; but I have employed this article much more often than Nitrate of Silver, Sulphate of Zinc, Sugar of Lead, and other astringents. I have never had occasion to prescribe the strong solution of Nitrate of Silver (grs. ten to fifteen to one ounce), for its effects can hardly be better than those obtained from Tannin, and since even its introducers admit that it sometimes causes severe and even violent symptoms, such as I have never seen in my treatment. When the inflammation is very severe, it is well to wait for its abatement before resorting to injections. —*Niemeyer's Practice of Medicine.*

tory which may readily be introduced. Other agents can not be used so easily, as the ordinary suppository has not sufficient consistence. Yet with a little care, I think it would be possible to use any agent heretofore named. A very good method is to make the suppository about one-half inch in length, and cutting an ordinary gum catheter, press the suppository upon the open end, and carry it up to the affected part; slight pressure with the finger, as the instrument is withdrawn, retains the suppository.

646. *Internal Remedies.* — Whilst some rely exclusively upon a local treatment, or only prescribe internal medicines to amuse the patient, others rely wholly upon internal remedies for the cure of the disease. The first claim a shorter time for the cure, the latter a more uniform success, less trouble and danger of infecting other parts, and an entire avoidance of the unpleasant sequelæ that sometimes will follow local means. Still a third class employ the two together, adapting them to the particular case in hand.

647. Veratrum and Gelseminum are the remedies for the acute gonorrhœal inflammation. If the passage of urine is free we prescribe the first alone; if there is scanty urine, and difficult passage, the two together. We prescribe them in the usual way: ℞ Tincture of Veratrum, gtts. x.; Tincture of Gelseminum, ʒj.; Water, ℥iv.; a teaspoonful every hour.

648. When the disease is less acute, or its intensity has been modified as above, Cannabis Indica is an excellent remedy, as: ℞ Tincture of Cannabis, gtts. x. to gtts. xx.; Water, ℥iv.; a teaspoonful every two or three hours.

649. Macrotys is the remedy where there is soreness or stiffness of the muscles, or muscular pain. We usually prescribe it with Aconite, especially if the pulse is small: ℞ Tincture of Macrotys, gtts. xxv.; Tincture of Aconite, gtts. v.; Water, ℥iv.; a teaspoonful every hour.

650. If the patient suffers unpleasant dragging pains in the perineum or urethra, I prescribe Staphysagria, ʒss.; Water, ℥iv.; a teaspoonful every three or four hours.

651. With general nervousness, and sense of formication along the urethra, Pulsatilla would be the remedy.

652. If the tongue shows a violet coloration, and the lips of the meatus are full, and show the same color when opened, Nitric Acid, gtts. xx.; Water, Syrup, aa. ℥j.; a teaspoonful every three hours.

653. Copaiba and Cubebs may be used when there is a sense of fullness and weight in the course of the urethra, with abundant yellowish muco-pus. I prefer Copaiba in capsules, and Cubebs in powder. I use Cubebs especially when the disease is prolonged, with a free discharge, the stimulation aiding the local remedies in checking the discharge, and lessening the intumescence of the mucous follicles and lacunæ.

654. We might supplement this by saying, that any remedy, markedly indicated by special symptoms, may be a remedy in gonorrhœa. In some cases we find need of, and marked benefit from a cathartic, a saline being preferable in some cases, the more active vegetable remedies in others. I have treated gonorrhœa with Podophyllin alone, with marked success, and yet I think if the patients had to choose they would prefer the gonorrhœa to the medicine. One case comes to mind, in my early practice, in which the near approach of the marriage day, made a speedy cure a matter of necessity—one grain of Podophyllin and two of Extract of Hyosciamus every four hours, as long as the patient could stand the remedy, effected a cure in forty-eight hours.

655. The urine becomes scanty in all cases, and in proportion as it is scanty it is acrid and irritating to the inflamed mucous membrane. Hence the benefit that follows the free use of diluents, whether of the simpler diuretics, or water. In some cases an abundant use of water with two or three drachms of Acetate of Potash during the day, gives relief.

656. Frequent micturition is a source of great annoyance and suffering, and intensifies the disease. The patient should be requested to make water at as long intervals as possible,

and in many cases will be able to control the desire. If not, and there is much tenesmus we will use an Opium suppository or injection into the rectum, or a hypodermic injection of Morphia.

CHORDEE.

657. The irritation of gonorrhœa not unfrequently causes sexual excitation, and involuntary erection, especially at night. This in consequence of the inflammation of the urethra, is quite painful, as it is impossible for the *corpus spongiosum* to become fully distended, or to take the length of the corpus cavernosum. Many crude theories have been held with regard to this unpleasantness. It has been claimed to result from over-distension of the corpora-cavernosa, they not being antagonized by the spongy body; or by an imperfect distension of the spongy body, owing to the inflammation. The true cause, inflammatory exudation into the structures of the urethra, seems to have been overlooked.

658. As is the intensity of the inflammation so is the severity of the chordee, at least in the majority of cases. Yet we find many times that the inflammation is very acute, and there is certainly much structural change in the urethra, and yet there is not chordee, for the simple reason there are no erections. In some persons the sexual function is very much excited, and erections will occur even in the day time. They will also come on frequently at night, waking the patient out of a sound sleep, with a pain so intense as to cause him to spring up on the floor. In some cases the erection speedily passes off when the patient is aroused, or by a cold application, but in others it persists for a considerable time. I have known cases of chordee so extreme that the patient would cry out in his agony, and the tension on the urethra would be so great as to cause hemorrhage.

659. TREATMENT.—In the olden time when Copaiba and Cubebs were prescribed for every case of gonorrhœa, chordee was a more constant attendant and required special means.

With a carefully selected treatment, as heretofore named, especially the internal remedies, it will give but little trouble. I should say, in any case, if there is severe and persistent chordee, the treatment is wrong—get a right treatment, and you will have the speediest relief from this unpleasant symptom. Since I have been careful in selecting my internal remedies, I have had no trouble from chordee.

660. If it requires means additional to those named, I should advise an injection (per rectum) of Tincture of Lobelia, Tincture of Opium, aa. ʒss.; Starch Water, ℥ss.; at bedtime. If it was still more severe, a hypodermic injection of Morphia will give speedy, and sometimes permanent relief. If we select internal remedies they will be Pulsatilla, Macrotys, or Staphysagria, as specific to the condition; or a pill of Opium and Camphor, aa. gr. j., as a palliative.

PHYMOSIS

661. As already mentioned, the prepuce occasionally becomes infiltrated with serum to such an extent as to produce phymosis. Usually I order a lotion of Acetate of Lead, the usual strength, keeping the parts well cleansed with soap and water. A strong decoction of Hydrastis, adding a small portion of Alum, does well. If it should be very perverse, it is recommended to make several incisions into the prepuce to permit the escape of the fluid.

HEMORRHAGE.

662. Hemorrhage from the urethra occasionally occurs as the result of chordee. Usually but little blood passes, but I have seen copious hemorrhage. Ligation of the penis temporarily arrests the flow; it may also be checked by the application of ice, or injections of ice water. If it persists and is severe, employ an injection of Persulphate of Iron, or of Alum.

ABSCESS.

663. Abscesses occasionally form along the urethra, and if allowed to run their course, sometimes terminate in urinary

abscess and fistula. If symptoms of such inflammation present, the part should be painted with equal parts of Tincture of Iodine and Tincture of Aconite; and if the abscess forms, it should be opened early. Occasionally the lymphatics of the groin become engorged, and inflammation ensues. In this case, the treatment will be that named hereafter for bubo.

UNPLEASANT SENSATIONS.

664. Unpleasant sensations of itching or pricking, or the feeling as if there was a drop of urine in the urethra, sometimes continues for a considerable time after the disease is arrested, causing uneasiness on the part of the patient. I usually order a Tincture of Pulsatilla, ℨj. to Water, ℥iv.; a teaspoonful four times a day. If it is persistent, the occasional passage of a bougie will prove serviceable.

ENURESIS.

665. Occasionally we find a case in which the gonorrhœa is attended with greater or less incontinence of urine. This is a very troublesome complication, as the continued passage of water keeps up a constant irritation. In addition to other treatment, I have obtained marked advantage from the use of Belladonna. I usually order it as follows: ℞ Fl. Extract of Belladonna, gtts. x.; Water, ℥iv.; a teaspoonful every three hours. The Tincture of Ergot may be used for the same purpose, in doses of half a drachm.

ISCHURIA.

666. Retention of urine during gonorrhœa is most usually caused by spasmodic stricture, and is met with most frequently in those who have previously had a diseased urethra. Though not often met with, it is a most troublesome symptom, and requires prompt treatment. It is of but little use to try to pass a catheter in some of these cases, though in others it passes without great difficulty. We will, however, have to depend principally upon medicines. A very good plan of treatment is to have the patient take a hot sitz-bath, and

drink freely of an infusion of Polygonum Punctatum; or Tincture of Gelseminum and Tincture of Lobelia in the usual doses may be given with good results. Or an enema of: ℞ Tincture of Gelseminum, Tincture of Opium, aa. ʒij. may be used. These measures are very effectual, and will not fail once in a hundred times.

667. Suppression of Urine occasionally occurs during gonorrhœa, but is rarely complete. The usual symptoms ensue, at first nervous irritability, then uræmic coma. It is a very grave occurrence, and is caused most frequently by irritating diuretics, though in one case I was called in to see, under the care of a Homœopath, it was the result of the disease. In the treatment of these cases, I have the bowels moved with a brisk purgative, hot applications applied continuously across the loins, and give internally Tinctnre of Gelseminum in the usual doses, Tincture of Veratrum in small doses. In a few hours mild, unirritating diuretics may be employed.

PROSTATITIS.

668. Gonorrhœal prostatitis is not of very frequent occurrence, but when the disease does extend to this gland, the symptoms are frequently severe. The patient complains of a dull, grinding or throbbing pain in the perineum, with sensation of fullness, desire to urinate, but the urine passes slowly and with shooting pain in the part. When the disease is severe the pain is intense, shooting to the anus, the back, and down the thighs, and the passage of water almost occasions spasms. If the part be examined, the prostate will be found swollen and tender on pressure.

669. In the treatment of this complication I would direct four or five leeches to the perineum, or active counter-irritation. For the latter the following will prove an excellent plan: ℞ Chloroform, Alcohol, aa. ʒj.; Benzine, ʒij.; wet a piece of lint in hot water, pour this liquid upon it, and press it firmly to the part. The burning is intense, far greater than would be produced with a hot iron, and of course the coun-

ter-irritation is proportionately efficient. After evacuating the bowels, I employ injections of a warm infusion of Lobelia, sometimes adding Opium or Gelseminum. Internally I prefer small doses of the Tincture of Staphysagria, or of Cannabis Indica, to all other means. In place of these, we would stimulate secretion from the skin, use relaxants and mild, diuretics.

CYSTITIS.

670. Rarely an acute gonorrhœa extends to the bladder but frequently chronic cystitis results. I have witnessed acute gonorrhœal cystitis, the symptoms being those usually described in the books. For symptoms and treatment the reader is referred to page 189.

ORCHITIS.

671. Gonorrhœal inflammation of the testicle, or epididymitis, is one of the most frequent complications of the disease. It does not differ materially from that heretofore described, yet the treatment will bear some relation to the disease of which it is an attendant. It has not yet been settled how the inflammation reaches the testicle. Some contend, that passing to the prostatic portion of the urethra, it makes its way along the mucous lining of the vas deferens. I am satisfied that this may occasionally be the case, as I have in two or three instances observed perineal pain, with tenderness and pain in the course of the spermatic cord, previous to the swelling of the testicle. But I have been just as well satisfied, in other cases, that there was no such extension of the disease, the gonorrhœa being confined to the anterior portion of the penis. In this case the orchitis was the result of abnormal innervation.

672. The symptoms of commencing orchitis are usually well marked. The patient feels a dragging pain in the scrotum and spermatic cord, with a sensation of tension and aching in the testicle. It sometimes enlarges rapidly, attaining the size of a goose-egg in a couple of days, but in other cases the swelling is more gradual. Frequently the pain is

intense, resembling that caused by a blow on the testicle, but at other times it is only when unsupported that it is thus painful, there being a constant dull aching and soreness at other times. The disease runs a very variable course, sometimes continuing for four or five weeks, if allowed to have its way, and occasionally terminating in suppuration and destruction of the testicle.

673. In some cases the inflammation and swelling declines, but does not entirely cease. There are dragging, unpleasant sensations, occasional soreness and pain, and the diseased testicle is larger than its fellow. In others, in addition to these unpleasant symptoms, the testicle seems to get injured frequently, the slightest blow or pressure producing pain. With this there may be a low grade of inflammation and gradual change in the structure of the organs. This might be called "irritable testis." In other cases the testicle remains permanently enlarged, and from its bulk annoys the patient.

674. Some writers seem to have thought that swelled testicle was a metastasis of the disease, and always associated with a more or less complete arrest of the gonorrhœal discharge. With these views they have urged the importance of re-establishing the discharge as a means of cure. I do not think that the premises are correct, at least my experience does not bear it out.

675. TREATMENT.—The most successful treatment in many cases is the judicious use of compression. For this purpose I employ the adhesive plaster, strapping the testicle firmly to the abdomen, as named under the head of orchitis previously. Dr. Howe straps the testicle and scrotum by itself, carrying the adhesive plaster around it like a roller. In either plan the straps must be applied equably, so as to produce equal compression, and renewed as often as they become loose. I have often seen a patient, after the application of the straps, get up and go about his business, when before he could hardly move without excruciating pain. If the case pro-

gresses favorably, we will observe the testicle getting smaller day by day until cured.

676. Though strapping answers, in a majority of cases, there are some that will not bear it. Here, in addition to the usual internal means, we use narcotics and sedatives locally. Equal parts of Tinctures of Belladonna, Stramonium, and Aconite, is an excellent local application; though other combinations may prove as efficient. Steaming the inflamed organ with a decoction of Tansy or Hops gives great relief, as does the application of hot fomentations. A poultice of pounded Peach leaves wet with water, is highly recommended. Occasionally the application of ice-water will give relief when warm applications increase the difficulty.

677. Internally, I prefer the use of the special sedatives, in small doses, associated with the use of the bath, and an occasional mild cathartic. If Copaiba and Cubebs have been used, they should be suspended, and the milder injections employed. In addition I would give a combination of: ℞ Ext. Conium, Iodide of Potassium, aa. ʒj.; Tinct. Macrotys, ℥ss.; Simple Syrup, ℥iijss.; a teaspoonful every three hours.

678. The treatment of irritative testes is a matter of considerable difficulty, as we have no remedies that act directly. Sometimes we will be successful by keeping the testicle well supported in an elastic suspensory bandage, and using a local application of one part of Pond's Extract of Hamamelis to three of water. The use of equal parts of Tincture of Iodine and Tincture of Muriate of Iron, applied locally over the spermatic cord and around the scrotum, is sometimes advantageous. Internally I prefer the Compound Tincture of Corydalis with Bromide of Potassium.

GONORRHŒAL OPHTHALMIA.

679. Gonorrhœal ophthalmia is never a metastasis of the disease, as some of the older physicians supposed, but is caused by bringing the virus in contact with the conjunctiva. It is strange, not that it should occur, but that its occurrence

is so seldom, witnessing as we do the want of care and disregard of cleanliness upon the part of persons affected with the disease. Statistics show that it only occurs once in about six hundred and twenty-eight cases; still it is a very formidable affection when met with.

680. Within twenty-four hours after the introduction of the virus, the patient will complain of a sensation of itching and burning in the eye, and feel a constant disposition to rub or wipe it. Succeeding this is a feeling as if sand was in the eye, with irritation when the lids are moved, accompanied by a flow of tears, and some intolerance of light. As the disease progresses rapidly, there will be a free secretion of muco-pus by the end of the second day, and by the third the disease is fully established. Now the patient can not bear the least light, the lids are swollen, there is a hot, burning sensation within the orbit, and circumorbital pains. The discharge of muco-pus is now abundant, and the eyelids glued together.

681. If we examine the eye—which we do by using warm water with a soft sponge to loosen the adhesions—we will find the conjunctiva uniformly red and swollen. When the affection is severe the conjunctiva surrounding the cornea is so swollen as almost to occlude it, and in some cases the eye is not visible at all—nothing but a fiery-red mass being seen when the lids are opened; this swelling surrounding the cornea is termed chemosis.

682. Progressing still further, ulceration of the conjunctiva occurs, and in other cases, *phlyctenula* of the cornea, which terminate in ulceration and sometimes perforation. In some cases the chemosis is so great as to strangulate the cornea, and it sloughs, discharging the contents of the eye. In others the cornea becomes weakened from imperfect nutrition, and possibly from ulceration, and the fluids of the eye pressing upon it causes it to project, forming staphyloma.

683. TREATMENT.—It is yet a matter of doubt which is the better plan of treatment—that looking to a removal of the

inflammatory action by the ordinary means, or the stronger local applications for the abortion of the disease. I will give the two plans, and the reader can adapt them to special cases.

684. If the disease is seen in the early stage, the patient should be put upon the use of the proper sedatives, Veratrum or Aconite, with Gelseminum or Belladonna, if indicated. The necessity of rest in a darkened room should be insisted upon, as well as frequent bathing in warm water to which a small portion of common salt, or Chlorate of Potash, has been added. Paint the lids with Tincture of Veratrum, and if necessary, keep the pupil dilated with a solution of Atropia. The bowels may be gently moved once a day, if thought necessary, and in some cases the alkaline diuretics will be of advantage.

685. In some cases I am satisfied that Rhus will be found an admirable remedy, as it is in purulent ophthalmia with phlyctenulæ, the sensation of burning being extreme. I would prescribe it with Aconite, as: ℞ Tincture of Rhus, gtts. v.; Tincture of Aconite, gtts. x.; Water, ℥iv.; a teaspoonful every hour.

686. As a local application use a solution of Tannic Acid, grs. x.; Glycerine, ℥ss.; Rose Water, ℥jss.; or: ℞ Chloride of Zinc, grs. j.; Water, ℥j.; adding Atropia, Morphia, or Gelseminum, when indicated. If we use the first it is usually in the proportion of one-half grain to the ounce; the second two to four grains to the ounce; and of the third, gtts. xx. to ʒij. to the ounce.

687. Counter-irritation amounts to but very little, if anything, in these cases, and it is not worth while wasting our time with it.

688. In the other plan of treatment we propose making a sharp impression, and destroy the specific character of the disease at once. In one of the two cases of the disease I have seen, I adopted Prof. Hill's treatment—the lids were everted and the eye filled with strong Tincture of Capsicum; the relief was speedy and permanent, and the pain was not so

severe as might have been expected, and in ten minutes the eyes were in a more comfortable condition than before using. The danger in this form of conjunctivitis is from arrest of circulation and sloughing, a want of stimulus, and the stimulation of Tincture of Capsicum or Myrrh can not be harmful.

689. Gross claims that a solution of the Bichloride of Mercury, is by far the most reliable remedy in these cases, especially where the disease is running a rapid course. He prescribed: ℞ Bichloride of Mercury, gr. ⅛; Solution of Opium, grs. ij.; Water, ℥j. I have seen it used in one case, in the practice of an acquaintance, with excellent results. Though my prejudices are very strong, if the question was put to me—Mercury or eyes, which? I should say, put in the Bichloride.

690. Chloride of Zinc, if it could be safely used of sufficient strength would be a good remedy, but when we increase the proportion beyond gr. j. to the ounce, and can not guide the application there is danger. Sulphate of Zinc may be employed of the strength of grs. v. to Water, ℥j.; Carbolic Acid, grs. v. to Glycerine and Water, aa. ℥ss.

691. Whatever is used, it is necessary that it should be thoroughly applied. The eye is extremely sensitive, and the swelling and involuntary contraction of the lids make the ordinary use of a collyrium impossible. Hence it is best to employ them with a syringe, carefully throwing the fluid under the lids from the outer and inner canthus. Before using the stronger fluids, the eye should be thoroughly washed with tepid water, or milk and water.

692. The swelling of the conjunctiva (chemosis) is what endangers the structure of the eye, and may cause sloughing of the cornea in a single day. A free use of the bistoury, will obviate this, and give marked relief, and should not be neglected.

693. As before remarked, counter-irritation does very little good in the acute stage, yet when the eyelids are enormously swollen, the disease running a slow course, the application of

a fly-blister to the lids is said to give relief. Gross gives it his recommendation, with the caution "that the surface be well protected with gauze, to prevent the fly falling into the eye." In a more advanced stage, benefit is sometimes experienced from the application of Oil of Amber around the orbit.

694. When the acute stage has passed, leaving a somewhat chronic purulent conjunctivitis, I should think of the solution of Sulphate of Hydrastia as likely to meet the indications. If the lids showed granulations, or there was corneal opacity, Prof. Howe's use of Nitric Acid, would probably prove best. He shapes his pine pencil with a smooth flat surface, dips it in the strong Nitric Acid, wipes it on paper, and passes it over the part. If the cornea is touched it is very rapid.

GONORRHŒAL INFLAMMATION OF THE NOSE.

695. I have seen a very severe form of inflammation of the mucous membrane of the nose, produced by the gonorrhœal virus. It may be confined to one side, or involve the entire nose, causing great suffering. At first the symptoms resemble, to some extent, a bad cold. The nose is dry, stops up, there is a feeling of itching and irritation, and some pain. Soon a discharge of muco-pus occurs, which in a day or two becomes profuse. There is pain and uneasiness, stopping of the nose, a feeling of fullness, and dull, aching pain in the forehead, and shooting pains in the face. The disease may go on in this way for two or three weeks, and finally decline into a chronic ozæna.

696. TREATMENT.—In this case we would adopt the constitutional treatment recommended in gonorrhœal ophthalmia. As a local application we will find the following to be efficient: ℞ Chlorate of Potash, ʒij.; Common Salt, ʒij.; Glycerine, ℥ij.; Water, Oj.; M. ℞ Permanganate of Potash, ʒss.; Water, Oj.; M. ℞ Decoction of Baptisia, Oj.; Common Salt, ℥ss.; M. ℞ Alnus Serrulata, ℞umex Crispus, Quercus Rubra, aa. ℥ss.; Boiling Water, Ojss.; infuse and

strain. ℞ Water, Oj.; Common Salt, ℥ss., may be used as a common wash to cleanse the parts. These washes may be used with a syringe, or with a hydrostatic apparatus. If a syringe is used, the pipe should be inserted into one nostril, which is pressed against it to prevent the fluids escaping, and the patient directed to breathe through the mouth, and the injection slowly thrown in.

697. A very ingenious apparatus, (Thudicum's nasal douche), used for chronic ozæna may be employed here. It consists of a holder; to the bottom of which is attached an india rubber pipe, a yard or two in length, terminating in a nozzle for the nose. The jar containing the fluid for injection, being placed upon a retort stand, one or two feet higher than the head, the fluid is permitted to flow into the nose by its own gravity. The patient *must* breathe through the mouth, when the fluid will flow into one side of the nose and out at the other; but if the mouth is closed for an instant it will flow down the throat.

GONORRHŒAL DISEASE OF THE RECTUM.

698. We meet with this affection most frequently in females, but it occasionally occurs in males. I have not yet satisfied myself whether it is a true gonorrhœal inflammation, or simply developed by position or sympathy. At any rate I look upon it as one of the most distressing accidents of this disease.

699. I have witnessed it in two forms, in one the symptoms being those common to hemorrhoids, but more severe, and in the other a species of dysentery. In the first case the patient feels an unpleasant sense of weight and heat in the rectum, with shooting pains from it. No position gives ease, both lying, sitting and standing being alike painful after a time. Any active exercise occasions severe suffering, which wears upon the general health. The bowels are constipated, though there is a desire to go to stool, and in some cases the passage of mucus. In the second case an irritation of the

rectum is set up with tenesmus, and discharge of muco-pus. The pain is tensive, and passes through the pelvis to the back and down the thighs. The bowels become affected with diarrhœal discharges, the appetite impaired, and the general health much affected. Not unfrequently the cellular tissue about the rectum becomes involved in the inflammation, and abscesses form which if not properly attended to result in fistula. In such cases the suffering is very intense, the pain tensive and throbbing, with more or less febrile action. I have known ten to fourteen days pass before there was distinct evidence of suppuration.

700. TREATMENT.—It is essential in this disease that the bowels be kept gently open, or if there is tendency to diarrhœa, that it be checked at the commencement. A very good combination to keep the bowels soluble is: ℞ Compound Tincture of Senna, f℥jss.; Essential Tincture of Leptandra, f℥ss.; in doses of a teaspoonful four times a day. If it produces griping a small quantity of Chloroform may be added. Should there be tendency to diarrhœa: ℞ Syrup of Rhubarb and Potash, f℥jss.; Essential Tincture of Leptandra, f℥ss.; Chloroform, fʒss. M. A teaspoonful every one or two hours. In addition to this I order: ℞ Essential Tincture of Hamamelis, f℥ss.; Tincture of Staphysagria, fʒj.; Simple Syrup, f℥iijss. M. In doses of a teaspoonful four times a day. When the pain is severe, and the patient restless and uneasy, we may prescribe Diaphoretic powder, grs. v.; Quinine, gr. j., every four hours, which is usually better than giving Morphine.

701. Locally I have been much pleased with the action of enemas of: ℞ Chlorate of Potash, grs. x.; Tincture of Opium, gtts. xx.; Glycerine, ℥ss.; Water, ℥ijss. A solution of Permanganate of Potash, gr. j. to grs. v. to the ounce of water is good, as is also a solution of Sulphite of Soda, grs. v. to Water, ℥j. A decoction of equal parts of Baptisia and Hydrastis, answers a very good purpose, and Opium or Mor-

phia may be added to it if necessary. One part of the Fluid Extract of Hamamelis to four of water will be our best local application, if the disease is slow, with torpid venous circulation. Sometimes injections will not be well borne, and we may then use suppositories in their place.

702. If symptoms of cellular inflammation come up, it is well to paint the skin around the anus with two parts of strong Tincture of Iodine and one part of Tincture of Aconite. When suppuration is manifestly progressing, relief is experienced by sitting over the vapor of a decoction of Hops, Stramonium or Tansy, or hot fomentations of these may be continuously applied. If the vapor is used, the part may be poulticed between times. As soon as evidence of accumulation of matter is had, the lancet should be passed down to it, and give exit to the pus. This relieves the pain, prevents the pus burrowing, and lessens the danger of fistula. If the pain continues after this, use an injection into the abscesses of a strong solution of Sesquicarbonate of Potash.

GONORRHŒAL RHEUMATISM.

703. Some writers have not been willing to admit any relation between gonorrhœa and rheumatism, claiming that the occurrence of the latter at this time was accidental, or dependent upon other causes. The majority, however, and especially late writers, recognize and describe the disease. The most rational account of the pathology of the affection I find in Chambers' "Renewal of Life:"

"Gonorrhœal Rheumatism is a convenient conventional term which we continue to employ, really for want of a better. It means a specific acute or subacute inflammation of joints and the neighboring white tissues, bearing in its external aspects a resemblance to sometimes one and sometimes another of the forms of the disease it is named after. But it has not the slightest other relation, either pathological or therapeutical, besides external similarity, to rheumatism.

"It is really due to a poison absorbed into the blood from

a mucous membrane affected with purulent gonorrhœa, and thus has more claim to be classed by the side of pyæmia than in the position where it is now placed. Like pyæmia, too, it has a strong tendency to disorganization of the affected part; pus and fibrin are formed and the tissues are destroyed in bad cases. Like pyæmia, too, it does not exhaust itself by the inflammations which arise; it is not an acute disease, in the sense of tending to recovery, but a chronic disease, getting worse and worse if not arrested. It is an accident of gonorrhœa, not an essential part of it, just as pyæmia is an accident of surgical operations on wounds.

"Its extreme rarity in the female sex is an additional evidence in favor of the poison being absorbed from the locally diseased part. In woman the mucous membrane principally affected by gonorrhœa is the vaginal, a tough, strong surface which bears a good deal of ill treatment without serious injury. Its diseases have but little influence on the general health. But the male urethra is a much more delicate part, and we can easily comprehend that it should oftener take up the gonorrhœal virus and communicate it to the rest of the body.

"Being an accident, it may occur at any period of the gonorrhœa, sometimes happening only a few days after the first commencement of the running; but by the simple doctrine of chances of course more likely in the longer period before the patient is free. Hence it often appears just as the urethra or vagina is getting well, and so has been reckoned an instance of metastasis. Metastasis, however, it is not, for often and often the discharge continues as bad as ever, or even grows worse, while the joints are swollen. And when the joints get better, there is no return or aggravation of the original ailment."

704. This is not merely a pathological question; for on the notion of metastasis it has been proposed to try and bring back the gonorrhœa to the genital organs by irritating injections. I have seen this actually done, but without any of the

desired effects on the arthritic affection. Even if it were a curative operation, I should be averse from practicing it, for the disease which you thus give the patient is not true gonorrhœa, but urethritis or vaginitis, and that of a chronic character—a much worse thing. I say it is a much worse thing, because it is so dangerous, so very difficult to cure, not rarely indeed proving quite incurable.

705. The symptoms of gonorrhœal rheumatism do not differ very materially from the sub-acute form usually met with. Some days or weeks after the discharge commences, the patient complains of pain and soreness in one or more joints, which become swollen, hot, red and painful. The tongue is coated white, the appetite impaired, and the secretions partially arrested. The constitutional disturbance is usually slight—sometimes entirely absent—but in rare cases it is very marked. The disease usually progresses slowly, and shows but little tendency to yield to the common treatment. Sometimes it becomes chronic, and the patient is permanently disabled.

So marked is the relation between the gonorrhœa and rheumatism, that we can safely assume in certain persons, that if they contract a gonorrhœa, rheumatism of the joints will follow.

706. TREATMENT.—If a gonorrhœa is treated according to *special* indications as named, I think rheumatism would be of very rare occurrence. In almost every case where rheumatism is developed as a complication or a sequel, there has been the special symptoms calling for Macrotys, which, if given, would have prevented this result.

707. In the majority of cases we would prescribe: ℞ Tincture of Aconite, gtts. v. to gtts. x.; Tincture of Macrotys, (green root), gtts. xx.; Water, ℥iv.; a teaspoonful every hour. If there was fullness of the general cellular tissue, or it showed itself in œdema of the feet or eyelids, I would advise:

℞ Tincture of Apocynum Canabinum, gtts. xx.; Water, ℥iv.; a teaspoonful every one or two hours.

708. In some cases the rheumatism is very persistent, and the role of anti-rheumatics is exhausted without any benefit. In these cases a careful examination will many times detect special indications for some one remedy. For instance, if the tongue is full and pallid, with a uniform dull white fur (calf's tongue), Iodide of Potash in doses of grs. v. to grs. xx. four times a day, will give a speedy cure. With the solid blue tongue I prescribe Tincture of Iron, with most excellent results. If there is violet coloration, Nitric Acid is the remedy. If the tongue is deep red, lemon juice, etc.

709. If the rheumatism has followed the sudden arrest of the discharge, and it resists treatment, it may be well sometimes to get a return of the urethral disease. In all cases, if Copaiba and Cubebs have been used, they must be suspended. Generally in these cases, the clap will come back in a few days, and the rheumatism will stop

GLEET.

710. Gleet is a chronic inflammation of the urethra, succeeding a gonorrhœa, attended with a muco-purulent discharge. Like all other chronic inflammations, it manifests little tendency to spontaneous recovery, and sometimes resists judicious treatment for a long time. In a majority of cases it follows gonorrhœa without any break in the symptoms—the pain, burning on passing water, and frequent micturition, passing off in some weeks or months—the discharge still continuing.

711. Examination of the urethra proves its inflammatory character—the mucous membrane presenting a similar condition to that found in chronic inflammation of other parts. Rokitansky thus describes its condition in gonorrhœa and gleet: "We find the anatomical characters to be those belonging to catarrh generally; in the acute stage there is, according to the violence of the process, redness, injection,

tumefaction of the urethral mucous membrane, enlargement of the follicles, relaxation of the sinuses, and a white or colorless secretion. The inflammation is either uniformly diffused over the urethra, or is limited to one or more spots. In genuine gonorrhœa of the male urethra, we find not only the navicular fossa, but every point as far as the prostatic portion, and especially the vicinity of the bulb of the urethra, liable to become the seat of the disease." In gleet, the inflammation is sometimes confined to the lacunæ of the navicular fossa, but in a majority and the more stubborn cases, it is situate at the bulb or at the prostatic portion.

712. The discharge in gleet varies greatly, even in the same person, at different times, and it may cease and recur at intervals. Most usually it is somewhat milky white, opaque and tenacious; but in other cases and at other times it is yellowish and creamy. The discharge varies in quantity—sometimes being abundant, at others just sufficient to keep the penis moist and stain the clothing. There is rarely any pain or uneasiness attending it, except an itching, pricking sensation before passing water, and sometimes whenever the mind is directed to it. It is surprising what an effect it has upon the general health, in many cases where the discharge is but a few drops daily. Persons become morbidly sensitive to the discharge, brood over it, examine the penis every opportunity, press it to see if any matter will pass, and thus keep the nervous system continuously upon the strain.

713. It is a matter of much importance sometimes, to determine whether a discharge from the urethra is contagious. This will frequently be pressed by the patient, who feels very anxious in regard to it, and who will have a direct answer. We have no means of determining this matter, and can not possibly tell when the contagiousness of a gonorrhœa ceases, and the gleety discharge is non-virulent, as there is no recognizable difference in the character of the muco-pus. I have seen a gonorrhœa lose its contagious character in a couple of months, and a gleet retain it for over a year.

714. On this subject Vidal remarks: "It is difficult to name the precise period at which a blenorrhagia ceases, and a blenorrhœa begins. Some authors maintain that the discharge is no longer blenorrhagia, but a gleet, when it ceases to be contagious; others regard it as a gleet when it is no longer troublesome, when the discharge is transparent and viscous, like mucus. But it is well known how difficult it is to establish contagion from an urethral discharge, and as regards its transparency and mucous character, this may change from day to day; indeed, a gleet which to-day may be transparent and mucous, to-morrow may be opaque and more or less purulent, and all this may come from the least imprudence in regimen." Bumstead remarks on this subject: "It may at the present moment be wholly mucous, and entirely innocent of contagious properties, and yet a short time hence be purulent, and in the highest degree dangerous. The fact is, no one can pronounce sexual congress safe, so long as a urethral discharge exists, and in replying to the frequent questions of patients on this point, the surgeon should not only avoid incurring the responsibility of allowing it, but do all in his power to dissuade from it."

715. As regards the *prognosis* of gleet, the surgeon should be very reserved. Some cases are readily amenable to appropriate treatment, while others are very stubborn. Not unfrequently the discharge ceases under the use of remedies, and we flatter ourselves that the patient is well, but a suspension of the medicine, or some indiscretion brings it back.

716. TREATMENT.—I have a stereotyped treatment for gleet that I always adopt at first; if it fails, then I try other means. It consists in the internal use of: ℞ Tincture of Staphysagria, f℥ij.; Water, f℥iv. M. ℞ Pond's Extract of Hamamelis, f℥ss.; Water, f℥iv. M. Each of these is taken in doses of a teaspoonful four times a day, the doses being alternated so that one will come midway between the other. An injection is used of: ℞ Acetate of Lead, grs. xx.; Quinia

Sul., grs. x.; Water, ℥iv.; used with a Tieman's universal syringe, so as to bring the fluid in contact with the inflamed part. Special attention must be paid to the general health, the bowels kept regular, the other secretions free, the appetite good, and a nutritious diet employed, avoiding stimulants.

717. In place of this treatment, a cure may, many times, be effected by strict attention to the general health, without special medication. The stomach should be placed in good condition, and digestion and nutrition improved by the use of Bitter Tonics and Iron. The compound Iodine pill, composed of: ℞ Iodine, Ext. Nux Vomica, aa. grs. vj.; Hydrastia, ʒss.; Ext. Macrotys, grs. xx. Mix, and make thirty pills; give one every three or four hours. Or the Compound Quinine Pill, composed of: ℞ Quinine, Hydrastia, aa. ʒj.; Ext. Nux Vomica, Podophyllin, aa. grs. vj. Make thirty pills, which may be given the same way. Tincture of Muriate of Iron seems to answer as well if not better than other preparations of Iron. Keeping the bowels regular, with slight action upon the liver, is an important part of the treatment. In addition to this, the patient should have a salt-water bath every day, with brisk friction the entire length of the spine.

718. Copaiba, Cubebs, Tincture of Cantharides, and remedies of like class, have been employed to considerable extent, but without any especial benefit that I have ever seen. In fact they many times do harm, by irritating the stomach and digestive canal, and keeping up too great excitement of the kidneys. Tincture of Cantharides may be employed for a short period, in small doses, in combination with the Tincture of Iron, with good effect; but its long use is not to be recommended.

719. Many agents are used for injections in this case. Sulphate of Zinc answers well, one to five grains to the ounce of water; Tannic Acid, grs. v. to x. to Water, ℥j.; Alum, ʒj. to Water, ℥viij.: Solution of Persulphate of Iron, ʒss. to Water, f℥vj.; Nitric Acid, gtts. xx. to xxx. to Water, ℥viij.; Permanganate of Potash, grs. vj. to Water, ℥iv.; Tincture of

Iodine, gtts. x. to Water, ℥vj. This list might be extended; but the remedies are of the same character. In using injections for the cure of gleet, Tieman's syringe with perforated tubes is indispensable, as the solution must be brought in direct contact with the parts diseased. Acton's glass syringe with long tubes may be used, if employed with care; or a common silver catheter may be perforated with fine holes and used as an attachment to a common syringe.

720. If the means first named fail, I place more confidence in the use of the bougie and blister than any other. The use of the bougie should be continued for some time in order to obtain its good effects, as at first it may increase the irritation and discharge. It may be passed once or twice daily, using as large a size as will pass easily. The blister is unpleasant, but it sometimes proves very serviceable. The Cantharides Plaster, about an inch in width, should be applied so as to cover the entire diseased structure. It may be reapplied every third or fourth day, so as to keep up constant irritation. I have no doubt but that the irritating plaster, applied after the first blister, would answer better, though I have never used it.

GONORRHŒAL SEQUELÆ.

721. The majority of writers claim that gonorrhœa is purely a local disease, and never produces constitutional disturbance of a chronic character. This is true to a certain extent, and of the majority of cases, yet there are some exceptions that need be noticed. It must not be understood, however, that the secondary results resemble syphilis, and it is possible that they are quite as frequently the result of the treatment as the disease.

722. We have already seen that there is a gonorrhœal rheumatism, which is sometimes very persistent, and may assume a chronic form. From this we may have various structural lesions of the articulations, and fibrous and muscular tissue. I have seen worse deformity from this cause than from secondary syphilis, if we except the destructive ulcera-

tion of the face. I can recall two cases of anchylosis, one of forced flexion of the knee, and one of paralysis, and I see daily a fearful example, in an almost complete loss of the lower extremities.

723. Structural heart disease has occasionally a gonorrhœal origin, as has the functional affection, and I think any one who has seen many cases, especially under the old treatment, will be able to recall an example.

724. Disease of the spinal-cord is still more rare, yet an ordinary practice will show cases where the nervous lesions, though not severe, will last for life.

725. It may be said that one who has suffered from gonorrhœa will usually have some reminder of it for months, if not for years. It may show itself in an irritable prepuce, and covering of the glans, with tendency to balanitis and posthitis; in an irritable urethra, bladder, or prostate gland; in a wrong of the vesiculæ seminales or testes; or especially in the tendency to aplastic deposits in the cellular tissue of the perineum.

726. The woman, as we have already seen, may suffer for years, or for life, various lesions of the reproductive organs, with morbid secretions, which will sometimes produce urethritis. So too we find that in men, a disease lurks in the lacunæ, and at times becomes sufficiently virulent to infect.

727. Thus it is claimed by a recent German writer, that some patients are never cured of gonorrhœa, and convey the infection in a modified form as long as they live. I know from experience, that this chronic gonorrhœa, as it might be called, is difficult of cure.

SYPHILIS.

728. The term syphilis is used to designate a class of diseases produced by a specific poison, which is generated during the disease and propagated by contact. As regards the character of the virus we know nothing, further than it clearly resembles the poison of other contagious diseases in many respects. It acts in the most minute quantity, as well as in large amount, and differs from the organic poisons of similar character, in that its influence is protracted and in some cases permanent, and instead of manifesting a definite set of phenomena, and being then eliminated, it seems to change its character with time, and gives rise to many different forms of disease.

729. Though the disease undoubtedly arises from prostitution, it is now generally admitted that it does not now arise *de nova*, but is invariably the result of inoculation with syphilitic virus. This virus is contained in pus, generated by syphilitic inflammation, and in no respect that we can discover does it differ from the product of ordinary inflammation. Thus the pus may be thin, thick, ropy, creamy, yellow, greenish, white, transparent, opaque, bland, acrid, plastic, amorphous, alkaline, acid, or neutral; each preserving the contagious element. This pus will retain its virulent properties for many weeks, if excluded from the air, and Sperlino gives a case where the matter, dried upon the lancet, was successfully inoculated after seven months.

730. It is generally supposed that this pus is only formed by primary sores, called chancres, and that other syphilitic lesions do not produce the virus. This, however, is a disputed point, and I am inclined to the opinion that it is not correct, though we will have more to say of this hereafter.

731. The syphilitic virus is communicated in different ways, but we will find, in a very large majority of cases, that patients get it in the *natural way*, by sexual intercourse. If,

however, the virus is brought in contact with a mucous membrane, or any abraded surface, syphilis will result, whether this has been done by the fingers, by linen, dressings, towels, surgical instruments, sponges, a privy seat, chamber utensil or bed covering. A surgeon meets with many cases in which the person denies having contracted the disease by connection, but it is only in rare cases where those other means have been the cause of it. I have known chancre of the hands contracted by dressing chancre of the penis, and by attendance upon a woman in labor suffering from the disease; chancre of the lip contracted from kissing; but these are exceptional cases, and we may safely assume that chancre of the genital organs is the result of sexual congress.

732. As regards its action at first, there is a difference of opinion. Some claim that it is at first purely a local disease, the syphilitic poison being confined to the ulcer, where it may be destroyed. Others contend that absorption of the poison first occurs, and that chancre is the manifestation of that poison from the blood. I take the first view of the question, and feel entirely convinced that it is the correct one. Still the syphilitic virus may be soon absorbed from the chancre, may in fact be absorbed from the mucous surface before the chancre is formed, and impregnation of the system thus occurs at a date so early as to render futile the usual abortive measures.

733. In the description of syphilis we may properly divide the disease into two forms, *primary* and *secondary*—the first embracing the period of the chancre or original sore; the second the constitutional effects of the syphilitic poison when absorbed.

PRIMARY SYPHILIS.

734. In the consideration of primary syphilis we are met with a difficulty at the very threshold of the subject. All good authorities have recognized two forms of chancre—the *soft* and *hard or indurated*, but of late it is urged that soft

chancre is an entirely distinct disease and does not give rise to secondary accidents

735. The reader may say, is not this a matter susceptible of proof, and could it not be determined in a short time? No man familiar with syphilis would put such a query, for we well know that many times it is difficult to determine whether a chancre is hard or soft; and the advocates of the new doctrine use the summary argument that has been so often applied to cancer: if it is a cancer, it is incurable; if you have cured it, it was no cancer. So in this case, they say, if the system was infected it was an indurated chancre, as soft chancre will not infect.

736. In many cases the sore has a specific character, by which it may be readily known as chancroid or chancre. The rapid development and entire want of induration in the case of the chancroid, its tendency to extend by erosion, and the acute engorgement and suppuration of the inguinal lymphatic glands, are characteristic. On the other hand, the prolonged incubation of the disease, the slowly formed chancre on an indurated base, the little tendency to erosion, and the slow engorgement and induration of the lymphatic glands, in the majority of cases, without suppuration, clearly defines the character of the lesion.

737. As a general rule, the local disease in chancroid is the severest. If you find phymosis, with swollen prepuce, much inflammatory action, a free discharge, a rapid extension of ulceration, you may suspect chancroid. The majority of cases of phagedenic chancre are non-infecting, as are the majority of those which give us most annoyance in treatment. On the contrary, though true chancre is frequently persistent, and heals with difficulty, it is sluggish in its movements, and does not give us so much annoyance.

738. But we have a far safer means of diagnosis, pointed out and insisted upon by Prof. Howe, for many years back. Probably he was not the first to call attention to it, but I am sure he was the first to present the subject in a clear light.

He insists that it is not the character of the sores, but their number, which should give diagnosis. If the sores are *multiple*, it is *chancroid* or non-infecting syphilis; but if there is *one* sore, it is true chancre and will be followed by constitutional syphilis. In his lectures he has been accustomed to impress this upon the minds of the class by the old Latin fable of the Fox and the Lioness.

739. If this is true, then the diagnosis becomes easy. If there are ulcers, it is non-infecting—chancroid. If there is but one ulcer it is true chancre. I believe it is true in the main, and the diagnosis based on the number of ulcers, rather than upon their character, is by far the most reliable. Yet there are exceptions, and it is well to get a clear idea of them. We have already seen that the three venereal diseases might exist in the same person at one time. A man or woman may contract true chancre, and during its incubation be again exposed, and contract chancroid, so that when seen by the physician he has the multiple ulcers, and yet suffers from the constitutional disease. I have known two cases of this kind; one in my own practice, in which the sores were so different in character, that the finger could detect it by passing it over the prepuce. Two of the ulcers healed readily by the application of Nitric Acid, and a simple dressing, the one persisted some four months; the two left no cicatrix, the one left cicatricial tissue that could be noticed three years after the attack. A second case was recently brought to my notice, in which a patient had a multiple chancre, a cluster of three small ones, at once arrested by the thorough use of Nitric Acid, and healed in five days. Nine days afterwards he presented himself with a single indurated chancre in nearly the same place, and has already shown a slight syphilitic eruption. In this case, the patient had connection with different women on alternate nights.

740. I am also well satisfied that I have seen cases of *single* chancroid, running their course in the usual way, with suppurating bubo. A treatment purely local was employed,

and there was no constitutional infection. These cases, so far as my memory serves, had the typical character of chancroid, without induration. I have also seen what was seemingly the simple irregular ulcer, formed from three primary points, presenting all the characteristics of chancroid, but which developed fearful secondary symptoms within six months.

741. But these are exceptions, and I think Prof. Howe's rule can be relied upon in the main. To assure myself of its truth, I have recently examined reports of cases, by close observers, and by those who have not had their attention called to the fact, for singular as it may seem, the best syphilographers have either not noticed it at all, or have placed very little reliance in it. Yet the cases all go to prove its truth. Thus in fifty-nine cases given by Ricord, forty-one cases of single ulcer were followed by constitutional infection; eight cases of single ulcer, which received general treatment from the commencement, did not show constitutional symptoms; four cases of multiple ulcer showed no constitutional infection; two cases of primary bubo gave constitutional infection; and but four cases of multiple ulcer gave constitutional disease. These cases give strong evidence in favor of Prof. Howe's theory—there are but four exceptions in fifty-nine cases, and it will be interesting to have the history of these:

742. The first was a case of *preposter venere.* "I examined the genital organs; they exhibited no evidence of former venereal ulcers nor discharge. The inguinal glands were engorged, indolent, elastic, and movable; the most external and most internal were also the largest. On inquiry of the patient if he had no affection of the anus, he replied that he had labored under hemorrhoids which, for six weeks, had given him great pain. On examination I found three ulcers in the anus. One was situated in the median line, one in the ano-perineal; and another in the ano-coccygeal region. Externally, they were semicircular, and extended toward the lower part of the rectum, as if they had been produced by those longitudinal fissures known by those who desire to re-

tain this faulty nomenclature, as *primary rhagades*. Their outer base was sharply defined, hard, elastic, indolent, and presenting a specific induration."

743. "P—— contracted in July two chancres: one on that part of the semi-mucous membrane reflected from the glans to the prepuce, and the other on the lower and cutaneous portion of the prepuce. They healed after a month with a simple application. Oct. 18th he presented the following condition: The chancres were completely cicatrized, but their cicatrix still presented well-marked specific induration. Several of the inguinal glands on both sides were swollen, hard, elastic, indolent and movable. The patient was ignorant of these swellings. The posterior, deep-seated, cervical glands were swollen hard, but little developed, and indolent, although the patient complained of uneasiness in the movements of his head. These intermittent and nocturnal headaches had become more intense. On the scalp were seen a large number of papulæ covered with impetiginous scabs.

744. "Four and a half years ago, P——, after sexual congress, perceived several ulcers on the glans and prepuce. These ulcers were unaccompanied with suppurating buboes. The patient was treated with mercurial pills, which produced slight salivation, and caused him to suspend their use after fifteen days. Soon after, there appeared at his anus painful pimples, which became excoriated, and discharged fetid pus. These pimples continued for a long time, and only yielded to some additional pills which he took. Accompanying the ulcers on the penis, he was affected with an urethral discharge, which was treated by astringent injections. From this date he enjoyed good health until three months ago, when he was attacked with the eruption for which he was admitted into the hospital. This eruption was seated on the skin of the penis, the scrotum, the internal surface of the thighs, and some parts of the trunk. It had commenced slowly by small maculæ, of a deep-red, followed by small,

suppurating pimples, arranged in circles more or less complete, and approximating each other closely."

745. "This was a young woman of twenty years of age, a brunette, robust, of a lymphatic temperament, having always enjoyed good health, and freedom from any cutaneous disease. After sexual commerce, she was attacked with ulceration of the vulva. The ulcers did not become very large, but their base soon indurated. When the patient applied for advice, the ulcers of the vulva had healed, but the specific induration was still observable. The inguinal glands did not appear to be engorged. The primary symptoms had existed nearly four months. She had not been treated, and the cutaneous affection had been present for two months."

746. I have thus presented these cases somewhat in detail that the reader may see the character of the exceptional cases. In each of them there was the characteristic induration, and also the indolent engorgement of the lymphatic glands. The sores were not only multiple, but the description shows clearly that each sore was a true chancre, and not chancroid and chancre together.

747. Of the eight cases of single chancre, not followed by constitutional infection, the history is not so clear. They were treated early, and with mercurials, which Ricord deemed specific, but so were the majority of the forty-nine that showed constitutional infection. Putting aside the treatment, we may conclude that some of them, at least, were chancroids.

748. I have deemed the evidence from Ricord more reliable than other authorities, for he had no theory to save, and presented cases of which he had the complete history to the constitutional disease. In the Hopital du Midi, of three hundred and twenty-seven patients diagnosed as chancroid, sixty-three patients had a single ulcer; fifty had two; one hundred and fifty-two, from three to six; forty-five from six to ten; eight from ten to fifteen; five from fifteen to twenty; six from twenty to twenty-four. In the Hospital at Lyons, of one hundred and eighteen cases, fifty had a single ulcer. Of the

remainder, twenty-two had two ulcers; eleven four ulcers; eleven five ulcers; seventeen six to ten ulcers; six eleven to fifteen ulcers; one twenty ulcers. Of four hundred and fifty-six cases of true chancre observed by Fournier, two hundred and twenty-six had but one; one hundred and fifteen several ulcers. Yet we have no means of knowing, and the observer did not think it necessary to specify, whether these multiple chancres were alike in physical characteristics, or whether there were not some who had the two diseases—chancroid and chancre—at the same time.

INOCULATION.

749. John Hunter proved by experiment that the virus of primary syphilis was inoculable, and proposed this as a means of distinguishing a specific from a non-specific ulcer, and the primary from the secondary disease. Ricord pursued these experiments with characteristic zeal, and at last taught the dogma that primary syphilis was always inoculable, and that no other form of the disease could be thus transmitted, and that if inoculation did not succeed, the disease was not syphilis. Inoculation thus became an important means of diagnosis, and was practiced to a very considerable extent.

750. But neither Hunter nor Ricord recognized the dual character of chancre, and many of their experiments were therefore worthless. Both chancroid and chancre are inoculable, but the first is particularly easy of propagation. The specific virus of a chancroid may be readily inoculated in the same person, as it can in another person. But the specific virus of true chancre can only be inoculated in the same person at a very early stage of the disease. If these are facts, and I do not think they will be disputed, the diagnosis by inoculation fails to distinguish true syphilis.

751. Very certainly the many recorded cases of inoculation in the same person are to be taken as representatives of the chancroid; whilst those of second persons may or may not have been true syphilis. If the virus of true syphilis, at

a very early period of the disease, be reintroduced into the same person, it will produce the characteristic sore, but after some days it has no influence. In this respect it is very much like the vaccine disease, which may also be re-inoculated before the system is fully impressed from the first virus, but which has no influence after the first vesicle shows its characteristic features.

752. Inoculation in the same person was successful with M. Puche in only ten per cent. of his cases; Poission obtained like results, and Laroyenne was unsuccessful in all of nineteen cases.

753. On the contrary, the chancroid may be reproduced in any number of places in the same person. It is this peculiarity of the disease that gives the multiple ulcer. Wherever the virus, discharged from a first ulcer, finds a part unprotected, it produces the specific ulceration. I saw some years since, a very singular illustration of this. A young man from the city, suffering from chancroid, went into the hay-field for a few hours, and in the exertion chafed his thigh at the point the penis rested upon it—the result was a beautiful crop of chancroid at this point.

754. In inoculation with the virus of chancroid, the period of inoculation is short, from two to five days, and it begins as a pustule. In inoculation with the virus of a true chancre, the period of inoculation is prolonged, from two to six weeks, and the initial lesion is in the form of a papule or tubercle. The inoculation from chancroid produces an open sore with irregular edges, free secretion, and tendency to erosion; the true chancre is indurated, indolent, and shows little tendency to the destruction of tissue.

755. The inoculation of chancroid is thus described by Niemeyer: "Upon introducing some of the secretion of a chancre beneath the epidermis, through a puncture from a lancet-point, no change takes place at the point of inoculation during the first twenty-four hours. At about the thirty-sixth hour a slight redness appears, and in forty-eight hours there

is a distinct, bright-red macula. In the course of the third day the macula rises into a flattish papule, and upon the fourth day the epidermis is raised, forming a vesicle, surrounded by a reddened areola. In the next day or two its contents become more yellow and purulent, the vesicle transforming into a pustule, which bursts between the fifth and eighth day; or else, together with its contents, dries up into a scab. After rupture of the pustule, or after removal of the scab, we see an ulcer of the size of a pin's head, or perhaps as large as a pea; it is almost circular, and penetrates into the corium in a manner disproportionate to its size. Its edge, which is œdematous from inflammation, has a puckered appearance. In the next few days, the base and edges of the sore are attacked, by a diphtheritic process, and it begins to enlarge. As the elements of the tissues are necrosed, and broken down into detritus, the base of the sore assumes a grayish, dirty, lardaceous appearance. As the diphtheritic destruction goes on irregularly at its periphery, the borders of the ulcer acquire a gnawed, ragged form. If the point of inoculation be destroyed by caustic within the first four days, the destructive process may generally be cut short. After the fourth day this is scarcely ever possible."

DIAGNOSIS OF CHANCRE AND CHANCROID.

756. I have already pointed out some of the principal elements of diagnosis, but it may be well to present them together, that they may be compared.

CHANCROID.	CHANCRE.
Origin. Produced by contact with the specific virus of chancroid; either from multiple ulcers, or the pus of a virulent bubo.	*Origin.* Produced by contact with the specific virus of an indurated ulcer, or by inoculation with the blood from one suffering from constitutional disease.
Incubation. The period of incubation is short, from two to six days, and the ulcer is rapidly developed, obtaining its usual size by the seventh day.	*Incubation* The period of incubation is prolonged; usually two or three weeks, but may be as much as six weeks.

CHANCROID.	CHANCRE.
Number. The chancroid is usually multiple, from two to a dozen or twenty. The proportion of single sores being, probably, not more than one in ten.	*Number.* Chancre is almost always single; as we have seen from Ricord's cases, the proportion of multiple sores being four in fifty-three.
Commencement. Commences by an elevation of the epidermis, presenting sometimes the character of a vesicle, sometimes a pustule, but always becoming pustular, the ulcer being formed when this ruptures or is broken.	*Commencement.* Commences with an engorgement of the skin, papular or tubercular, erosion of the epithelium, and the formation of one ulcer.
Induration. Never indurated; there may be inflammatory engorgement of the tissues, but its character is readily determined, the cellular tissues being as much affected as the skin or mucous membrane.	*Induration.* Springing from an induration, this persists during the progress of the disease as a characteristic feature. The ulcer with its base has a cartilaginous feel, and may be freely moved upon the tissue beneath.
General Appearance. The edges are sharply defined, and show the tendency to erosion. The bottom is covered with a white or grayish pultaceous secretion; and the discharge is usually free.	*General Appearance.* The edges are adherent, sloping or flat, and seem to be a part of the induration. The floor may be covered by a grayish film of secretion; but if exposed, it is red, livid, or copper colored.
Sensibility. Is painful, and as it progresses, a source of much uneasiness, with considerable change of adjacent parts.	*Sensibility.* Is not sensitive, and may be carried weeks or months, without the patient's knowledge.
Progress. Increases continually in size, until its specific character is destroyed.	*Progress.* Remains very nearly the same, after the first eight or ten days.
Inflammation. Is frequently the cause of severe inflammation of adjacent parts.	*Inflammation.* Is very rarely associated with inflammation.
Destruction of Tissue. Is that form of ulcer which assumes a phagedenic character, and occasionally is very destructive.	*Destruction of Tissue.* Very rarely proves destructive.
Bubo. Rapid engorgement of the glands of the groin, followed by inflammation and suppuration.	*Bubo.* Induration of the inguinal lymphatics, without suppuration.

757. I think a careful comparison of the two, as presented above, will enable every one to make a correct diagnosis. The superficial observer would perhaps jump at conclusions from the number of the sores, or some other single characteristic, but as we have already seen, there is no safety except in a careful examination and analysis of the symptoms. There are abundant reasons why the diagnosis should be carefully made, as there is not only the endless train of constitutional symptoms to be looked after in true syphilis, but there is a difference in the therapeutics of the local disease.

CHANCROID.

758. The chancroid is purely a local disease, and never produces constitutional infection; but as a local disease it is many times far more serious than chancre, always more painful, unpleasant from swelling and excess of secretion, and in some cases is associated with violent inflammation, and rapid erosion of tissues. We say it *never* produces constitutional infection, but we must be understood as having reference to the disease and not to the treatment, for the latter is not unfrequently a cause of life-long disease and suffering. I have witnessed this in both the Old School and Eclectic practice. The one would administer mercurials for months, under the mistaken idea that he was preventing constitutional infection. The other would drench his patients with Compound Syrups, and defibrinate his blood with Iodide of Potassium, deranging the digestive organs with purgatives, under the same mistaken notion. One of the severest cases of constitutional disease, involving the bones, that ever came to my knowledge, was produced by mercury given in and after chancroid, and I have no doubt that there are hundreds and thousands of like cases.

759. It is essential, therefore, that we know this disease, if for no other reason than that we may avoid doing an injury with general remedies, bearing in mind that there is no mean in the action of drugs—they either do good or harm. We

find an additional reason in the increased care necessary in the management of the local disease.

760. The period of incubation in chancroid is very brief.* Sometimes the person will notice an irritation the day succeeding a suspicious connection; or at farthest within a week. Upon this appears a vesicle or pustule within twenty-four hours, and the distinct ulcer by the third day. This ulcer presents the characteristic features of chancroid from the commencement. Its edges are distinct and clear cut, and sufficiently irregular and "worm-eaten" to show the tendency to erosion. It already furnishes an abundant secretion, which under the microscope shows an abundance of pus-globules. The sores are irritable and painful, and quite early the tendency to inflammatory engorgement is manifest.

761. If we see the case early, there may be but one ulcer, or there may be more from the first, but we notice a tendency to their reproduction from contact with the secretion, and usually in that situation which is continuously bathed in the secretion from the sore. But whether one or many, they increase in size from day to day, growing deeper as well as larger in circumference.

---

*Fournier reports fifty two cases in which the disease was first noticed as follows:

	CASES.
The first day after exposure	6
The second day after exposure	2
The third day after exposure	9
From the third to the fourth day	4
The fourth day	3
The fifth day	1
The sixth day	3
From the seventh to the eighth day	13
The ninth day	1
The tenth day	2
The eleventh day	1
The thirteenth day	2
From the thirteenth to the fourteenth	8
From the seventeenth to the twentieth	2
Total	52

762. The situation of the chancroid varies in different cases, though the majority will be found upon the prepuce. In four hundred and forty-five cases classified by Fournier, they were distributed as follows:

FOURNIER'S TABLE (MEN).

Chancroids of the glans or prepuce	347
" on the sheath of the penis	21
" on various parts of the penis, as, for instance, occupying the prepuce and sheath, the sheath and the glans, etc.	24
" on the penis (exact situation not recorded)	25
" on the meatus	11
" within the urethra	5
" of the scrotum	3
" on the pubes	3
" on the fingers	2
" on the upper and inner portions of the thighs	2
" of the anus	1
" of the anterior thoracic region	1
Total	445

763. If on the prepuce, there is many times an infiltration of its cellular tissue, and if there are several sores this may go on until the opening of the prepuce is so contracted that it can not be drawn back. This condition of phymosis is very unpleasant, as the ulcers are concealed from view, and it is difficult to keep the parts properly cleansed, or to make local applications.

764. The same trouble may come from an active inflammation set up in the prepuce, the parts becoming very much swollen, red, hot, and painful. In both cases the discharge will be free, and may be mistaken for gonorrhœa upon superficial examination.

765. The chancroid is most painful when situated in the sulcus immediately behind, or sometimes eroding the *corona glandis*. The ulcer in the fold of the frænum is also very irritable, and not unfrequently perforates the fold of membrane, and spreads on each side. When thus perforated, the least

tension on the frænum produces exquisite suffering. Chancroid of the meatus is also exceedingly irritable in some cases. The chancroid behind the *corona* may sometimes perforate the mucous covering, and have its base in the body of the organ.

766. Commencing as a point not larger than a pin's head, the ordinary chancroid attains the size of a silver three or five cent piece, and continuing for about three weeks, it terminates spontaneously, seemingly from the exhaustion of the virulence of the specific contagion. It is not to be understood that the disease can not be arrested short of this time by local treatment, or that all cases of chancroid will terminate in a given time.

767. So long as the edges of the sore have the ragged, eroded appearance, it retains its specific character, and can be transmitted by inoculation; and so long as the floor of the ulcer is bathed in pus, with some fibrillation of the secretion, there is no tendency to reparation. The reparative tendency is shown first in a cleaner appearance of the sore, laudable pus covering a rosy granular floor. The edges lose their irregular form, become more consistent, and are less elevated, and are sloping.

768. The specific virus in chancroid seems to reside in the pus globules, and not in the remainder of the secretion, and is thus the reverse of true chancre. This has been proven by filtering the secretion, and thus removing the globules, when the remainder inoculated would no longer produce infection.

769. *Inflammatory Chancroid.*—Inflammation occurs most frequently when the ulcers are upon or near the prepuce. From the commencement the sores have been quite sensitive, and surrounded with more or less redness. Suddenly, seemingly sometimes from treatment, at others from over-exertion or some indiscretion, the parts swell rapidly, become red and hot, and quite painful. In a few hours there is phymosis, and as the swelling increases the contraction of the prepuce is more marked. Sometimes within twenty-four hours, the

tissues become distended to their utmost capacity, and if not relieved, soon show the effects of impaired circulation, in dusky discoloration, and tendency to gangrene. In some cases there is but little tendency to sloughing, the inflammation doing but little harm—further than it prevents treatment. In other cases, it runs the usual course of inflammation of cellular tissue, and terminates in suppuration. The pus may be laudable, if there is no communication between the chancroid and the abscess; but if the abscess is inoculated from the dressings, then its secretion will be virulent—it is indeed transformed into a specific ulcer.

770. As already named, sloughing is indicated by impairment of the circulation, marked by dark discoloration, and sometimes by an elevation of the epidermis in the form of a blister. Usually the slough gives away rapidly, exposing a foul surface, and leaving very ragged edges, and a tendency to phagedena. There have been rare cases in which the gangrene thus set up continued to the destruction of the glans, and even the entire organs, and rarely proving destructive to life.

771. *Phagedenic Chancroids.*—In the ordinary phagedenic chancroid, there is simply an increase in the ordinary tendency to erosion. We see it manifest in the irregular, ragged, worm-eaten edges of the ulcer, which seem somewhat excoriated and loose; soon the tendency to erosion in a particular direction is marked, and the ulcer becomes irregular in form, and the tissues seem to melt down before it until the sore is of very large size—and yet it has not lost the peculiar features of a chancroid.

772. In other cases, the sore is covered with a peculiar dark, shreddy, pultaceous material, seemingly the debris of connective tissue. The erosion goes on under the edges of the sore, which assume a dark color, and fall in. In depth it reaches the body of the organ, and sometimes the destructive process goes on in this. In the glans, there seems to be an infiltration of tissue, dark discoloration, a thin, dark, ichorous

secretion, and the tissues seem to melt away before the destructive process.

773. *Serpiginous Chancroid.*—This will hardly be mistaken for the *serpiginous* ulceration of constitutional syphilis, as it is here associated with the primary ulcer, and commences sometimes as early as the second or third week from its formation.

774. Usually before the end of the first week the eroded loose edges of the sore give evidence of a tendency to phagedena or sloughing. When this character is assumed, the ulcer having penetrated the skin or mucous surface, destroys the connective cellular tissue, so that the edges of the ulcer are detached, and may be raised up like flaps. As it progresses, they lose vitality, and are perforated at many points like a carbuncle, and finally sloughing, or sometimes melting away. The floor of the ulcer is covered with a gray, fibrinous, pultaceous material, very like the covering of a carbuncle, which the disease somewhat resembles. In this way they may dissect up and destroy the entire integument of the penis, and extend to scrotum, perineum, abdomen and thighs.

775. This serpiginous ulceration may commence in a virulent bubo, and dissect up and destroy the integument of the groin, the abdomen and thigh, for some distance. I have seen one case in which the entire inguinal region, and one side of the scrotum was thus denuded by this form of ulcer.

776. TREATMENT.—The treatment of chancroid will vary in different cases, and as has been already remarked, will prove successful in proportion as it is adapted to the special condition of the patient.

777. In the simpler forms of the disease, the treatment is almost wholly local. We endeavor to destroy the specific character of the ulcer, keeping the parts free from the secretion, and protected from irritation.

778. The escharotics in most common use to destroy the specific character of the ulceration are: Nitrate of Silver, the acid solution of Nitrate of Mercury, Nitric Acid, Sulphuric

Acid, Chloride of Zinc, and the Potassa cum Calce. We need hardly class with them Carbolic Acid, Permanganate of Potash, and Tincture of Iron, though each has been employed and recommended.

779. Nitrate of Silver is frequently used, and fails to accomplish the object in nine out of ten cases. It is hardly worth while to repeat, that these applications must be thorough, and reach every pus globule, as well as the tissue cells that are being transformed. If this agent is used, the stick should be pointed, and pressed into every nook and crevice of the sore, giving sufficient time to it to make the work thorough.

780. Nitrate of Mercury, though used by many and strongly recommended, possesses no advantage over Nitric Acid: this is now conceded by the best authorities. In the nature of the disease there is not the least occasion for the topical or general use of Mercury, even if it is conceded a specific influence in some forms of syphilis. But there is this objection, that it can not be handled so easily, it may impair the life of adjacent tissues, and will sometimes produce salivation. I will give Bumstead as an authority for the last statement.

781. Nitric Acid is a favorite remedy with me, and I think it can be so used as to accomplish the object with very great certainty. We use it with a pine pencil, shaped to suit the conformation and situation of the ulcer. This being charged with the acid, and wiped, is thoroughly pressed into every portion of the sore. It is well to take sufficient time to this, recharging the pencil, and going over the ground until we are certain that every portion is reached. It is very easy with free acid to coat the ulcer with a white film of changed pus and tissue, the virulent secretion being covered up, not destroyed.

782. Sulphuric Acid is best used in the form of the "carbo-sulphuric paste," as recommended by Ricord and Cullerier. It is formed by saturating willow charcoal with Sul-

phuric Acid, in a glass-stoppered bottle. The paste is most commonly applied with a glass rod, though the pine pencil will answer well. The application should be thorough to the ulcer, but *not* to adjacent structures, as is the failing with some practitioners. Its advantage is, in its searching character, reaching every part of the diseased surface.

783. Chloride of Zinc has been used and recommended by many surgeons. It was first employed in the form of a paste, made by mixing equal parts of the Zinc and flower (Canquoine's paste.) We usually make this paste with powdered Gum Arabic. In using it the sore should be thoroughly cleansed, and the paste carefully pressed into it with a probe or the pine pencil, then covering with a small piece of adhesive plaster; it may remain for five to fifteen minutes.

784. The Potassa cum Calce may be used in the form of the sticks of Filhos, or made into a paste with a little Alcohol. In either case the application should be thorough, and continued for ten or fifteen minutes.

785. Carbolic Acid may, in some rare cases, prove sufficient, but only in the early stage, and even here I should not advise it. The same may be said of Permanganate of Potash, and of Tincture of Iron, recommended by some of our School—the less said, or used, the better.

786. In selecting the remedy, I should advise the Nitric Acid where the secretion was thick and not too profuse. The Sulphuric Acid paste, when the parts were tumid, and the secretion profuse. And the Potassa cum Calce where the edges were ragged and worm-eaten, showing a tendency to phagedena. In using either the Chloride of Zinc or the Potassa, the adjacent surface should be protected, and the patient should be kept still, until its action was complete, and the surplus removed.

787. Having thus effectually destroyed the specific character of the sore by a first cauterization if possible, or by subsequent ones if found necessary, we have to decide upon a proper dressing. It is well to bear in mind that cleanliness is

essential, and that protection from irritation is important. In some cases, these are the essential elements of choice, in others there is some special object to be accomplished, as sedation, stimulation, etc.

788. A dressing of dry lint picked fine, answers a very good purpose in some cases, and it is well to bear in mind that lint is best adapted for the application of almost all of the remedies we are likely to use. In using dry lint, we find that it absorbs the secretions, and when changed frequently, keeps the parts clean.

789. When the part needs stimulation, we may dress it with Aromatic Wine; when the tissues are relaxed, a solution of Tannic Acid, ʒss., Water, ℥vj., will be found a good application; if stimulation is thought desirable with this, we may substitute Port Wine for the water. In some cases water acidulated with Nitric Acid does very well (gtts. x.; Water, ℥viij.) Lime Water is sometimes a good dressing, or it may be used with an equal part of Olive Oil.

790. When Iron is indicated, I prefer the paste made by throwing the Hydrated Sesqui-Oxide on filtering paper, until it has the proper consistence. Permanganate of Potash may be employed where the discharges are very fetid, in the proportion of grs. v. to Water, ℥j. Carbolic Acid may also be used, in the proportion of grs. x. to Water and Glycerine, aa. ℥ij. The two last will sometimes be found excellent dressings when the parts are very sensitive and painful.

791. Occasionally we find that a dry dressing is preferable to the wet. The dry lint has already been mentioned, but occasionally dusting the ulcer with Sub-Nitrate of Bismuth, is much better.

792. After giving the above list, I may say that a good Mayer's Ointment is my preference in the majority of cases. It is spread upon lint or soft cotton rag, placed upon the sore and the prepuce drawn down over it. It should be changed sufficiently often to remove the secretion.

793. In the *concealed* chancroid from swelling and contraction of the prepuce (phymosis), we can not use the escharotics, and are obliged to rely on such local applications as we can make. I have generally treated them by the use of a weak solution of Carbolic Acid with Glycerine and water, Chlorinated Lime, or Chlorate of Potash, used with a syringe, for cleanliness, and Mayer's ointment carried up to the diseased surfaces. This dressing, it is true, is not a very agreeable one, but it has answered a better purpose than any others in my practice.

794. If the progress of the ulceration, and the constriction of the prepuce is such, that the integrity of the tissues are endangered, we have to take into consideration the propriety of dividing the prepuce with scissors or bistoury, as heretofore named. The danger is, that the wound becoming impregnated with the specific pus, is transformed into an immense chancroid. To prevent this, the part should be thoroughly cleansed, and cauterized, the edges of the wound included.

795. If *inflammation* springs up in the case of a chancroid, we employ the same general and local means that we would, if it was located in any other part. The patient should be enjoined to keep quiet, and we prescribe the special sedatives in the usual dose. Here is an excellent field for the exercise of skill in the selection of remedies. Whatever may be indicated by special symptoms, will be found a remedy. I had a very marked illustration of this in a case the past Winter. The inflammation was violent, the phymosed prepuce of a vivid red, with burning heat, and the formation of a few vesicles. Rhus was prescribed with Aconite, and the inflammation yielded in forty-eight hours.

796. The local dressings will vary in different cases. In some it will be a wet dressing with Aconite. In others we pencil the part with Tincture of Veratrum. In some a poultice of powdered Hydrastis. Thus we may take the range of the common topical remedies in such cases.

797. The tendency to sloughing will always be associated with general symptoms indicating special remedies. In some it will be for Sulphite of Soda, Sulphurous Acid, Baptisia, Chlorate of Potash, Iron, Quinine, etc. The local applications will be Sulphurous Acid diluted, and Permanganate of Potash in the proportion of ʒj. to water, Oj. I think these two remedies will be found adapted to the majority of cases.

798. In the early stage of *phagedena*, a very thorough cauterization may arrest the progress of the disease. But if but the smallest spot escapes, furnishing the specific virus, the disease will progress just as soon as the eschar is removed, and we will have accomplished nothing but an increased size of the sore. Notwithstanding such untoward results, it is to be commended as good treatment.

799. If we conclude not to use the escharotics, we will have to choose between Permanganate of Potash, Sulphurous Acid, Sulphate of Zinc, and Tilden's Bromo-Chloralum, as a dressing. Either of these will be found to answer the purpose in some cases; in others, we will find that one after another fails, and we only succeed in arresting the progress of the ulcer when we have reached the disease by internal remedies.

800. The internal treatment will consist in the use of such remedies as may be specifically indicated, with the ordinary restoratives. Iron has been employed in many cases with advantage, and Ricord deemed it a specific for phagedæna. He employed the Potassio-Tartrate, which may be administered in syrup, in the dose of grs. v. to grs. x., three or four times a day. The Tincture of Muriate of Iron, in common use, will answer quite as well, when it is kindly received by the stomach. Here we will find the same indications for the use of Sulphurous Acid, Sulphite of Soda, Baptisia, Chlorate of Potash, Hydrochloric Acid, etc., as in other diseases, and their good effects, when indicated, will be quite as marked.

801. In some cases Quinine is used with good results, as is Opium. Once in a while we find a pill of Opium, at bed

time, will relieve pain, give refreshing sleep, and improve the appearance of the ulcer.

BUBO.

802. By the term bubo we understand an engorgement of the lymphatic glands, first above the seat of the chancre, attended with more or less inflammation. As the common seat of the chancre is upon the external genitals, we find the bubo located in the groin, and as it is so generally associated with syphilis, many persons think that any affection of the glands of this region must be venereal. This, however, is not the case, as they may become affected from common irritation or inflammation of adjacent parts.

803. In chancre upon the penis or vulva, the bubo most generally appears upon the affected side, but not always, for we occasionally see it upon the opposite side. In chancre of the hand, the bubo or enlarged gland will be found at the elbow, and in chancre of the lip, it will be found under the inferior maxillary.

804. It is claimed by late writers on syphilis, that as a general rule the bubo of *chancroid* always suppurates; but that of the hard chancre very rarely does so, but simply remains indurated for a considerable time. And carrying the doctrine still further, some have claimed that chancre with suppurating bubo does not infect the system, while if it is indurated and does not suppurate, the system will surely be affected.

805. These doctrines, though containing some truth, can not be depended upon, though by specious arguments they have seemed to gain ground. I am positive that I have known infection from soft chancre when there was no bubo, and when there was, and it suppurated. Of course no man has had experience that would prove non-infection from non-suppurating bubo. The facts are, that soft chancre is usually attended with such a high grade of inflammatory action of the lymphatic glands, that the tendency to suppuration is very strong, while in hard chancre the tendency is to effusion

of lymph; yet suppuration does frequently occur, and sometimes is very severe.

806. The symptoms of bubo are usually very plain. Some five or six days after the commencement of the sore, if the finger is passed over the inguinal region, a slight enlargement of one or more glands will be observed. They are not adherent to adjacent tissue, but move freely under the skin, and are generally slightly tender on pressure. They enlarge with greater or less rapidity; in some cases a week or more will elapse before inflammation fairly sets in, while in others it progresses with great rapidity.

807. When the glands attain the size of a cherry, inflammation is set up, they are tender on pressure, and painful when the patient is on his feet or walking. In soft chancre the inflammation increases rapidly; adjacent glands become involved, until the swelling will in a week attain the size of a hen's or goose's egg, very sensitive to pressure, painful in walking, or sometimes when lying still. If the part is examined it will be found red, sometimes dusky or livid, and the temperature and sensibility increased. In some cases the inflammation is very high, and all the symptoms severe, the patient suffering very much and being confined to his room. In no case can we determine with much exactness as to the future progress of the disease. Sometimes suppuration is very rapid and only a few days elapse before the pus points; but in others week after week will drag along, and when the abscess is opened suppuration is but partial.

808. In some cases the pus formed resembles laudable pus, and when discharged either by natural process or by puncture, the pain, soreness and inflammatory symptoms subside, and the abscess heals kindly. In others the pus discharged is thin, serous, flocculent, and keeps flowing away without very much abatement of symptoms or tendency to heal. In still others, the swelling of adjacent glands and structures remain, and a process of ulceration goes on until a large foul ulcer is formed in the groin. Occasionally suppuration occurs

at different points, and pus is discharged from several openings, giving, in bad cases, a honeycombed appearance to the groin. In these severe cases the disease at this point may continue for three or four weeks, or as many months.

809. In *indurated chancre*, as has been already remarked, there is not the same tendency to active inflammation, and a simple enlargement and hardness of the glands, lasting for a month or two, is all that is observed. At other times the glands enlarge more, become tender on pressure, and cause pain in walking, but finally with the cure of the chancre the enlargement subsides. In others, inflammation becomes active after a time, and suppuration occurs, presenting the same symptoms as heretofore named.

810. Buboes may be divided into two classes, specific or virulent, and non-specific or inflammatory, though it is impossible to make the diagnosis in many cases. The first arises during the progress of a chancroid, and the connection between the two is usually quite clear. The second may arise from any injury of the parts sending lymphatic vessels to the inguinal glands.

811. Whilst the virulent bubo is usually produced during the progress of the ulcer, this is not always the case, for we sometimes find that the progress of the sore is arrested and it is healing before the glands are much enlarged.

812. It is yet a disputed question whether we may have a primary bubo or not. It is my impression that there are such cases, though they are not frequent. One came under my care in which no ulcer or abrasion of the genitals had been noticed. The bubo formed rapidly, was livid, and gave a simple purulent discharge, but in the course of a week opened deeper, and furnished a specific pus, which was inoculable, and gave rise to a very unpleasant ulceration in the groin.

813. The non-virulent bubo may be caused by any irritation, and is not necessarily the result of impure intercourse. Occurring in the inguinal region, this is always suspected, and a careful examination is made to detect the primary lesion.

814. As before remarked, we have no means of determining a specific from an inflammatory bubo, and we may have either the one or the other from a chancroid. There is first the enlargement of the gland; it then becomes tender and sensitive to pressure; then comes the evidences of heat, pain, redness, and rapid enlargement principally from deposit outside of the gland; and finally suppuration.

815. In the simple inflammatory disease, there is but one abscess, and when the pus is discharged it is inclined to heal readily. In the virulent bubo, however, when the abscess is lanced, it does not run out freely, there is still something at the bottom which rising up closes the opening, and a careful examination will determine that this something is an engorged gland. After a longer or shorter time this also breaks and discharges pus, which is inoculable. Frequently up to this time nothing unpleasant in the appearance of the part has been noticed. Now the edges of the opening become thin and discolored, and a process of erosion is set up, which increases the size of the opening many times, and sometimes exposes the chain of lymphatics lying at the bottom of the abscess.

816. We have to distinguish bubo from hernia, both inguinal and femoral, and though generally easy, sometimes difficulty will be experienced. If the case is seen at an early day, the mobility of the gland, and the absence of succussion upon coughing is sufficient. At an advanced stage, the dusky redness or lividity, thinness of the skin, and long duration of the disease are sufficient. The presence of a chancre, or evidences of there having been one, is the best proof of the syphilitic character of the glandular disease. The presence of a boil, wound, injury, or local inflammation of a part near, or having lymphatic connection with the glands, is evidence of its simple nature. There are cases, however, in which the best observer will be at fault, and will have to wait the development of symptoms before giving a decided opinion.

TREATMENT OF BUBO.

817. Taking the ground that the non-suppurating bubo is followed by constitutional symptoms, some practitioners use means to favor suppuration rather than to discuss the enlargement. It is an error in practice readily accounted for by the nature of the disease, as has been heretofore named, the soft chancre giving rise to suppurating bubo, the hard chancre to indurated bubo. I take the ground that it is good practice to discuss the swelling in all cases, as the patient can not be benefited by the suppurative process in the groin. If the system becomes infected at all, this occurs at the commencement of the swelling, and both experience and analogy teach us that the most minute quantity of syphilitic virus is equivalent, when introduced into the blood, to the total secretion of the chancre. And as no person claims that the suppuration of the glands removes the poison already introduced, there can be no good reason for not arresting it, if possible.

818. Various plans for aborting a bubo have been recommended, but I prefer one of the following: The application of Collodion so as to shield it from the air, is very efficient: I order ℞ Best Collodion, ℥j.; Chloroform, ʒj. to ʒij. Shave the part, and apply the liquid over a space of two or three inches with a camel's hair-brush, until a thick coating is formed. In a couple of days this may be removed and the Collodion reapplied. Another very good application is made by dissolving Gutta Percha in Chloroform, and applying it in the same manner. Or, in the first stage, we may frequently effect its removal by the use of revulsives, as: ℞ Chloroform, Benzine, aa. ℥j.; Alcohol, ℥ij.; two or three thicknesses of lint or cotton cloth being wrung out of hot water, this lotion is sprinkled on it and pressed firmly over the bubo. The most common practice is the repeated application of Tincture of Iodine over the bubo; when I employ it I add half a part of Tincture of Aconite root.

819. The means named should be assiduously employed while there is hope of success. And in addition we use such

general means as experience teaches will counteract the inflammatory process, keeping the bowels open, strict attention to the skin, the alkaline diuretics are important, and we must not forget that rest of the part is indispensable in the severer cases.

820. If, however, the inflammatory process progresses notwithstanding these means, for four or five days, especially if the skin covering the bubo becomes dusky-red or purplish, and thinned, we need not hope to succeed, and we adopt measures to promote suppuration. Some practitioners employ fomentations, others prefer poultices, each of which will prove beneficial. As a poultice we may use Ulmus Fulva, flaxseed, bread and milk, or other simple agents. If we wish to hurry the process, we will find nothing better than grated carrot mixed with milk or water, or we may add a portion of powdered charcoal. If the inflammation is extensive, a decoction of Cornus thickened with wheat bran answers a good purpose.

821. As before remarked, the suppurative process is not unfrequently very slow, and we will often find that suppuration takes place at a limited point, while the inflammatory process progresses around it. I hold it to be good practice to open the abscess as soon as evidence of accumulation of pus is observed, and not wait for the suppurative process in other parts. In most cases we will find that by thus early discharging the pus, the inflammation gradually subsides, and but a small portion of the structures are broken down, while if we had waited there would have been great destruction and a large abscess difficult to heal.

822. As a dressing, after lancing the part, we may use Mayer's Ointment, spread on soft muslin or leather of considerable size, a hole being cut opposite the opening of the abscess. Dr. McCarthy's Soothing Ointment is also an excellent application, and as it is one of our best preparations, I will give the formula for it: ℞ Simple Cerate, Resin, Beeswax, aa. ℥j., melt together in a vessel, and when thoroughly

mixed pour in a porcelain mortar; and, while cooling, add of Gum Camphor, ℥j.; Tincture of Opium, ʒiij.; Turpentine, ʒij.; Oil of Peppermint, gtts. xv.; stirring until cool. The Elder Ointment, or Black Salve, may be used in the same way as the Mayer's Ointment, with good results.

823. As a general rule, if the treatment has been conducted as I have described, the case will progress without trouble; but occasionally it is difficult to manage. Suppuration having occurred, and the abscess opened, adjacent parts break down, the opening increases in size, the skin thins around it, with the entire abscess in a sloughy condition; we may thus in time have a foul ulcer an inch or two in diameter, showing no tendency to heal. It has been recommended to use the Sesquicarbonate of Potash or Sulphate of Zinc, in strong solution, in these cases; but, though sometimes successful, I do not like the practice. Let the part be kept thoroughly cleansed with Soap and Water, give the attention to the general health heretofore directed, and apply the Mayer's or Soothing Ointment, and you will succeed well in very severe cases. If more is needed, paint the edges, or even the entire ulcer, with equal parts of Tincture of Iodine and Tincture of Muriate of Iron, or a solution of one part of Carbolic Acid to eight parts of Water, or a solution of Permanganate of Potash, five grains to the ounce of Water. These last may be used as an injection also. A strong decoction of Baptisia, Cornus or Hydrastis, sometimes answers a good purpose.

824. The lividity and induration remaining after the healing of the bubo is got rid of slowly — sometimes months elapsing before its removal, at others years. To facilitate this process, it has been recommended to use an ointment composed of Simple Cerate, Camphor, and Iodide of Potassium, or the Elder Ointment with the addition of Camphor.

SYPHILITIC VEGETATIONS.

825. We have already noticed the fact that vegetations about the genitals may be the result of gonorrhœal irritation,

or indeed from any persistent irritation of the parts. In these cases the vegetations may propagate themselves both in the individual and in others by contact. Certain of these gonorrhœal growths may retain the specific contagion for a long time, especially in the female.

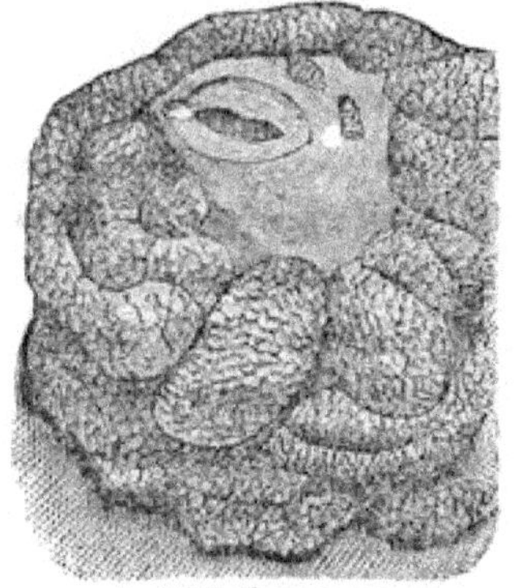
Syphilitic Vegetations.

826. We also find such growths following chancroid, sometimes springing up before the sores are fairly healed. In these cases the warts may be simple, or they may retain the chancroid virus, retaining the inoculable property for many months.

827. Whilst in the majority of cases they are confined to the mucous lining of the genitals, in some they spring up on the skin of the penis, scrotum, perineum, nates, thighs, etc.,

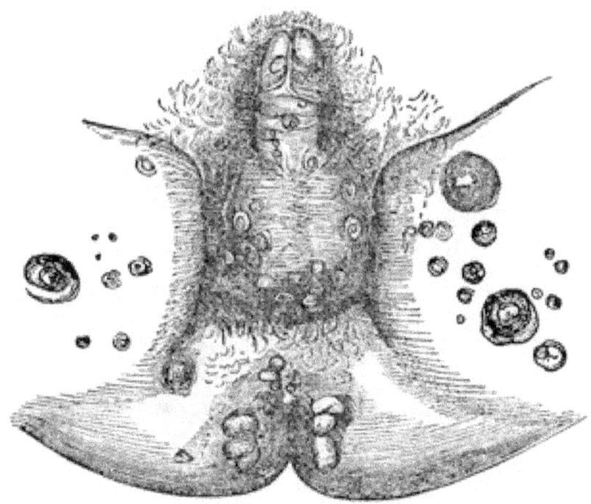
Condylomata.

as in the accompanying illustration. Even in these cases, the growths may be non-venereal, and propagate themselves like similar growths upon the hands. It is safe to conclude, however, that in the majority of cases, they result from impure connection or venereal excesses.

828. TREATMENT.—The treatment will not differ materially from that already given. The careful use of Chromic Acid will destroy the growths, as will the Nitric, Muriatic and Sulphuric Acids. In some cases, the Chloride of Zinc paste may be used, and if the principal growth is thoroughly destroyed, the others will disappear. In the condylomata of the glans and prepuce, the use of the Irritating Plaster to free suppuration, will be found the most effective treatment.

829. When the patient has suffered from syphilis, especially if there are still evidences of disease, the treatment must be directed to this. Alternations of Cod-Oil and Arsenic one week, with Iodide of Potash another, answer an excellent purpose in many of these cases.

CHANCRE.

830. The initial lesion of syphilis has a well marked period of incubation, ranging from two to six weeks. In some cases we will find patients expressing surprise at the appearance of an ulcer, when they have almost forgotten the time of exposure; or when it has appeared after a recent connection with one that they would not suspect, forgetting a previous exposure.

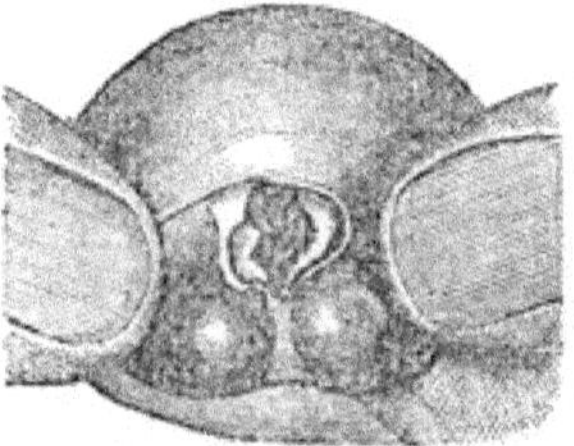

Chancre of the Meatus.

831. The situation of the chancre varies as greatly as in chancroid, and both are more frequent on the prepuce. In four hundred and seventy-one cases observed by Fournier, they were distributed as follows:

Chancres on the glans and prepuce - - - - - -	314
" on the skin of the penis - - - - - - -	60
" on various parts of the penis - - - - -	11
" involving the meatus - - - - - - - -	32
" within the urethra (not visible on forced separation of the lips of the meatus, but recognized by palpation, inflammation of the lymphatics, etc.) -	17

Chancres on the scrotum and peno-scrotal angle	- - - -	11
" of the anus	- - - - - - - - - -	6
" of the lips	- - - - - - - - - - -	12
" of the tongue	- - - - - - - - -	8
" of the nose	- - - - - - - - - - -	1
" of the pituitary membrane	- - - - - -	1
" of the eyelid	- - - - - - - - - -	1
" of the fingers	- - - - - - - - - -	1
" of the leg	- - - - - - - - - - -	1
Total	- - - - -	471

832. As we have already seen the typical chancre makes its appearance as a papule or tubercle, and not as a vesicle or pustule. This nodular engorgement may sometimes be noticed before ulceration, but usually when the patient presents himself for treatment, there is erosion of the epithelium, and secretion of pus. This sore runs a very slow course, does not secrete freely, is not very sensitive, and occasions but little uneasiness. The induration is within the skin or mucous membrane, and rarely involves the connective tissue, hence the ulcer and induration are freely movable upon the tissues below.

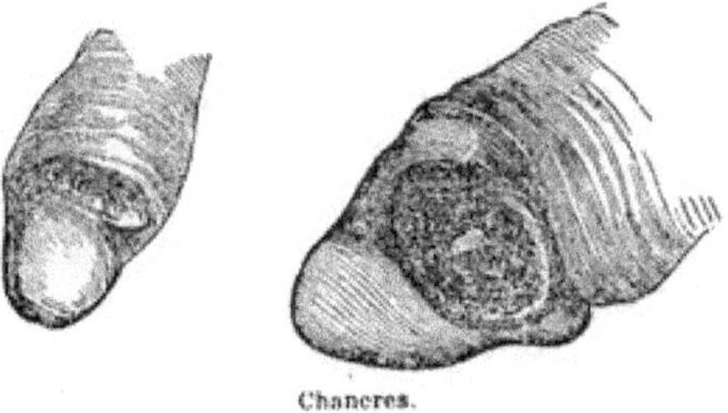

Chancres.

INDURATED OR HUNTERIAN CHANCRE.

833. The induration is distinct from the adjacent tissues, in which it seems imbedded, in shape and size very much like a split pea, and is somewhat elastic like cartilage. If upon the prepuce, it may be grasped and moved in any direction, seeming more like a tubercle than anything else. In a majority of cases it assumes a circular form, is very rarely irregular, and its cavity is cup-shaped, with smooth edges,

sometimes slightly overhanging. It secretes but little pus; in many cases the bottom of the ulcer is covered with a grayish, plastic matter, but in others the entire surface is smooth, and with scarcely any secretion. The edges are sloping, hard and elastic.

In one form of the disease the chancre seems raised above the adjacent tissues, *ulcus elevatum*. According to Vidal, "the base is raised by a kind of vegetation of the form of a rounded or oval basin, of a fungous nature. They occur frequently upon the edge of a prepuce, furnish a sero-purulent matter, generally not painful, and their borders and base but little painful."

834. The quotation from Mr. Erichsen* describes a majority of chancres met with. They are not the typical indurated chancre, and yet there is some induration, which is manifest after the sixth day. They do not furnish the abundant secre-

*"When chancres are caught in connection, they usually commence with a small excoriation, which appears to have been directly inoculated with the specific poison. In other cases, again, though more rarely, they may be seen at first in the shape of a small pointed pustule, which speedily breaks, leaving an ulcer of a specific character in its site. Very generally, however, this pustule escapes observation, and the disease is presented in the first instance as an ulcer. The chancrous ulcer, whatever form it assumes, seldom makes its appearance until a few days—five or six—after connection. In some cases, however, I have observed it, evidently from the infection of a fissure or crack, on the day following impure intercourse, and occasionally, in rare instances, it does not occur until a much later period than that which has been mentioned.

"Whatever may be the appearances presented by a chancre, there can no longer be any doubt that the disease arises from one kind of virus only, the modifications in the sore depending on its situation, the constitution of the patient, and occasionally on that of the individual who communicates the infection. That this is so, is evident from the fact that any chancre, when inoculated, reverts to one typical form, and that, however much chancres may ultimately differ, they all present the same characters during their early stages. The progress of a chancre that has been artificially inoculated on any part of the cutaneous surface is as follows, and its study will serve to elucidate what takes place under other circumstances. During the first twenty-four

tion of soft chancre, and yet are constantly bathed in pus, which is not the case in the typical chancres above described.

835. The hard chancre almost always leaves some induration after it has healed, marking its situation for months, sometimes for years. The common form in which the induration is less marked, may or may not leave induration, depending somewhat upon the treatment. The chancroid rarely if ever leaves induration.

836. It might seem from what has been said that the diagnosis of chancre is easy, and so it is to the expert who has made the disease a special study. But to others it is sometimes a matter of much difficulty. Ulceration simulating chancre sometimes occurs in balano-posthitis, and occasionally ulceration of the follicles back of the corona, resembles it. If, however, the part be closely examined, bearing in mind the description of the disease as above given, a

---

hours after the introduction of the specific pus into the skin on the point of a lancet, we find that some inflammation is set up around the puncture, which becomes hot, red, and itchy. About the third or fourth day, a pointed pustule is produced, which is at first deep-set, but becomes on the following day more superficial, with some depression in the center, resembling pretty closely a smallpox pustule; on close examination this will be found not to be a true pustule, but rather a mass of epithelial scales and pus not included in a distinct wall. On the fifth day it has become hard at the base, apparently from the infiltration of plastic matter, and on the sixth, it has usually dried, forming a small round scab, and leaving an ulcer, which presents the typical characters of a true chancre, being circular and depressed, with a foul, grayish surface that can not be cleansed, sharp cut edges, a hard base, and an angry looking red areola around it. This is the typical chancre, and these are the appearances that every true syphilitic sore on the skin will present, about the fifth or sixth day after inoculation; from this time it may diverge more or less completely from these characters, but will yet, if inoculated at any time during the poisonous stage, produce an ulcer that will run the specific course up to the same period, after which it may in its turn again deviate into one or other of the special forms that chancres occasionally assume. When inoculated on a mucous surface, chancres do not so early assume an indurated character around their base."

mistake can not occur. To avoid error, it is best to treat all suspicious sores upon the genitals, as if they were syphilitic. Secondary syphilitic ulceration may be determined by the existence of other symptoms of constitutional infection.

837. In urethral chancres mistakes are frequently made, as the disease simulates gonorrhœa. Yet in this case it will be noticed that many of the symptoms of gonorrhœa are absent, the discharge is not so great, and close examination will detect induration. In other, though rare cases, a chancre of the lip, hand, or anus, may not be recognized, for the simple reason that the disease is not looked for in those places.

838. Occasionally a case will present itself in which the patient has decided secondary symptoms, without ever having been aware of having had the primary disease. In some of these cases, the chancre is small, secretes but little, is not noticed, and in a week or so nothing but a slight induration can be detected by the practiced eye. In others, the virus is no doubt absorbed without ulceration, and the only evidence of the primary disease is induration of the lymphatic glands, sometimes very slight.

839. Thus, we must agree with Vidal when he says: "Sometimes it must be acknowledged, that notwithstanding the most minute attention to details, and the greatest power of grouping them in one assemblage, which shall represent their diagnosis, the latter still remains obscure, and our doubts are removed only by the appearance of certain consecutive accidents. The young practitioner should therefore be very cautious in announcing his opinion, especially in courts of justice. It is important that he be forewarned, not only that observation may lead to mistakes, but that he should also understand the errors which may result from experiments.*

---

*FORMS OF SYPHILITIC OR INFECTING SORE.—1. *The dry papule* is the rarest form seen by the surgeon; for usually that stage has passed before advice is sought. It is a papular protuberance, varying in size from a pin's head to that of a sixpence, at the point of contamination, of a dark-brown, red, or

840. This chancre is very variable in its duration. It may heal spontaneously in three weeks, and it may be destroyed earlier than this with escharotics and healed at once. But in some cases it will persist for months, despite the treatment.

841. As we have already noticed, there are cases in which the chancre can not be diagnosed from chancroid; this is especially the case with women. I have seen them with sharply cut edges, deep erosion, secreting pus freely, sensitive, complicated with inflammation, attended with suppurating bubo, and not presenting any or but little of the characteristic induration. Such sores may be rare, and yet the fact that they

---

purplish color, round or oval, firm and elastic, sometimes covered with white scales of epithelium or scurf—hence, sometimes it is called a *desquamating papule*.

The induration and the papule sometimes both disappear by resolution or absorption, without ulceration, just as the gummy tumors or nodes disappear in the same way. The induration loses its resistance and elasticity, diminishes in extent and volume, becomes gelatinous, finally subsides, and leaves behind a slight violet, copper, or black depression. These are the most insidious cases; and when secondary phenomena appear, the existence of a primary sore is generally denied, as never having been considered of sufficient importance to attract attention. It may, in fact, never have been seen or noticed in any way.

2. *The syphilitic or hard chancre erosion.* This is the most frequent form in which primary syphilis presents itself. *Patchy excoriation*, or *superficial ulcer* of primary syphilis, or *parchment-like chancre* (Ricord's *chancre parchemine*) are other names by which this form has been described. It commences as a copper-red spot, scarcely raised, papular, and dry. It is covered with a crust or thin scales, which desquamate, and finally the spot becomes eroded or slightly ulcerated on the surface.

The ulceration is circumscribed within the induration, and presents a *flat*, rose-colored surface, projecting on a level with the summit of the swollen part; and is prominent in proportion to the amount of increased volume and induration. If it is pinched up between the finger and thumb, it imparts a feeling as if a bit of parchment had been inserted beneath the surface of the ulcer.

It discharges a small quantity of serous fluid from a diffused base, which is indurated on its surface, rather than deeply. This sore is often so slight, the discharge so little abundant, cicatrization so rapid, that, in the absence of in-are occasionally seen should make us careful in examination and treatment.

842. The period of constitutional infection is not determined. Some authorities claim that syphilis commences by an absorption of the specific virus, and that the chancre is but the first manifestation of the disease from the blood. That being thus constitutional from its commencement, there can be no such thing as an abortion of the disease by local treatment. Others claim that for a short time after the formation of the chancre it should be regarded as strictly a local disease, and that proper means for the destruction of the sore will prevent constitutional infection. The period named in

---

duration of the sore, diagnosis must be doubtful, till some secondary result demonstrates contamination of the system.

This lesion lasts about two months, terminates by resolution and cicatrization, and generally leaves a slight induration, with the corresponding ganglia hard and indolent.

When the papule opens and becomes a sore, the fluid discharged from its open surface has been shown by Hubbenet, Lee and Rollet, to furnish a diagnostic test of the kind of disease, and of the sore from which it proceeds. Sigmund does not go so far as this. He does not consider the sores or chancres so different in form or character as to be at once distinguishable the one from the other. *He waits to see the virus produce* PART *of its effect* upon the system beyond the site of inoculation before he decides as to the nature of the sore. He waits to see the lymphatics indurate. He believes that then, and not till then, the distinction can be absolutely drawn between a sore which will infect the system and one which will not. He believes—(1.) That if induration of the lymphatics does *not* take place within six or eight weeks, and (2) That if repeated successful auto-inoculations can be made on the bearer of the chancre during this period, then it is certain that the sore will not infect the system. If on the contrary, the lymphatics indurate, and auto-inoculations can not then be effected, the sore is assuredly an "infecting" chancre.

The addition to our means of diagnosis from the nature of the discharge—pus from the one, not from the other—is one of great value when it can be made, because the diagnosis as to the probability of subsequent infection may in some cases be made earlier. The distinction, however, is considered by Dr. Berkeley Hill to be untrustworthy, for the following reasons: *First*, the syphilitic virus may be present in a patient suffering with local ulcers also,

which such local abortive treatment will prove successful, is from two to eight days. For my own part I believe there is constitutional infection from the day of exposure, if the person is infected, and though an early arrest of the local disease is desirable, it will not prevent secondary symptoms.

843. TREATMENT.—If there is but one chancre—and this is small and situated on the prepuce—the simplest and best plan is to remove it by excision. Cleansing the chancre thoroughly with soap and water and clean towel, grasp it with the finger and thumb nail below the induration, and excise it with a sharp bistoury. Of course strict attention must

---

and the pus of those ulcers might be inoculable, notwithstanding the presence of general syphilis. *Secondly*, the thin discharge of the ulcerated papule of syphilis is not inoculable on its bearer; nevertheless, if the papule is made to suppurate by any kind of irritation, the pus from it sometimes becomes freely inoculable. The test is therefore considered useless as a guide in diagnosis.

3. *The indurated sore of syphilis—non-suppurating chancre—Hunterian chancre (ulcus vallatum).* Induration is the primary lesion, first as a papule, over which a crust may form, and underneath this crust a cup-shaped ulcer of greater or less depth rapidly develops itself. It is indolent in its progress, and having the appearance of being scooped out; it presents raised and rounded edges, a glossy iridescent surface, a base generally grayish or lardaceous-like, bathed with a serous or watery-like secretion, not reinoculable, and not pus.

This is the most characteristic lesion of commencing syphilis. The induration, which forms the bed of the lesion and base of the ulcer, extends beyond its circumference, and has been compared to the half of a dried pea for hardness. It is elastic, resistent, and cartilage-like, quite different from cicatricial hardness or œdema.

This condition of ulcer lasts about three to six weeks, when the edges of the chancre begin to empty themselves and collapse. The granular particles which covered its base become eliminated or absorbed. At any rate the false membrane-like surface disappears, granulations form, and cicatrization commences from circumference to centre. The resulting cicatrix is round and slightly depressed, and is the seat of induration, sometimes persistent. For a long time it is of a dark-brown or bronze color, and finally all color disappears, and an unnatural whiteness takes its place. *Aitken.*

be paid to cleansing the parts, for if the minutest portion of virus comes in contact with the excised surface, the chancre would be reproduced in a much more severe form. But when done according to direction it must succeed, and the wound heals as speedily as any other clean incision.

844. Escharotics are the means usually made use of to abort the disease, and to accomplish this they must be employed before absorption takes place, and entirely destroy the specific character of the sore. It is most absurd to be continually using caustics after the second week, or when enlargement of the glands is felt, unless it is done for the purpose of more speedily healing the ulcer; and yet we find such practice frequently extending over a period of months. If a first thorough cauterization does not remove the induration, and change the chancre to a simple ulcer, it will not usually be accomplished by repetition.

845. In these cases I prefer one of the three following remedies: Chloride of Zinc Paste, Potassa-cum-Calce, or Nitric Acid. They are used as directed for chancroid, carrying their action so far as to entirely destroy chancre and induration. It is bad practice to half cauterize these chancres, as the specific sore is not destroyed, but rendered more perverse and less amenable to remedies, the induration being increased. It will sometimes require more than one application to accomplish the purpose, but if it is well used, one will generally suffice.

846. A water-dressing, or a poultice, may be employed while the slough is separating, or the sore may be dressed with Mayer's Ointment. After this, we treat it as has been named for soft chancre. Some cases get along better with the use of the wine lotions, others require dry dressings, with Bismuth, and still others heal rapidly under the application of Mayer's Ointment. If cicatrization progresses slowly, and the circulation is sluggish, or the granulations too large, the occasional use of the stick Nitrate of Silver will be found useful.

847. In the *elevated* chancre I employ the Chloride of Zinc paste, to thoroughly destroy it, and then dress it with Mayer's Ointment, occasionally using the solution of Carbolic Acid, or Permanganate of Potash. In the *serpiginous* form, the solution of Persulphate of Iron, or Tincture of Muriate of Iron, will be found good, and as a common dressing a solution of Potassio-Tartrate of Iron, ʒv., to Water, Oj. Tincture of Iodine sometimes proves useful in these cases, or we may combine it with an equal part of Tincture of Iron. Especial attention to the general health is necessary in this form, Quinine, Iron, and a nutritious diet being indispensable.

848. GENERAL TREATMENT. — While we did not consider special medication necessary in soft chancre, in this form of the disease we consider it of prime importance. We have already seen that the constitution becomes affected at least by the eighth day, and that after this the abortive treatment is useless. If this is so, and it can not be disputed, we have something more to do, than simply heal the chancre, as many imagine. We must stimulate the removal of the virus from the system, or destroy it within; the first can be readily ac-accomplished, but we have no specific that will effect the second.

849. Medical men like a treatment that requires no thought, and will adapt itself to every condition. Our Old School friends, many of them, are loth to believe that Mercury is not a specific for syphilis, it was so easy to administer the remedy, which was adapted to all cases, and would grapple with the disease in any part of the body. Those who reject Mercury, replace it with the class of alteratives which they suppose will find the poison and remove it in some inexplicable manner.

850. If we are to succeed in the treatment of syphilis, we must have some well defined plan of action, and give remedies for the accomplishment of certain results. We have no just grounds to look upon any remedy in our Materia Medica

as a specific to the poison of syphilis, and the sooner we realize this fact the better for our practice. What then are the indications, and how may we best fulfill them?

851. Like all other animal poisons the virus of syphilis is removed by the excretory organs, and as in analogous cases the poison affects those tissues, the vitality of which is impaired, rapid metamorphosis of tissue should be stimulated that these parts may be removed, and replaced by new material. All the evidence that has accumulated on the subject of syphilis goes to prove the truth of these propositions, and they are acted upon by the most successful practitioners in this disease.

852. To accomplish the objects named, I would put the patient upon the use of a pill composed of: ℞ Podophyllin, grs. x.; Hydrastin, grs. xx.; Quinine, grs. v.; Extract Nux Vomica, grs. iij.; Vallett's Mass., ʒss. Make twenty pills, of which one may be taken two, three, or four times a day, so as to give a couple of actions from the bowels daily. Let the patient take a daily bath, using soap and water with brisk friction, and if this is not sufficient to get good action from the skin, use the vapor bath two or three times weekly. If the kidneys act well, this will be sufficient; if not, give ʒss. Acetate of Potash in a tumbler of cold water three times a day. In some cases the pills will have to be suspended from time to time, and the patient placed on the use of the Restorative Wine Bitters, with Iron, or Nichols' Elixir of Peruvian Bark and Iron.

853. Under this treatment the patient should have increased appetite and power of digestion, and to replace the rapid waste, a highly nutritious diet should be advised, of beefsteak broiled, roast beef, mutton chops, soft boiled eggs, milk, etc. We intend to renew the body as rapidly as possible, and to obtain as high a degree of health as is possible, and by the time the chancres are healed, the patient will be in vigorous condition, and the syphilitic poison thoroughly removed.

854. I wish it understood, that I object decidedly to the use of alterative syrups and Iodide of Potassium in this stage of the disease, as inefficient to effect the objects named, and a waste of invaluable time to the patient. They will, however, be recommended hereafter in their proper places.

SECONDARY OR CONSTITUTIONAL SYPHILIS.

855. Syphilis, as we have already seen, is, in a majority of cases, a constitutional disease from the first; if not, in a longer or shorter time, the virus is absorbed by the lymphatics or bloodvessels, and the entire system becomes infected. It is sometimes difficult to account for it, as parties protest that they never had chancre, and no marks of it can be found. Yet if we bear in mind, that many times the infecting chancre is small, superficial, and causes no uneasiness, we may readily see that it may have escaped the person's notice, or have been regarded as a simple abrasion. Many cases of chancre get well in a few days without treatment, or they may continue as a slight indurated sore for months, without secretion, or causing the person any uneasiness, and, when unacquainted with the affection, any thought of syphilis. In other cases the primary sore is concealed, situated within the urethra, or a fold of the vulva or anus, or in some situation where it would not be suspected, as upon the lip, hand, etc.; in such cases it may run a regular course without suspicion.

856. The evidence, however, is growing stronger, that secondary symptoms may be transmitted from one to another, under peculiar circumstances. Thus it is now claimed that a party having the constitutional infection may have intercourse with another for a long period without injury, but that some local irritation of the parts from other causes will so concentrate the syphilitic infection that it will be contagious. Thus Vidal remarks: "As to the transmissibility of the secondary accidents, aside from hereditary descent, the doctrine is proved by the fact of the infection of the nurse by the child affected with consecutive tubercles, and the contagiousness of

the mucous tubercle in the adult; it has been proved by the experiments of M. Cazenave, Wallace, Walter, M. Bouley, M. Richett, M. Litthman, by my own, and by those of other experimenters. Under the head of mucous tubercles, experiments have already been mentioned, and when we come to treat of the pustular syphilida we shall find certain facts which leave no doubt on the subject. The distinction, therefore, between the primary and secondary accidents, which rest on their transmissibility—a distinction to which so much importance has been attached—is destroyed both by experiment and clinical observation. Both primary and secondary accidents are inoculable."

857. The virus of syphilis, like other contagious diseases, has a period of incubation in which some of its effects are manifested. If no general treatment has been employed, the first of the secondary symptoms occur, at a somewhat regular period, the mean being about fifty days. In fifty-two cases recorded by Diday, the earliest symptoms appeared in twenty-five days; the greatest length of time elapsing was one hundred and five days. In one hundred and seven cases reported by Bassereau, fourteen occurred between twenty and thirty days, sixty-six between thirty and forty, twenty-three between sixty and ninety, three between ninety and one hundred and twenty, and one in the fifth month.

858. General treatment modifies the disease so much in some cases that this period is greatly protracted, sometimes to months, at others to years. The first symptoms are sometimes so slight and evanescent that they are not recognized by the patient, and this is also a source of error. The following table compiled by Mr. Martin, will show the usual development of the more common syphilitic lesions:

SYMPTOMS.	Date of usual development.	Date of earl'st development.	Date of latest development.
Roseola	45th day.	25th day.	12th month
Papular eruption	65th "	28th "	12th "
Mucous patches	70th "	30th "	18th "
Secondary affections of the fauces	70th "	50th "	18th "
Vesicular eruption	90th "	55th "	6th "
Pustular eruption	80th "	45th "	4 years
Rupia	2 years.	7th month.	4 "
Iritis	6th month.	60th day.	13th month
Syphilitic sarcocele	12th "	6th month.	34th "
Periostitis	6th "	4th "	2 years.
Tubercular eruption	3 to 5 years	3 years.	20 "
Serpiginous eruption	3 to 5 "	3 "	20 "
Gummy tumors	4 to 6 "	4 "	15 "
Onychia	4 to 6 "	3 "	22 "
True exostosis	4 to 6 "	2 "	20 "
Ostitis, changes in the bones and cartilages.	3 to 4 "	2 "	41 "
Perforation or destruction of velum palati.	3 to 4 "	2 "	20 "

859. DIAGNOSIS.—The different manifestations of secondary syphilis will be considered in detail hereafter, and we now wish to consider only the general characteristics of the disease. In a large majority of cases, the first manifestation of it is in the form of an exanthematous eruption upon the skin, frequently as an erythema or roseola, which may be attended with fever. This eruption fades in the course of from two to six days, and leaves the skin dingy, dusky, or dirty. Following this are *maculæ*, at first dusky red, but assuming soon more or less coppery discoloration. They appear first upon the cheeks, nose, forehead, inside of the arms and thighs, and upon the back. Shortly they are associated with lesion of the mucous membrane, as sore throat, passing to ulceration, small excoriations of the lips and edges of the tongue. At a later stage, the hair commences to fall—alopecia, and other of the accidents hereafter named. Dr. Tilbury Fox gives the following points as aids to diagnosis:

860. "The syphilitic poison once introduced into the system is apt to be followed by certain eruptive manifestations: these are only the naked-eye evidences of a deep-seated change in the system at large. The functions of various organs are deranged, the blood is charged with a poisonous principle, and all the organs and structures supplied with that blood suffer to a greater or less extent. The brain evinces its

suffering by mental dejection ; the nerves by a general feeling of prostration and debility . . . . there is often a neuralgia (nocturnal) . . . the pulse is quickened . . . the tongue coated, white, broad, and indented by the teeth. The fauces are more or less congested, the tonsils and soft palate being frequently swollen ; there is irritation of the larynx, producing a mucous cough and often nausea . . . the conjunctiva is congested and muddy, and the whole skin remarkable for its yellowish and dirty appearance, looking as if saturated with impure and discolored humors.

861. "Syphilitic eruptions have certain peculiarities :

"1. There is *a history of syphilitic inoculation*, which tells its tale by the numerous symptoms (due to the circulation of the poison), noticed at the opening of this chapter : and, in addition, by the presence of cicatrices, indurations, scars, and stains about the penis and groin.

"2. *Their color.*—It is described as copper colored ; in reality '*a reddish-yellow brown*' (Wilson). It is dull red at first, and becomes coppery after awhile, and as the eruptions vanish, a dull red or yellowish dirty stain remains for a varying length of time. In the early stages of disease the tint may be violet, but this soon becomes replaced by the coppery hue.

"3. *Their form*, which is peculiarly circular. This feature is not perhaps of much moment, *per se*, but in conjunction with other points is of some aid in a diagnostic sense. It may be destroyed or prevented by the confluence of other patches, but even then the typical form can be recognized in the component parts of the patch of disease. Syphilitic *scaly* eruptions are composed usually of small circular spots. Scales or squamæ are thin, oftentimes very fine, gray, and a few in number ; fewer and lighter than in the typical aspects of eruption. Crusts are thick, greenish, or black, and firmly adherent. Vesicles are flattish, and do not readily rupture. Ulceration is a common feature ; the ulcerated surface is ashy gray, covered with a pultaceous substance, and bounded by sharply cut edges. Cicatrices are whitish and reticulated, or dull and brownish, leaving in their place on disappearance a yellowish stain. Fissuring is marked in the squamous forms.

"4. *The Absence of Pain or Itching.*—With the exception of mucous tubercles and some forms (moist) of infautile syphilis, syphilodermata are generally unaccompanied by heat or pruritis during their existence. In their tubercular forms, just prior to ulceration, a process of softening, apparently depending upon a low kind of inflammation, goes on, and the tubercles may be painful and tender.

"5. *Their Polymorphism.*—This is very characteristic of syphilitic disease. Several different kinds of eruption may co-exist, and this is a rule of general applicability, if we except the squamous class of eruption. It is no unusual thing to see papules, pustules and squamæ co-existent on the same syphilitic subject."—*Dr. Fox on Skin Diseases, p.* 267.

862. PROGNOSIS.—The most important question in the consideration of secondary syphilis is, whether the poison can be entirely removed from the system, so as to leave the person without a taint. Some writers claim that this can not be accomplished; that the present symptoms may be cured, but that sooner or later they will reappear, or at least the system will remain contaminated. I admit that under a mercurial treatment this is the case, for Mercury acts as a mordaunt and fixes the disease in the system, sometimes beyond the possibility of removal. But under the treatment that I shall name, I am satisfied that the virus can be entirely removed, and the patient will be as well as before contracting the disease.

It is even claimed by good observers, that the natural powers of the system, if not interfered with, are sufficient to effect the removal of syphilis. Thus Dr. Bennett says: "For my own part, I believe that the virus of syphilis, if left to itself, and if the health of the patient be attended to, will generally wear itself out. Unfortunately we are only commencing to observe the natural progress of syphilis, and consequently we are unable to determine how long, under ordinary circumstances, it takes to accomplish this."

863. GENERAL TREATMENT.—We take up the constitutional treatment of the disease here, because it will be nearly the same for all syphilitic lesions, and in considering these separately we will notice the necessary modification of it, and the local means to be employed.

864. The poison of syphilis continually reproduces itself, and affects those parts, the molecular life of which is feeble. Thus those persons are most severely affected whose health is impaired, and who contain the largest amount of worn out or devitalized material. We may then claim that it can be removed by getting rid of these old materials, which form its *nidus*, and replacing them with new and highly vitalized material. Experience proves that resistance to diseased action is directly proportionate to the vitality of tissue.

865. The reader will find an explanation of many phenomena of syphilis in my Principles of Medicine, p. 208. It is a disease that involves the nutrition of the entire body, and must therefore be associated with blood making. The germs of the blood are furnished by the lymph, and as is this product so will be the blood and the tissues.

"The syphilitic poison always gains entrance through the lymphatics, and some of the earlier and more constant phenomena are of this system of vessels and glands. I claim that the reason why the disease is so general, so obstinate, and causes such varied and sometimes fearful lesions of nutrition is, because it is a disease of the lymphatic system, and poisons the fountain from which the blood is drawn. I have made a number of examinations upon the cadaver in persons who were suffering from constitutional syphilis, and in every case I found perceptible lesions of the lymphatic glands. In one severe case, in which there was ulceration, nodes, and syphilitic psoriasis, there was not a sound lymphatic gland in the body. This person had died of the syphilitic cachexia.

So confident am I of the correctness of these statements, that I will risk my reputation that no case of secondary or constitutional syphilis can be found in which disease of the lymphatic system is not present.

"If we examine the matter closely, we will see that there is no other way in which we can rationally account for the continuance of the disease as a permanent part of the life of the individual. The ordinary supposition that it is a morbid material in the blood, and governed by the same laws that control other animal miasms, is untenable; for it would be an exception to the rule, that after a longer or shorter time they are *always* removed by the excretory organs. On the contrary, we find that remedies that simply increase secretion do not influence this virus, but, on the contrary, it requires remedies that influence the lymphatic system. So true is it that the lymphatic system is the seat of the disease, that many physicians at once examine certain parts of the body, to determine the condition of the glands, whenever a new case presents. A friend of mine claims that in a very extensive experience, extending over many years, he has never seen a case in which there was not enlargement of the *occipital lymphatic* glands."

866. The indications of cure in secondary syphilis are, then: 1st, To stimulate the excretory organs to increased activity, and promote the removal of worn-out tissues, the seat of the syphilitic poison; and 2d, To replace this material by other products of a high degree of vitality and well formed. As Chambers well remarks, "It is a renewal of life."

Bearing in mind these principles, we will consider separately the various agencies employed in the treatment of the disease.

MERCURY.

867. From the days of Paracelsus it has been claimed that Mercury is an antidote to the poison of syphilis, and the only remedy that can be depended upon for the removal of the poison. Different practitioners have employed different pre-

20

parations of the mineral; thus some use the Bichloride, others the Iodide or Proto-Iodide, some soluble Mercury, some Calomel; it is employed by mouth, by inunction, and as a fumigation. We object decidedly to the employment of mercurials in any case, though admitting that certain symptoms yield speedily to their influence. We ground our objections on the facts: 1st, That it is now clearly proven that Mercury will not cure syphilis; 2d, That it tends to fix the syphilitic poison in the system, and prevents its removal by other remedies; and, 3d, It produces symptoms far worse and more permanent than the disease for which it is given. I might give pages of evidence from Old School men in proof of these propositions, if space would permit, but I will only make a quotation from Dr. Bennett:

868. "The idea that Mercury is a specific for syphilitic poison, and the incalculable mischief it has occasioned, will constitute a curious episode in the history of medicine at some future day. It is now well known that the poison of Mercury produces a cachectic disease and secondary sores in the body, which have been to a great extent mistaken for those of syphilis. It consequently has happened that Mercury, given to cure primary sores, has produced a constitutional disorder closely resembling that of syphilis; more Mercury has then been administered, increasing the mischief, and so the disease has been perpetuated. The real fact, however, is, that the syphilitic poison is no exception to the general rule, which informs us that all contagious diseases of the blood run a certain course, and that we have not yet discovered a specific cure for one of them. The great proof of this is, that the intensity of the disease in modern times has declined exactly in proportion as its treatment by Mercury has diminished, and the disorder been left to follow its natural course. When we treat syphilis on the same principles that we do scarlatina and smallpox, it will prove infinitely less fatal than those disorders."

With reference to the *simple* and *mercurial* methods he remarks:

869. "Both kinds of treatment have now been extensively tested. In the year 1822, the Royal Council of Health in Sweden having been charged by the king to conduct a series of experiments upon the different modes of treating venereal diseases, reports from all the civil and military hospitals were ordered to be drawn up annually. These reports establish the inconveniences of the mercurial system, and the superior advantages of the simple treatment. In the various hospitals of Sweden, 40,000 cases had been under treatment, one-half by the simple method, the remaining half by Mercury; the proportion of relapses had been, in the first class, seven and a half, in the second thirteen and two-thirds, in one hundred. Dr. Fricke's experiments in the Hamburg General Hospital were first made public in 1828. In four years, out of 1649 patients of both sexes, 582 were treated by a mild mercurial course, and 1067 without Mercury; the mean duration of the latter method was fifty-one days, and that by Mercury eighty-five. He found that relapses were more frequent, and secondary syphilis more severe when Mercury had been given. When the non-mercurial treatment was followed, they rarely occurred, and were more simple and mild when met with. He tells us that he has treated more than 5,000 patients without Mercury, and has yet to seek cases in which that remedy may be advantageously employed. He has never observed caries, loss of the hair, or pains in the bones follow his treatment, and in all such cases which have come under his care, much Mercury had been given.

870. "In 1833, the French Council of Health published the reports sent in by the physicians and surgeons attached to regiments and military hospitals in various parts of France. Some of the reports are in favor of a mild mercurial course, others in favor of simple treatment. They all agree in stating the cure by Mercury to be one-third longer than by the other treatment. At Strasburg, Mercury was only given to very

obstinate cases. Between 1831 and 1834, 5271 patients had been thus treated, and the number of relapses and secondary affections calling for the employment of Mercury was very small. No case of caries, and only one or two instances of exostosis, had been observed. Full reliance may be placed on these facts, as regiments remain in garrison at Strasburg for five or six years.

871. "In the various reports now published, more than 80,000 cases have been submitted to experiment, by means of which it has been perfectly established that syphilis is cured in a shorter time, and with less probability of inducing secondary syphilis, by the simple than by the mercurial treatment."

872. Mercury partly fulfills one of the requisites of a remedy for syphilis—it breaks down devitalized tissue; when it increases secretion to such an extent as to cause its removal, it fulfills the first indication of cure. Acting in this way it may as is claimed, assist in the cure of an indurated chancre, when common means fail. The second indication of cure it does not fulfill in any degree, but in many cases retards the nutritive process.

873. But however much we may object to the general use of Mercury, or the common use of the drug in syphilis, we can not shut our eyes to the fact that it sometimes accomplishes results that are not attained by other means. I have known many practitioners who had been educated to believe that the non-mercurial treatment was not only the safest, but the most successful, try those remedies without effect, and see the cases pass into the hands of a neighboring physician who gave speedy relief with small doses of his Proto-Iodide of Mercury. The chagrin that follows such an experience is not very pleasant, and the young doctor will not unfrequently reach the conclusion that he has been imperfectly taught, or willfully deceived.

874. These experiences come in part from imperfect teaching, and recipe practice—" Here is the disease, *secondary*

syphilis, and for this you should give *Compound Syrup of Stillingia and Iodide of Potash.*" This is followed by a peroration on the wonders of the Eclectic practice, and denunciation of Mercury as the bane of life, the intensifier of syphilitic disease, and probably the cause of all its horrors. The means proposed for the cure of such a protean malady is ridiculous, and must of necessity lead to failure; and though the denunciation of Mercury is just in the main, having reference to its indiscriminate use, it is soon seen to be overdrawn, when the student is enabled to use his own eyes. I doubt whether any good comes from such teaching, and I propose to state clearly what results may be witnessed from the administration of Mercury in syphilis, always premising that they may be obtained quite as well or better in the majority of cases, by a skillful use of other remedies.

875. In the case of an indurated chancre, that will not heal, and probably is already associated with syphilitic maculæ, and ulceration of mouth and throat, Proto-Iodide of Mercury, to the amount of one to three grains daily, will sometimes relieve all the unpleasant symptoms in two or three weeks, and the sore heals without trouble. In some of the unpleasant skin diseases we meet, as early secondary symptoms, the ordinary remedies fail, the patient presents an unpleasant appearance, and becomes discouraged—small doses of Mercury give speedy relief, and the skin resumes its natural condition. In this way we might go through the entire catalogue of secondary syphilitic lesions.

876. Reverse the picture, and you will see results the very opposite. The chancre becomes more persistent, the lymphatics more involved, the skin disease grows rapidly on the mercurial diet, the hair falls out, the throat ulcerates, and there is tendency to destruction of the soft palate, and in the nasal cavities, nodes spring up and become very painful, syphilitic periostitis results, and presently we have the destructive lesions of the bones. The evidence that Mercury

has intensified all these lesions, is quite as marked in this case as that it proved curative in the other.

877. What shall we say to a drug of this character? Most certainly wisdom would dictate that it should not be employed until it was possible to determine the cases in which it would prove curative, from those in which it proves harmful. Such a study has not yet been made, indeed it has not been attempted by those who use Mercury as a specific for syphilis, though it would seem to be an easy matter as we study the action of drugs.

878. So far as my observation goes, I would say that the anti-syphilitic action of Mercury is manifest only when there is strength of circulation, and good nutrition, secretion, and innervation. Such a condition would be marked by a strong pulse, moderately hard, florid mucous membranes, and a free secretion of urine containing abundance of urea. The unpleasant symptoms come in those cases marked by atony of mucous membranes, impaired nutrition and secretion, and an enfeebled circulation. Given a broad, full, pallid tongue (leaden pallor), and Mercury will develop the most fearful symptoms. Given a full, oppressed pulse, with evidence of enfeebled capillary circulation, and there is no bad result catalogued that you can not obtain from Mercury. Given a cloudy urine containing an excess of phosphates, mucus, or albumen, and Mercury will give constitutional symptoms rapidly.

879. This is the study of one who does not employ the drug, or recommend it; if those who believe it is the *specific* for syphilis will continue it until they can tell us definitely the cases in which it will prove curative, they will have accomplished a very desirable object in the therapeutics of syphilis.

PREPARATIONS OF IODINE.

880. It is claimed that Iodine and some of its preparations are *anti-syphilitic*, or, in other words, act as antidotes to the poison. As heretofore stated, there are no specifics for the

disease, and we must see how it fulfills the indications of cure before named. These remedies facilitate the metamorphosis of tissue, breaking down imperfectly vitalized material, and in a marked manner they stimulate secretion. We thus see that they accomplish the first object of cure. In some cases they stimulate digestion and nutrition, and then they would fulfill all the requirements of remedies for the disease. They fail in their action—first, by not stimulating the excretory organs in the proportion that they break down tissue, and hence we have to aid them by such of the vegetable alteratives as do promote secretion. Second, in many cases they impair the nutritive processes, and in these it is necessary to use the bitter tonics, Iron, and a highly nutritious diet.

881. If these remedies had been studied with sufficient care we might point out the special indications for the class, and for the individual agents. As used at present, they may often do much harm, and I have seen quite serious disease result from the abuse of Iodide of Potassium, as well as from Mercury.

882. Iodide of Potassium seems to exert a specific influence in those cases which show pallidity of mucous membranes, especially when the tongue is full, doughy, with a leaden pallor. The full atonic skin with leaden pallor is also a very good indication for this Iodide. In such cases I would advise its use in the proportion of grs. v. to grs. xxx., four times a day. It need not be admixed with any "compound syrup," or unpleasant vehicle, and serves its purpose quite as well when prescribed in powder, to be solved in considerable water when taken.

883. The Iodide of Ammonium is io be preferred, where nutrition is enfeebled, and especially where there is impaired innervation. Given, pain as a symptom of syphilis, and we always think of this iodide. Especially is this the case with nocturnal pains, hemicrania, nodes, etc. There is a peculiar curled tongue, which may be regarded as an indication for this remedy.

884. The Iodide of Lime, Iodide of Starch, Iodide of Iron and Iodoform, have each their use in the direction first pointed out, but we are not able to point out special indications for their use.

SALINE DIURETICS.

885 In some cases we find that the system is more rapidly freed from the syphilitic poison by the class of renal depurants. The cases are those in which the nutritive processes are active, and the principal object is to increase retrograde metamorphosis and excretion. These cases will be marked by a free circulation, a healthy appearance of mucous membrane, and good capillary circulation. In some of them there is excitation of the pulse demanding Veratrum, and it should precede, or be used with this class of remedies.

Acetate of Potash may be taken as the type of the renal depurants, and may be used in the proportion of two to six drachms daily, with an abundance of water.

THE WATER CURE.

886. We cure some cases of syphilis with diluents alone, applying the water inside instead of out, or as well as out. There is no mistake but that the syphilitic poison may be washed out of the body, and much of the benefit of the old-fashioned decoctions depended upon this. The cases are those in which the vegetative functions are well performed, and any excess of fluid is rapidly removed by action of the skin and kidneys.

887. In some of these cases simple cold water will answer the purpose as well as anything else, especially in the Summer time. The patient has a bath in the morning, and is then thoroughly rubbed, and continues to drink freely through the day. This may be alternated with some diaphoretic infusion (weak), as of Asclepias, one day, and a diuretic, as Eupatorium Purpurea, the next day, water the third day, and so on.

888. Many of the so-called vegetable alteratives are only beneficial when given in weak infusion, and in large quantity. I had a curiosity once to try a "Zittman's decoction," without the Mercury, and found that the two pints daily had quite as good an influence as the original. So it is with Sarsaparilla, Stillingia, Corydalis, Scrofularia, Iris, etc.; in the ordinary sirup these are almost worthless.

889. We not only find an important use for water internally, but we also employ it externally as a curative means. The wet-sheet pack, with cold douche and brisk rubbing will be found a valuable adjunct in any form of treatment, where the circulation of the skin is vigorous. The hot-blanket pack is successfully used, in some other cases, when an increased activity of skin is desirable. In some cases, we employ an alkaline bath, in others an acid bath, being governed by the usual indications.

VEGETABLE ALTERATIVES.

890. All of this class of remedies that have proven useful in syphilis, stimulate the secretions in a greater or less degree. They favor metamorphosis of tissue, but do not exert the same influence in breaking it down as the agents heretofore considered. Many of them also improve the nutritive processes, and aid in renewing the structures of the body. It will thus be seen that they fulfill all the indications in the cure of syphilis, and were they sufficiently active we would need no other remedies. The fact is—and we may just as well recognize it—that their action is feeble in all these aspects, and must be assisted by other means. Thus we render their action on the excretory organs more decided, by remedies that act in this way; by the addition of the Salts of Iodine or Potash we give them greater power over the worn-out tissues; and by the addition of tonics and stimulants we renew the tissues more rapidly.

891. They will cure syphilis without any aid, but many times their action is so slow as not to be available in practice,

if used alone. Hence the importance of a judicious combination of other remedies with them. If we desire their greatest influence, I am satisfied that they must be employed in infusion, as their action is much more decided when employed with considerable quantities of water. This class of remedies is quite large, and we have not space to consider all of them. More is not necessary, for every practitioner has his Dispensatory or Materia Medica at his elbow. I will therefore name the more important.

892. I place Podophyllum and its preparations at the head of the class, as being more generally useful, and fulfilling the indications to a greater extent than most others. It may be employed in powder, in doses just sufficient to act on the bowels; or first give sufficient to produce its full action, and afterward in small doses. I would prefer it, however, in the following or similar form: ℞ Podophyllum, Hydrastin, Spearmint, aa. ℥ss.; Boiling Water, Ojss. Let it digest for two hours, and give in wineglassful doses sufficiently often to act gently on the bowels. Other alteratives may be combined with it, and it is well to get it of such strength that the patient may take a pint in the twenty-four hours. Of course, it is not pleasant medication to thus use infusions, but it is very successful. Podophyllin is much employed in syphilis, the internal treatment recommended for indurated chancre being one of the most successful practiced in all forms of the disease. The following formula for its use will be found as good as any: ℞ Podophyllin, grs. xx.; Hydrastin, grs. xl.; Quinine, grs. x.; Extract of Conium, ℨj. Make forty pills, the dose being one, two or three times a day.

893. Corydalis, Stillingia, Alnus, Scrofularia, Rumex, Ampelopsis, Phytolacca and Kalmia, are among our best alteratives in this disease. In severe cases I employ them in infusion, one or more together, alternating them from week to week. We use them associated with the salts of Iodine and Potash, and with bitter tonics and restoratives.

TONICS AND RESTORATIVES.

894. These are very important means in the treatment of secondary syphilis, fulfilling the second indication of cure, the renewal of the structures of the body. It must not be supposed, however, that they are useful alone—there must first have been a breaking down of tissue—then its removal, before these remedies are indicated; or they may be employed together. After a long course of vegetable alteratives and Iodide of Potassium, which seems to do but little good, the administration of Hydrastin, Quinine, Nux Vomica and Iron, will effect a rapid cure. Iron is of especial importance in depraved states of the system, or when the blood is dark colored in the veins, and should be used freely. Cod-liver Oil answers a good purpose in the worst of these cases.

895. Any of the bitter tonics may be employed; in fact, we will find use for many of them, as the remedies are best alternated every week or so. With the improvement of the appetite and digestion, let the patient have a highly nutritious diet, taken in moderation, but proscribe all pastry and indigestible food.

896. In the treatment of most forms of chronic disease the bitter tonics play a very important part. In fact, the treatment frequently resolves itself into the use of means to establish secretion from the skin, kidneys, and bowels, and the bitter tonics to improve the appetite and digestion; and just in proportion as these are accomplished is the recovery of the patient. The cure of disease is really a renewal of life. This will be more apparent if we reflect that all action is resultant from change of matter, and vital action from change in organic forms. A healthy organization must give rise to healthy action, as a defective organization will cause diseased action. If this is so, we may expect abnormal nutritive changes whenever we find morbid action.

897. Reasoning from these premises, we would adopt such plan of treatment as would remove old structures and replace

them by new, and in this way obtain healthy action by having healthy tissues. In many diseases, a systematic treatment looking to these ends accomplishes wonderful results. The man literally rotten with syphilitic disease has his flesh restored as in childhood, and is freed from all his aches and pains; the scrofulous child becomes hale and robust, and the consumptive, even, gains new life and vigor.

898. It is necessary that the old tissues be removed in a quiet manner, so as to create but little disturbance of function, and at the same time that the digestive organs shall well prepare material for its replacement. In health the soft tissues are renewed as often as every four or five months; in disease this process of renewal is checked to a greater or less extent. In proportion as it is checked are the tissues old, effete, and unfitted for use. And not only so, but in enfeebled states of the system, the nutritive processes being enfeebled, the tissues then made must possess a lower vitality than in health. Thus, as disease progresses, we have first molecular debility, sickness and death, until finally the power to resist decomposition is so enfeebled that entire death results.

899. If the tongue is persistently coated, somewhat broad and pasty, I premise the use of tonics with a thorough emetic, and follow with laxative doses of Podophyllin and Leptandrin. Occasionally, in a very stubborn case, the emetic will have to be repeated once or twice a week for some time. If the coating is not so constant, we may attain the desired end by the use of Sulphite of Soda, or Acetate of Potash, or even Bicarbonate of Soda.

900. If, however, the tongue is red and slick, as we find it in another class of stubborn cases, I generally give the liquor Bismuth, a teaspoonful every three or four hours. I have never employed a remedy that has given more satisfactory results than this. It is applicable, no matter what the condition of the bowels, but is especially useful if there is a ten-

dency to diarrhœa. In its stead I might use an infusion of Epilobium, or of Peach Tree Bark.

901. One of the best, and at the same time the cheapest, tonic preparations is: ℞ Hydrastis (powd.), ℥ss.; Carbonate of Iron, ʒj.; Tincture of Xanthoxylum, ʒij.; Water, ℥xiv. M. Shake well, and give a tablespoonful four times a day. As a stomachic, especially in atonic conditions of the stomach, I have never seen its superior; and, though seemingly unpleasant and crude, the stomach will tolerate it better than most remedies of the same kind, or than any other preparations of Hydrastis.

902. An excellent preparation of Hydrastis will be found in the following: ℞ Hydrastis, Cornus, Prunus Vir., Matricaria Chamomilla, crushed, aa. ℔j. Put in a percolator, and pour on four pints of Dilute Alcohol; then add Boiling Water until the fluid measures one and a half gallons. Bring this to the boiling point, and add Sugar, six pounds. The dose is from a tablespoonful to a wineglassful.

903. When there is great irritability of the stomach I like the action of the Matricaria Chamomilla. It is very mild, rarely disagrees with the stomach, and is yet quite effective. Occasionally a cold infusion will be found an excellent vehicle for the administration of the stronger tonics. A cold infusion of Prunus possesses somewhat similar properties, as does an infusion of the common Peach Tree Bark.

904. The Collinsonia is a favorite of mine, especially in dyspepsia, diseases of the heart, respiratory organs, and kidneys. I generally order: ℞ Fluid Extract of Collinsonia, Simple Syrup, aa. ʒij. A teaspoonful four times a day. It controls irritation of the pneumogastric nerves in a very marked manner; hence its importance in diseases of organs supplied by this nerve. A form of laryngeal disease, very persistent, and which I have called irritative laryngitis, is most effectually relieved by this remedy. The affection is attended by irritation, tickling cough, and huskiness of voice, from singing, public speaking, etc.

905. We then have cases which demand stronger remedies than these, especially those which give increased innervation; Quinine, Strychnine, Iron, and Phosphorus, variously combined, answer a good purpose. The following will be found a good formula: ℞ Quinia Sul., grs. xx.; Strychnia, gr. j.; Sulphate of Iron, ʒss.; Dilute Sulphuric Acid, ʒij.; Syrup to ℥iv. Or: ℞ Quinia Sul., grs. xx.; Solution of Strychnia, ʒij.; Dilute Phosphoric Acid, ʒss.; Phosphate of Iron, ʒj.; Syrup to ℥iv. Either of these formula will answer an excellent purpose, and will be found especially useful in malarious regions, as the Quinine in this form, associated with Strychnia, is an excellent prophylactic, as well as curative.

906. We have also used this formula very largely, especially in syphilitic diseases, as well as those of a malarious character. It is the most powerful combination for this purpose we have ever employed, and has but one objection—its cost.: ℞ Ferri Sulph., ʒi.; Soda Phos., ʒvi.; Quinia Sul., grs. 192; Sul. Acid Dil., q. s.; Aqua Ammonia, q. s.; Strychnia, grs. vi.; Acid Phos. Dil., fʒxiv.; Sacch. Alba, ʒxiv. Dissolve the Sul. Iron in ʒi. of Boiling Water, and the Phos. Soda in ʒij. of Boiling Water. Mix the solutions and wash the Precip. Phos. Iron until the washing is tasteless. With q. s. Dil. Sul. Acid dissolve the Quinine in ʒij. of Water, precipitate the Quinine with Ammonia and carefully wash. Dissolve the Phos. Iron and the Quinine thus obtained, as also the Strychnia, in the Dil. Phos. Acid, and then add the Sugar, and dissolve the whole without heat.

907. I employ Strychnia quite frequently, and value it highly for its tonic, stomachic, and stimulating properties. I use the solution in this form: ℞ Strychnia, gr. ij.; Acetic Acid, gtts. x.; Dilute Alcohol, fʒss. In prescribing it I order of this, fʒi. to fʒij. of Syrup, the dose being from one-half to one teaspoonful four times a day. The Citrate of Iron may be added to the solution as in this formula: ℞ Solution of Strychnine, ʒj.; Citrate of Iron, ʒj.; Water, ʒiv. Dose, a teaspoonful every four hours.

NITRIC ACID.

908. I have used, and recommended Nitric Acid in some cases of syphilis with excellent results. The special indication for the remedy with me, is a violet color of tongue, or whereever arterial blood shows itself. It is given in the usual proportion: ℞ Nitric Acid, gtts. xl.; Water, Sirup, aa. ℥ij.; a teaspoonful every three hours. This was employed in the olden time with good results, as the following quotation from Dr. Good will show:

"How far it exercises a chemical power upon the syphilitic virus, and forms a new and blander substance with it, is uncertain. Its general effects are, as we might expect them to be, tonic and sedative; whenever the appetite is increased, a greater rigidity or firmness is given to the living fibre, and a greater density to the coagulable lymph; the action of the bowels, and even of the bladder, being diminished. Besides these, it has a particular effect on the mouth approaching to that of ptyalism, for the gums are rendered slightly sore, the mouth and tongue become moist. Under this change the syphilitic symptoms assume a better appearance, and especially those belonging to the primary set."

ARSENIC.

909. Arsenic is only employed in a later stage of the disease, when the symptoms are very stubborn, the general health much impaired, and the nutritive processes feeble. Though objectionable, it is less so than Mercury, as its influence is but temporary, and it does not produce those grave lesions that have rendered Mercury such a fearful agent. It is claimed that when the assimilative processes are very feeble, and there is strong tendency to molecular death, it acts as a powerful tonic and restorative. However this may be, those who employ it only claim that it assists in the cure, aiding the action of vegetable alteratives, bitter tonics, and Iron.

910. In *small* doses, and when indicated, Arsenic may be regarded as a vital stimulant, and one of the most powerful of this class. But we must not forget that the dose *must* be small, and there *must* be special indications for its use. What are these indications?

911. In that condition of the blood, and of nutrition, where there is a tendency to the deposit of a low or imperfect albuminoid material—yellow tubercle, caseous deposits—or degeneration of tissue, Arsenic may be used as a blood-maker, and especially to improve nutrition.

912. A class of skin diseases depending upon such deposits, or an enfeebled nutrition, is cured by Arsenic. Among these are the more chronic affections—the squamæ, the chronic vesiculæ, some of the pustulæ, and the tuberculæ. It will not cure all cases, it will do harm if injudiciously used, but it affords relief in many otherwise intractable.

913. But it should never be employed where there is irritability of the nerve centers, and especially of the sympathetic. This rule I think is absolute, and must be constantly regarded. Arsenic is a *nerve-stimulant;* quite as much so as Phosphorus, with this addition—that its action is greatly intensified when there is already erythism of the nerve centers.

914. It has been successfully employed in some cases of phthisis, presenting the conditions above named. Prof. Howe uses it in combination with Veratrum, and there is no doubt that this renders the system tolerant of Arsenic where it could not otherwise be employed.

915. Arsenic is topically employed to destroy malignant growths. The majority of the "cancer specialists" use it in some form, and their preparations differ only in the inert material with which it is combined. The preparation now employed most frequently is made as follows: Take Hydrated Sesquioxide of Iron a sufficient quantity, throw it on a paper filter, and when of the consistence of an ointment, add an equal part of Lard. To this add Arsenious Acid, in the proportion of ʒss. to ʒj. to the ounce.

916. Arsenic may be employed in the treatment of some cases of intermittent fever with excellent results. They are those marked by impairment of sympathetic innervation, and with a general want of nervous excitability. The dose should be very small, gtts. v. to x. of Fowler's Solution to ℥iv. of Water; a teaspoonful every two to three hours. I have used the Homœopathic pellets, medicated with Fowler's Solution, and though the dose was not more than the twentieth to the one-hundredth of a drop, the effect was marked, where specially indicated.

917. It is also used with advantage in atonic diarrhœa, with indigestion, the conditions being as above named. Especial benefit has been observed in those cases in which there were periods of great depression, followed by hectic fever.

918. I need hardly say in conclusion, that Arsenic is one of those agents that will do either good or harm. Good if given in a proper case, and in medicinal doses; harm if not indicated by special symptoms, or contra-indicated as above named, or if given in poisonous doses.

919. Fowler's Solution is the preparation to be preferred. Dose from the fraction of a drop to two drops.

CHLORIDE OF GOLD AND SODA.

920. If a practitioner of our School finds a case in which he would like to try a mercurial, but is restrained by prejudice, he generally uses this salt. I doubt whether its influence is different from the Proto-Iodide or Bichloride of Mercury, other than it is not so active. A single case coming to my notice in which the drug had been pushed to its poisonous action, showed clearly that it had an influence for evil as well as good. Prof. King thus describes its use:

"The Chloride of Gold and Soda, in large doses, is a corrosive poison, in small medicinal doses it is endowed with general stimulant and diuretic properties, acting also as an energetic alterative. It has been highly recommended in primary and secondary syphilis, scrofulous and herpetic affections, goitre, scirrhous tumors, ophthalmic affections, dropsy, etc. It is principally used among physicians as an antisyphilitic; in which it is of decided efficacy. In four cases where some of the virus from chancres had accidentally lodged in the eye, producing symptoms threatening a loss of that organ, I saved the eyes by bathing them several times a day, with a wash made by dissolving seven grains of the Chloride of Gold and Soda in a fluid ounce of distilled water; likewise using the salt internally. The dose internally is from one-twelfth to one-thirtieth of a grain, which may be given in pill form or in solution, thus,—Dissolve two grains of Mur. Gold and Soda in a fluid ounce of water, of which the dose is ten or fifteen drops every two or three hours. For pills, mix two grains of the Salt of Gold, with one drachm of powdered Starch, Lycopodium, or Orris Root, and form into a pill mass with a sufficient quantity of Gum Arabic in solution; divide into forty pills, each of which contains one-twentieth of a grain of the Gold-Salt. Or, it may be given in powder made by rubbing together one grain of the Salt with one drachm of White Sugar, or Sugar of Milk, and dividing into twelve, fifteen, or twenty powders, according to the dose required. It has, however, been given in doses of from one-sixth to one-half a grain, three times a day, and without any unpleasant consequences; but when such doses are prescribed, its action should be carefully watched, and its administration be suspended for a time. Its effects upon the system in over doses, or when the patient contracts cold while under its influence, are said to be equally as severe and dangerous as those following the use of Corrosive Sublimate, under the same circumstances. Externally, it may be applied to scrofulous and syphilitic ulcers, in solution, or made into an ointment with prepared Lard, in the proportion of seven or nine grains to the ounce of Water or Lard."

BATHS.

921. The employment of appropriate baths does much to assist the cure. The skin being one of the most important emunctories of the body, and the part through which the largest portion of the poison is removed, as is manifest by its frequent disease, we may readily see how much may be effected in this way. The object is to keep the skin continually active, but not to so stimulate it as to lead to exhaustion. We sometimes employ Soap and Water, Saleratus Water, or Salt, using the bath daily, or less frequently. If the skin is dry and harsh, oleaginous frictions at night, with Soap and Water in the morning, answer an excellent purpose. If relaxed and flabby, a decoction of Hydrastis, Cornus, or Oak Bark, with or without stimulants, is appropriate treatment.

922. In severe cases, especially where the skin is affected, vapor, hot-air and medicated baths prove serviceable. A vapor bath is very easily given. Take a bucket of hot water, or what is much better in these cases, a strong decoction of Tansy or Smartweed, put it under a wooden bottomed chair, on which the patient is seated, draw a blanket around him, and put a hot iron or brick in the water to produce the amount of steam required. Alteratives may be employed in this way with good advantage in skin disease. The hot-air bath is the spirit-vapor bath heretofore described. A medicated vapor bath is often of service. A very convenient way to give them is to have a wire frame attached to a spirit lamp, to hold the tin or iron plate two or three inches above the flame. The patient being stripped and placed on a wooden bottomed chair, is surrounded with a blanket, fastened closely around the neck and dropping to the floor. Alcohol is burned under him until perspiration is started, when the plate containing the medicine is placed over the flame. Sulphur is an excellent stimulant to the skin when used in this way, and we obtain an excellent influence from Iodine.

923. The means I have named are associated in varying proportion, according to the condition of the patient and the effect desired. I have refrained from giving formula, as I do not wish to place any obstacle in the way of a rational practice in this disease, preferring to present plainly the indications of cure and the action of those remedies that we employ to effect it. I can vouch for the success of the plan named, as it is based upon an extended experience in my own practice and that of others, and feel satisfied that it will meet the expectations of our practitioners.

LESIONS OF SECONDARY SYPHILIS.

924. Most writers upon the subject have divided the symptoms of constitutional syphilis into two forms, *secondary* and *tertiary;* but I have never been able to see the importance of such classification. The syphilitic poison is single in its nature, and although, as time passes, it manifests itself in different forms, it still requires the same general treatment.

925. In its pathology it approximates the degenerations, and may be properly classed with them. It is the opinion of the best observers, that the initial lesion of secondary syphilis is of the lymphatic system, and from this the entire mass of the blood, and eventually all the tissues of the body become syphilized. My opinion with regard to this will be found in the quotation from my Principles of Medicine, already given.

926. But whether this is true or not, the disease of the blood which all admit, must work a continuous depravation of the tissues. As is the life and development of the blood, so is the life and development of the tissues. If the blood is good, and contains a good albumen for nutrition, the tissues will be good. If the blood is depraved, or its organization lessened or imperfect, the tissues will be depraved and imperfect.

927. Thus as the syphilitic virus influences the blood more and more, and the materials of repair become syphilized, the tissues built of this material become syphilitic. This is not

only good in theory, but observation of the symptoms shows that it is true in fact.

928. The symptoms of syphilis, in many cases, are evidently those of degeneration. The skin has the unpleasant, sallow color, and loses its elasticity. The muscular system shows it in every movement of the body, and many times we will find all the tissues of the body sitting upon the bones like an ill-fitting suit of clothes. The movements and expressions of the patient will frequently tell the story of degeneration, as he walks into the office, and before he has opened his mouth.

SYPHILITIC FEVER.

929. I believe observation will show that the manifestations of secondary syphilis are always preceded by febrile phenomena, more or less distinct. This we should suspect, from an examination of the pathology of the disease. Whether the absorption of the virus is by the lymphatics, or the capillary blood-vessels, the ultimate lesion is one of the blood, and the influence is to impair this fluid. Such impairment always, so far as we know, produces febrile symptoms.

930. Since my attention has been called to this subject. I have examined three cases of syphilis with the thermometer, and in each the secondary symptoms were announced by an elevation in temperature; in two to 101½° and 103° respectively. In the three there was evidence of impaired digestion, blood-making, nutrition, excretion, and innervation corresponding to the increase of temperature, and such as we might expect in ordinary fevers.

931. In so far as my memory serves me, I do not recollect a single case in which the usual impairment of the vegetative functions common to the prodroma of fever, did not precede the recognized outbreak. In some it was not noticed, because many times so slight that patients do not apply to the physician, until there is a distinct syphilitic manifestation.

932. I conclude farther, that the earlier syphilitic skin diseases may be classed with the eruptive fevers, the blood being partially freed from the morbid material by such eruption. I do not wish to be understood as ignoring the *specific* character of the virus, or its specific results, or the necessity of special means in its treatment, but I think it well to point out these features of the disease as suggestive of the character of an early treatment.

933. As above stated, the outbreak of secondary syphilis is preceded by an impairment of the functions of vegetative life. The patient feels languid and depressed, the tongue is coated, the appetite poor or variable, bowels inclined to constipation, urine scanty, or changed in character, skin dry, pulse increased in frequency, and temperature elevated. There is, in some cases, sensations of chilliness, but in the majority this will not be noticed. In the majority, the temperature will be higher in the afternoon than in the morning.

934. These symptoms may continue for one, two, or three weeks, and terminate with the appearance of an eruption; or there may result a still more distinct febrile reaction. In some cases they are of but a few hours' duration.

935. In the more advanced stages of the disease we have sometimes a condition of the system analogous to hectic fever. The skin is dry and harsh, dark-colored and wanting elasticity; the digestive organs suffer, and their function is impaired; the nervous system is irritable, and the patient suffers much from this source; the secretions of kidneys and bowels are impaired; the circulation is impaired, and pulse frequently shows an increase of 10 to 30 beats per minute; temperature constantly elevated. With such symptoms, the local manifestations of syphilitic disease, whatever they may be, are very intractable.

936. TREATMENT.—In the majority of cases the objects of treatment will be to correct the lesion of the circulation, and establish free excretion, then using any antisyphilitic that

may be indicated. I believe that treatment in this stage will give satisfactory results, and that permanent and radical cures may be effected.

937. Select the proper sedative, as in every form of fever, and give it as frequently and persistently as if it was the ordinary acute disease of the country. It is well for the patient to give the treatment two or three days of time, that nothing may interfere with its success. With the sedative, we employ means to establish secretion from the skin—sometimes the ordinary sponge-bath, sometimes the hot vapor-bath, and sometimes the wet-pack. I like the action of the cold wet-pack in some of these cases, and think that it will be found a much better antisyphilitic than many suppose.

938. The bowels may be gently moved with a saline or vegetable laxative, as may be indicated, active cathartics being avoided. A small portion of Bitartrate of Potash, Crab Orchard Salts, or Citrate of Magnesia, will answer well; or if there is an indication for Podophyllin, we give it thoroughly triturated 1-10 1-100, or small doses of the Fluid Extract of Jalap and Senna.

939. Diluents are *the* diuretics. You may wash the syphilitic virus out with water, when it can not be driven out with drugs. A weak infusion of some of the vegetable alteratives that go out by way of the kidneys—as the Alnus, Scrofularia, Sarsaparilla, etc., given freely. Or, a solution of Acetate of Potash given in the same way. Or, if deemed best, the proper Iodide may be largely diluted, and we may use it for its direct, as well as this indirect action.

940. Let this treatment be followed by the proper antisyphilitic remedies, associated with tonics and restoratives, and it will be found very satisfactory.

941. But we have another class of cases in which special remedies are distinctly indicated, and we will find most marked benefit from their use. It is hardly worth while to point out the special indications for the different remedies, as they are the same here, as in the treatment of ordinary dis-

eases. We have special indications for the use of Sulphite of Soda, Sulphurous Acid, Chlorate of Potash, Iodide of Potassium, Iodide of Ammonium, Rhus, Macrotys, Phytolacca, Nitric Acid, Belladonna, etc., and we obtain very marked results from their use when so indicated. This is not only true of syphilitic fever, but of the treatment of all syphilitic lesions, and I advise a careful examination of the patient to the end of determining such indications where they exist.

942. In the treatment of the chronic or hectic fever of ad-advanced syphilis, we find Veratrum, Cod-Oil and Arsenic occupying important places. In some of these cases Veratrum is *par excellence* the remedy, preparatory to the use of the Iodides, or other means that may be deemed antisyphilitic. Cod-Oil is not only restorative, but it is sometimes the only means of permanently reducing the temperature to a normal standard. Arsenic stands among the first of vital stimulants, when the vegetative processes have been long diseased, and the tissues are thoroughly syphilized.

AFFECTIONS OF THE SKIN AND ITS APPENDAGES.

943. Affections of the skin are of more frequent occurrence than any other lesions, and are among our best evidences of the disease. In many cases they are also an index to the success of our remedies, and when entirely removed and the skin natural and healthy, we have good reason to suppose our patient cured.

ERYTHEMA.

944. This is the earliest as well as the most frequent of the syphilitic eruptions. It makes its appearance as rose-colored spots, irregular in form, and like simple erythema or roseola, is effaced by pressure. They are sometimes so grouped together as to cover large surfaces, as the greater portion of the abdomen, breast, or arms. It is not attended with fever, nor is there any unpleasant sensations, so that many times its discovery is accidental.

PAPULÆ.

945. Syphilitic *lichen* comes out as small pimples of a coppery-reddish color. They appear most frequently upon the back, shoulders and neck, though they may be found on any portion of the body. They are usually preceded by some derangement of the system, as loss of appetite, arrest of secretion, headache, etc. The eruption frequently does not continue more than two or three weeks, and passing off, leaves slight blotches, and desquamation of the cuticle. A broad papular eruption is sometimes seen, thus described by Vidal: "Sometimes we observe them of a firm consistence, very prominent, and of a decided copper color; at another point, we find little elevations already faded, less prominent, of softer consistence, and of a paler tint; on one side are yellowish spots, with a rosy tint, which are in process of being converted into papules; on the other, they are of a grayish shade, more depressed than the latter, and the marks left by the papules which have disappeared. They are separated by intervals, at which the skin is of a peculiar earthy color, giving to the whole a very characteristic aspect.

SQUAMÆ.

946. Of syphilitic squamæ we have three varieties—lepra, pityriasis, and psoriasis. It may be remarked that all syphilitic skin diseases are scaly to some extent, this being a characteristic symptom; but these possess the features of the diseases named, in fact are the same diseases modified by the syphilitic poison.

947. Lepra appears in the form of small, coppery-red, shining spots, a little elevated above the skin. In a short time they lose their smooth appearance, and become covered with thin scales, which are constantly falling off and being renewed. They increase in size, maintaining a circular form, until they are two or three inches in diameter, and the skin becoming thick and hard, movements of the part are impeded and painful. In some cases ulceration occurs, the result being

the formation of very unpleasant sores. The disease may be confined to the extremities and about the joints, but in some cases it extends to every part of the body.

948. Pityriasis is most usually confined to the scalp. It makes its appearance in the form of coppery-red discolorations, with but little change in the skin, but continued exfoliation of the epidermis. It may or may not be attended with the falling of the hair.

949. Psoriasis may appear in four forms. First, in the form of small coppery or dusky-red patches, irregularly rounded, and elevated above the adjacent skin. These soon become covered with thin scales, which are continually cast off. In other cases it occurs in the form of flat, angular, irregular patches, which, as the disease progresses, form continuous surfaces, covered with thick, dirty-white, and pretty adherent scaly incrustations. The margins of these spots have the characteristic dirty-yellow or coppery color, and when the incrustations are removed, the part presents a livid appearance. In the severer cases the skin becomes thick, hard, hypertrophied, and fissured in various directions. On pinching up the skin it is found to be much altered in structure, rough, hard and uneven. The disease occasionally appears about the eyes, and gives rise to much irritation, and about the lips, which are dry and present fissures which are irritable and painful. The most frequent form is psoriasis palmaris. It makes its appearance in the form of one or more red blotches or papules, exfoliation of the epidermis occurs, leaving a coppery-red and tender surface. At a later stage these become tender, crack, and when used, frequently bleed. Sooner or later the disease involves the tips of the fingers passing under the edges of the nails, and may cause their entire removal.

950. In the treatment of this form of the disease I employ the vegetable alteratives in infusion, using them freely, and bathing the surface with the same. If the patient's health is not much broken down, give Iodide of Ammonium or Potas-

sium, and after two or three weeks, put the patient upon the use of Tonics and Iron. These are the cases in which Arsenic has been employed with such marked benefit, both internally and locally, but I would only recommend it where the skin is dry and harsh, and has lost its tonicity; then it proves a valuable stimulant.

951. In addition to the means named, we will frequently derive much benefit from vapor baths, followed with fumigations of Sulphur, or Iodine. Sulphite of Soda, ʒij. to Water, ℥iij.; Glycerine, ℥j.; is an excellent local application. Or: ℞ Glycerine, ℥j.; Benzoic Acid, ʒij.; Oxide of Zinc, ʒj.; Water, ℥ij. M. My favorite local application in this, as well as some other of these affections, is: ℞ Iodide of Ammonium, ʒj.; Water, ℥iv.; Glycerine, ℥j. I have also employed the Glycerole of Tar with very good results.

VESICULÆ.

952. Syphilodermata rarely appears in the vesicular form, and when it is met with it is an early symptom. It most frequently takes the form of simple eczema, appearing upon the back, face and extremities. In many severe cases it answers the character of *eczema* impetignodes, the skin being swollen, the vesicles large, which when ruptured form a scab, which is cast off and renewed for several weeks, leaving coppery discolorations or cicatrices.

BULLÆ.

953. Of this we have two varieties, *pemphigus* and *rupia*, the first being of rare occurrence, while the second is a quite frequent form of syphilitic skin disease. Pemphigus is most usually seen in congenital syphilis, and is evidence of grave impairment of vitality. It makes its appearance in the form of large blebs or blisters, ovoid in form, situate on a violet-colored base, and filled with a straw colored fluid. When they rupture, thin, brownish crusts form, which may be renewed for some time.

954. Rupia is one of the later symptoms of constitutional syphilis, and is almost invariably associated with poverty of the blood, and enfeebled vitality. It commences by the formation of large vesicles, upon a reddish base, sometimes filled with a yellowish serum, at others the fluid is bloody. By the third to the sixth day its contents dessicate and form a scab, covering a superficial ulcer, which is violet in its color when the scab is removed. The constant secretion of purulent matter adds to the under surface of the scab, and it becomes more and more prominent, until it is half an inch or more in thickness. The scab is yellowish brown, or almost black, and the skin surrounding it presents a coppery-red areola.

955. The treatment for these forms will be similar to that directed for the squamæ, especial attention being paid to the digestive organs, and the administration of Bitter Tonics and Iron. The Compound Tincture of Corydalis proves a good remedy in this case, associated with Hydrastis and Iodide of Iron. An infusion of Corydalis or of equal parts of Corydalis, Alnus and Rumex is also an efficient treatment.

956. As a local application, we will find equal parts of Tincture of Muriate of Iron and Glycerine to answer well in some cases. The Hydrated Oxide of Iron, with an equal part of Lard, is good, as is the Glycerine and Oxide of Zinc, previously mentioned. In quite severe cases I have obtained good results from an application of a strong decoction of Alnus, Rumex and Cornus. If single points of rupia are very persistent, I sometimes apply the Chloride of Zinc Paste to produce a slight slough, and then dress the sore with Mayer's or Mild Zinc Ointment.

PUSTULÆ.

957. Pustular eruption is a frequent form of syphilitic skin disease, when the poison has thoroughly impregnated the system. We recognize three varieties — ecthyma, impetigo, and acne, each of which possesses many of the characteristics of the non-syphilitic affection.

958. Ecthyma is of most frequent occurrence. It makes its appearance as small, red, indurated spots, which soon suppurate, and a pustule is formed in the center. When severe, the skin is much inflamed, swollen, and of a dark color, and the pustule is blackish and infiltrated with blood. In the first form, when the pustule ruptures, a brownish scab is formed, which may be renewed for some time; the surface, when it is removed, has a coppery-red color, and when healed it leaves a slight cicatrix. In the second form, a thick, dark scab results, which is very adherent; progressing further, a process of ulceration is set up, which increases its size, and at last terminates in the formation of an open ulcer.

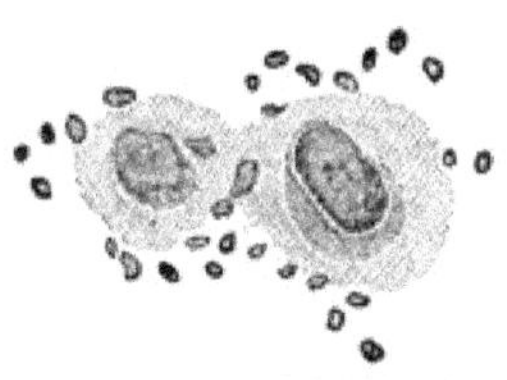
Vesiculo-Pustular Syphilida.

959. Impetigo appears as slightly raised, red patches, upon which soon appear numerous pustules, flat, and of variable size, manifesting a tendency to run together. The fluid is abundant and soon dries, forming thick, yellow incrustations, and when thrown off, the pit is coppery-red and tender. The eruption extending by new eruptions of pustules, may extend over a considerable portion of the body. The disease is occasionally very severe, especially about the mouth and nose, the pustules being large, and forming thick, yellowish-green or brown crusts. In a later stage of the disease, the pustules arrange themselves in circles, and the crusts are thick, yellowish brown, and cover considerable surfaces. The cicatrices left are of a dull white color, and permanent.

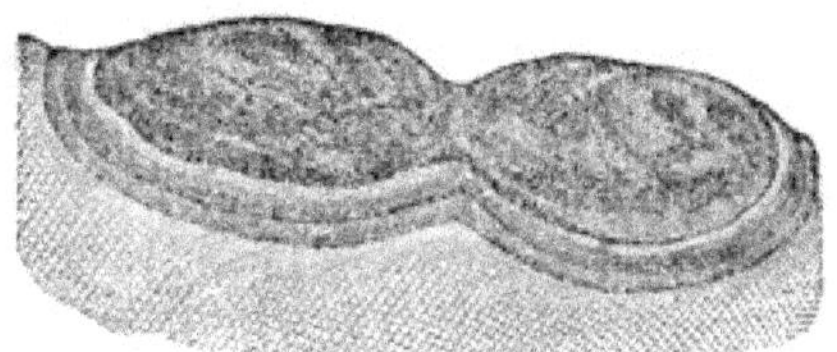
Pustulo-Crustaceous Syphilida.

960. In syphilitic acne, the pustules are of small size, situated upon red indurations; remaining stationary for some time, they become covered with a thin scab, which when removed leaves a slight coppery redness. In other cases, the disease assumes the indurated form. It commences as livid, red, indurated tumors, which are painful when pressed upon. Suppuration proceeds slowly, and small scabs are formed upon the surface; in some cases the cellular tissue is involved, and the induration remains for some weeks.

961. The treatment in these cases will not differ materially from that recommended for rupia. Sulphite of Soda sometimes answers an excellent purpose, in doses of twenty grains four times a day, and a strong solution may be employed as a wash.

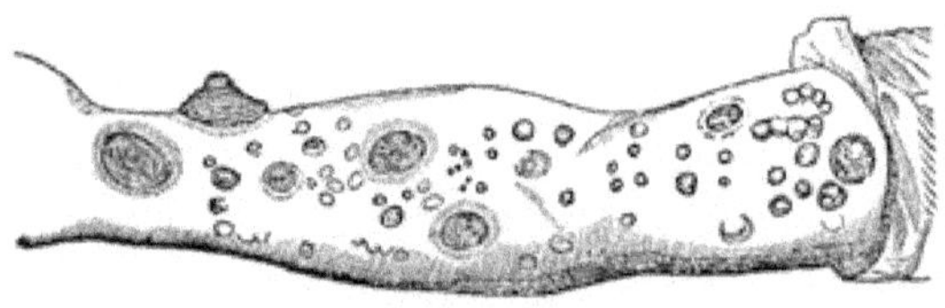

Syphilitic Rupia.

TUBERCULÆ.

962. "Syphilitic tubercles," says Langston Parker, "are deep-seated, solid, circumscribed elevations, containing neither lymph nor pus; they differ from the papulæ in their size, being much larger, more prominent, and better defined. Syphilitic tubercles are either isolated or grouped, of a shining red, livid or brown color, surrounded by an areola of a dark-red or coppery appearance. These tubercles are prone to become ulcerated, and form excavated sores with thick and elevated edges, and a foul surface, secreting an offensive pus, which, drying up, is transformed into gray or dark colored scales or crusts. The syphilitic tubercle forms the connecting link between the secondary and tertiary symptoms of M. Ricord: it is the first of that class of syphilitic diseases in which the virus appears to have penetrated more deeply into the economy, and to have produced a disorganization in tis-

sues, which those forms hitherto considered have left untouched.

963. "The flat tubercle of M. Cullerier, or the tuberculous pustules of Alibert, sometimes occurs as a primitive affection, but more commonly as a symptom of constitutional syphilis; in the former instance it is observed on the scrotum, the labia, the vicinity of the anus, or the mammæ. The surface of these tubercles is smooth and flat, of a deep red or copper color, varying from the size of a sixpence to that of a shilling; they are not so much disposed to ulcerate as the other varieties.

964. "The more common forms of tubercles are conical, or round elevations, dispersed here and there over the skin, or assembled in groups or clusters, which are also irregularly distributed. The size of these varies from that of a pea to that of a large hazel nut or filbert; they are more commonly situated on the anterior surface of the chest, or the abdomen, or the neck, or the internal part of the arms.

965. "Another variety of tubercle is situated more commonly on the alæ or lobule of the nose, or on the forehead; frequently, also, upon the neck of the uterus, or upon the tongue, when they may be mistaken for cancerous affections. These tubercles are commonly assembled in circular groups of variable size; they are so prone to ulcerate, that this termination appears to be one of their natural characters; when in this condition, they are frequently described under the name of syphilitic lupus. The tubercular syphilida are commonly complicated with a scrofulous, scorbutic, or herpetic tendency or diathesis; their progress is slow, and generally without pain; they gradually increase in size till they terminate in softening or ulceration. They are the most formidable of all the forms of constitutional syphilis, producing great deformity in all the parts invaded by ulceration, and exceedingly difficult to cure."

966. In the treatment of syphilitic pustules, the remedies should be carefully selected. If Iodide of Potash is indicated

as heretofore named, it will sometimes effect a speedy cure, and the same is the case with Nitric Acid, Arsenic and Cod-Oil, The vapor bath every other day, with Sulphur, proves a valuable aid to the treatment.

967. If the tubercles become painful, and show a tendency to suppuration, we may employ emollient applications, or sedatives and narcotics. I like the action of the following: ℞ Extract of Conium, ℥ss.; Extract of Aconite, ʒij.; Glycerine sufficient to form a paste. In some cases an application of equal parts of Tincture of Iodine and Tincture of Muriate of Iron will prove serviceable, or they may be covered with the Collodion or Gutta Percha mentioned under the head of Bubo. When they are indolent, we sometimes obtain good results from a continuous application of Mayer's Ointment.

ULCERS.

968. Ulceration may be the result of the vesiculæ, pústulæ, or tuberculæ, as already described, or it may even occur from the long continuance of the papulæ or squamæ. These ulcers possess all the characteristics of those arising from other causes—being *irritable, indolent, corroding*, etc. They also vary greatly in size, from that less in size than a three cent piece to one that covers a surface as large as the hand. When arising from the vesiculæ or pustulæ, there is usually a constant tendency to incrustation, no matter what their size; but when caused by suppuration of tubercles or gummy tumors they are usually open.

969. We will find them presenting every variety of form—round, oval, and irregular—at times superficial and without effusion into adjacent tissues, at others deep and surrounded by a wall of adventitious tissue. Whatever may be their shape or size, there is the coppery discoloration around them, or in the cicatrices of former ulcers, which gives their history.

970. The treatment will not differ from that already laid down, as the open ulcer is but a continuance of the prior disease. I believe it is the experience of all practitioners, that

syphilitic ulceration heals as readily as the simple, when the constitutional affection is removed. They may be healed before this, by the use of the local applications that have been named, if the general health is good. If there is general debility and impoverishment of the blood, they will sometimes heal rapidly under the use of tonics, Iron and nutritious diet.

971. Mayer's Ointment, made strictly according to the Dispensatory, is an excellent dressing, as is the Ointment of Elder, the Ointment of Baptisia, and the Ointment of Nitric Acid. The decoction of Alnus, Rumex and Cornus—heretofore named—proves useful when the ulcers are indolent. If the secretion is profuse, we may use a decoction of equal parts of Baptisia and Cornus, or a Solution of Permanganate of Potash, one or two grains to the ounce of Water, or of Carbolic Acid one part to forty parts of Water; or, what is better: ℞ Carbolic Acid, ʒss.; Glycerine, ℥iv. If the ulcers are sluggish and will not heal under these applications, we sometimes apply the Chloride of Zinc Paste to destroy the imperfect structure of their edges and base, when they heal as simple ulcers. The Ointment of Iron—made by precipitating the Solution of Persulphate with Ammonia, and combining with half a part of Lard—answers a good purpose in the same cases.

MUCOUS TUBERCLE.

972. Mucous patches may be an early or late symptom of syphilis, occurring as early as the twentieth day, or not for two or three years. It is even claimed that they may be a primary symptom, taking the place of a chancre, and transmitting the primary disease by their secretion. I am satisfied that when appearing thus early, that they have their origin from an irritation of the surface produced by the syphilitic virus, or as we have seen, from the chancre itself, and in such cases the secretion is the specific virus.

973. They are also transmissible when really secondary symptoms, and not only will the growth spring up, but the constitution will be infected. They may be propagated from

point to point of the same person by contact with the virus, and this is probably the means of their extensive distribution in some cases.

974. Mucous tubercles most usually make their appearance at points where the mucous membrane joins the skin, though they will be found on the mucous membrane proper, or upon the skin, as the scrotum, perineum, groin, axillæ, between the toes, the inside of the thighs, etc. They most frequently present themselves at the margin of the anus, or just behind the corona-glandis, and in the female upon the vulva; and from these parts they may extend so as to involve a considerable portion of the genital organs, and the perineal fissure. They may also be found at the lips, the inside of the cheeks, tonsils, the nose, etc.

975. They first appear as one or more red spots, slightly elevated above the surface. Their growth is usually rapid, so that in a short time they are one-fourth or one-half inch in height. When grouped together they resemble a bunch of red raspberries. Their color is a bright vivid red, and they bleed freely when their covering is ruptured. The secretion is usually thin and muco-purulent, but if from friction or other cause ulceration occurs, it is purulent and abundant. At times the secretion from them becomes so ichorous as to excoriate adjacent parts. When situated on the skin, their color is brownish-red, and when upon the mucous membrane of the mouth, a blanched white, like the eschar of Nitrate of Silver.

976. As in other forms of constitutional syphilis, we expect to remove this symptom, by eradicating the general disease upon which it depends. And although local treatment will effect their removal in some cases, without internal remedies, it should always be held subservient to the latter.

977. Various local means have been employed in this case, sometimes with and at others without success. I have seen the strongest escharotic used for their removal, and the re-appearance of the mucous tubercles before the part had healed.

So I have seen the hot iron applied to the entire perineal fissure until the patient could not be seen for the smoke produced by the burning, and in two weeks they were as abundant and prominent as ever. If this teaches us anything, it should cause us to rely upon constitutional measures.

978. I have obtained good results from cauterization with Chromic Acid, as named under the head of gonorrhœal vegetations, but I would only employ it when the patches were small. A strong solution of Permanganate of Potash has also answered a good purpose. And I am informed that Carbolic Acid has been successfully used. Dusting the patches with equal parts of Sub-Nitrate of Bismuth and Oxide of Zinc, being careful to separate the folds and apply the powder between, is a very good plan. In other cases we may use a saturated solution of Tannin, freely applied. The extract of Red Clover has also been recommended.

GUMMY TUMORS.

979. Gummy tumor is a late symptom of syphilis, not usually appearing for two or three years or more. They are generally found in the cellular tissue under the skin, but the same development may take place in the muscles, or even in tendinous structures. They make their appearance as hardened masses, freely movable under the skin, from the size ot a cherry to a hen's egg. They frequently remain without change for months, giving the patient but little uneasiness, further than the sensation of an adventitious body. At last they become tender on pressure, form adhesions to the skin, which become dark-red, or livid and coppery, and at last thinned and ulcerated, discharging an ichorous pus. Suppuration usually commences at their center, and as it progresses a large foul ulcer is formed. No tendency to healing is manifest until all the formation has been removed, with subsequent adventitious deposit, and at last when healed a permanent cicatrix of a dull white color remains.

980. The treatment will not vary from that heretofore described, but it needs to be very thorough, as the presence of these tumors is evidence of grave syphilitic cachexia.

ALOPECIA.

981. Falling of the hair is an early symptom of constitutional syphilis, and will usually be found associated with the exanthemata, and with redness of the fauces. At its commencement it seems a minor affair, the hair coming out in small quantities, but as it progresses the hair has so frail a tenure that it comes out in quantities on slight traction. Thus if it progresses the patient will become nearly or quite bald, and in some cases will lose the eyebrows and eyelashes also, giving him a very singular and uncomfortable appearance. Usually there is but little apparent disease of the scalp; occasionally there is pityriasis, and again the pustules and scabs of impetigo.

982. Caused by the syphilitic infection of the system, the constitutional treatment is mainly to be depended upon, and when the person is brought under the influence of the proper remedies, the hair ceases to fall out. To gratify the patient, we usually prescribe local remedies, which to some extent check the falling of the hair. The following formula will be found as good as any: ℞ Tincture of Cantharides, f℥j.; Castor Oil, f℥iv.; Alcohol, f℥xij.; Oil of Bergamot, Oil of Lemon, Oil of Lavender, aa. ʒij. Mix. Let it be applied with slight friction once or twice daily. Dupuytren's Pomade is frequently used: ℞ Medullæ Ossium Bovis, ℥j.; Tincture of Cantharidis, ℥j. Add: Plumbi Acetatis, ℈j.; Bal. Peruviani, ʒiij.; Olei Carophylli, Olei Canellæ, aa. gtts. xv. Mix.

ONYCHIA.

983. Not only does the skin suffer in its nutrition, independent of the eruptive diseases named, but as we have seen, its appendages become diseased. Affections of the hair are far more common than of the nails, but in protracted syphilis

we will always find these presenting some evidences of disease.

984. In the majority of cases, the nails have lost their bright, fresh appearance, and look dull and opaque. They are inclined to incurve, become brittle, break and scale off. Becoming more diseased, we find that the matrix and edges of the skin surrounding them become swollen and tender, the nail grows thick, rough, opaque, and dark colored, looking somewhat like the crust of rupia prominens. After a time the matrix and edges ulcerate, and the entire nail may be thrown off by this process. As would be supposed, it is a very unpleasant and painful manifestation of the disease.

985. The general treatmant will be, of course, for the constitutional infection, and if anything is suggested here it will be the use of Cod-Oil and Arsenic, or in some cases, Phosphorus or Sulphur. The local means will vary. In some Permanganate of Potash will be the best local application, in others Carbolic Acid. Whenever the eruption at the edges of the nail is eczematous, I would advise the Brown Citrine Ointment, at first of full strength, afterwards one part to three of Simple Cerate.

DISEASES OF THE RESPIRATORY APPARATUS.

AFFECTIONS OF THE NASAL CAVITIES.

986. Disease of the nose is usually a late symptom, though we may observe erythema with catarrhal symptoms, associated with the disease of the throat. It commences with the symptoms of catarrh, and continuing for a time, we will find the mucous membrane swollen, dusky red, and at last presenting points of ulceration. At first there is diminished secretion, but after a time, masses of inspissated mucus, with blood and pus, are, from time to time, discharged. Progressing still further, this secretion becomes more abundant, the patient complains of a fullness, sense of tension, and aching in the nose, which is frequently somewhat swollen at the lower mar-

gin of the nasal bones. The ulceration progressing further, the bones become affected, and there is frequent discharge of fetid muco-pus, scabs, inspissated mucus, and the debris of bone.

987. Points of ulceration may be visible to the eye, when they present the same appearances as those described in the throat. But the middle and posterior parts of the nose seem to be the favorite locality, and it there commits its greatest ravages. The turbinated bones are frequently affected, and are first cast off. The vomer becoming involved, the support of the outer nose is destroyed, and we have that peculiar sinking of it so characteristic of syphilis, or it may continue to the destruction of the cartilaginous septum, the nose becoming flat. Passing upward it destroys the superior turbinated with the lateral masses of the ethmoid, and backward it erodes the soft palate, and at last destroys more or less of the palatine arch. We thus find in some cases that the mouth and nose is but one cavity, all the superior structures as far as the orbits, and base of the cranium, having been removed by the ulcerative process.

988. In the earlier stages, the disease yields readily to treatment, but when the bones become involved much care is required to arrest it. Select internal remedies, so as to remove the constitutional affection without producing debility or impoverishing the blood. Iodide of Ammonium with the vegetable alteratives, and the employment of Bitter Tonics and Iron to improve digestion and assimilation, will be the best treatment. The prolonged use of Iodide of Potassium frequently does much harm.

989. Local means are of much importance. They are used to best advantage in the fluid form, either with syringe or the new method of hydrostatic pressure. In either case they should be used in considerable quantity, to clear the cavities of accumulated secretions, and to thoroughly reach the affected parts. It has been shown that if the patient breathes through the mouth exclusively during their use, the

soft palate closes the posterior nares, so that a fluid thrown into one nostril will pass out at the other. If a syringe is used, it should contain four to six ounces, work easily, and have a large nozzle; having filled it, let the fluid be forced slowly into the nose until it is thoroughly washed out. In the other method, a jar or funnel, resembling a bottle with its bottom removed, is placed on a retort stand. To the small lower extremity a piece of rubber tubing, three or four feet long, is attached. Now filling the jar, which is higher than the patient's head, the tube is inserted into one nostril and the fluid flows through and out at the other. Any amount of fluid may be thus used.

990. To wash the nose out, we may use a solution of Common Salt, ℥ss. to Water, Oj.; or of Permanganate of Potash, ℥j. to Water, Oj. A very good lotion for relieving irritation is composed of: ℞ Chlorate of Potash, ʒij.; Glycerine, f℥iv.; Water, f℥xij. We may sometimes substitute, with advantage, a decoction of equal parts of Alnus, Rumex and Cornus, with or without a portion of Glycerine. A solution of the Permanganate of Potash, alternated with the infusion just named, is the remedy I have obtained the best results from.

991. I have used the inhaling apparatus, or atomizer, of Dr. Seigle, in these cases, as well as in syphilitic sore throat, and laryngitis, with marked advantage. The instrument consists of a copper boiler, resting on a tin frame work, which also incloses the spirit lamp by which the boiler is heated; passing from the top of the boiler is a glass tube, bent at a right angle and terminating in a small opening, and at right angles to this a similar one, which passes into a small cup holding the medicated fluid. The instrument works well, is automatic, and not liable to get out of order.

992. In using it, fill the boiler half full of water, light the alcohol lamp, and in three minutes a jet of steam will pass out of the glass tube. Place the fluid to be inhaled in the small glass cup, and as the jet of steam passes over the small

tube leading from the cup, a vacuum is formed in it, and the medicated fluid rises and is carried off in the current. With the vaporization of one drachm of water in the boiler, two drachms of the medicated fluid will be atomized and carried off.

993. Any remedy in solution may thus be carried to the part affected. I use decoctions of Chamomile, Hydrastis, Baptisia, etc., and solutions of Chlorate of Potash, Permanganate of Potash, Sulphite of Soda, Chlorinated Soda, and Nitrate of Silver.

SYPHILITIC LARYNGITIS.

994. Among the serious lesions of syphilis, disease of the larynx occupies a prominent place, and is one of the most common causes of death. Chronic laryngitis is at all times an unpleasant affection, but especially so when it goes on to ulceration. Intractable and with difficulty arrested in ordinary cases, this difficulty is greatly increased in the specific form of the disease by the depraved condition of the blood.

995. In the early stages of secondary syphilis, with throat disease, we will frequently observe a roughening of the voice, and a disposition to a short cough to clear the throat. This usually passes away without special treatment, as the general disease yields.

996. In a further stage of the disease, the voice is roughened, and the patient finds it somewhat difficult at times to control it as he wishes, and the throat requires frequent clearing in speaking. The cough is especially for the removal of increased secretion, and becomes worse when this increases, better when it decreases. As yet there is no evidence of ulceration, but there is secretion of mucus or muco-pus.

997. With commencing ulceration the patient suffers from local pain in the larynx, and considerable irritation. There is not unfrequently some difficulty in breathing, from contraction of the intrinsic muscles, the result of the irritation. If the ulceration is upon or near the vocal cords, the voice is markedly changed, and its use becomes very painful. The

sputa is now characteristic, at least in many cases. The secretion of the ulcer remains for a time, sometimes partially dessicates, and is then brought up in a mass, its surface being tinged with blood.

998. At a still more advanced stage of the disease, the patient suffers continuously and severely with his throat. There is no time that he breathes with ease, and when the larynx becomes irritated he suffers as a child would with croup. The voice is rough and hoarse, and he can talk but little without causing severe irritation. The matter expectorated is an unpleasant, greenish pus, and is sometimes discharged in large quantities. Hemorrhage is also of frequent occurrence.

999. The impairment of the general health keeps pace with the local disease. With the first symptoms it is distinct, and as the local disease runs its course as above named, we find the patient losing flesh and strength, until in the latter stages he presents the appearance of one in the advanced stages of phthisis, and has hectic fever, night sweats, colliquative diarrhœa, etc.

1000. Post-mortem examination shows all phases of disease, from simple thickening of the mucous membrane, to ulceration involving and destroying the mucous membrane, vocal cords, and even the cartilages of the larynx.

1001. Treatment in the early stage of the disease will, in the majority of cases, prove very satisfactory. If the irritation is marked, and acute, with erythematous redness of the fauces, I would prescribe: ℞ Tincture of Aconite, gtts. v. to gtts. x.; Water, ℥iv.; a teaspoonful every two hours; the wet vinegar pack to the throat at night, and cold sponging in the morning. In very severe cases the use of Aconite with the spray apparatus, will give speediest results; either the steam apparatus, or the air bulbs, may be employed. If the throat shows the peculiar fibrinous exudation, covering it like a film, or in streaks or patches, especially if diphtheritic, I would prefer Phytolacca, as: ℞ Tincture of Phytolacca, (green root), ℨss.; Water, ℥iv.; a teaspoonful every two hours. If the disease is more slowly developed, with roughening of the voice, I would advise Collinsonia, in the usual dose: ℞ Tincture of Collinsonia, ℨj.; Simple Sirup, ℥iij.; a teaspoonful four times a day.

1002. The wet pack at night, and cold sponging in the morning, will be found markedly beneficial in the majority of cases. But in some it does harm rather than good, and in these I would use the perpetual blister on each side of the larynx, covering a spot from the size of a dime to that of a twenty-five cent piece.

1003. In the more advanced stages of the disease we use local applications, principally with a spray apparatus, of Iodine, Iodoform, Carbolic Acid, Tannic Acid, Nitrate of Silver, etc., but further than palliating the disease, I have never seen them do much good.

1004. Very much will depend upon the careful selection of remedies for the constitutional disease in these grave cases. If we persist in giving Iodide of Potash, when not indicated, defibrinizing the blood with it, and impairing nutrition, we will see our patient grow worse rapidly. In the majority of these cases, especially the more advanced, a restorative treatment is of the utmost importance, and should not be neglected. In some it will consist of the Bitter Tonics, as the Triple Phosphate of Quinine, Strychnine and Iron, (Compound Tonic Mixture); in others of the Hypophosphites; in others of Cod-Oil; in others of Arsenic; in all of an abundance of good, nutritious food.

1005. There is an occasional case of these grave lesions, marked by a small, incurved tongue, with prominent red papilla, in which I should give small doses of Donovan's Solution, say gtts. ij. to gtts. iij., three or four times daily; to be followed after three or four days, with Cod-Oil

SYPHILITIC DISEASE OF BRONCHIÆ AND LUNGS.

1006. Among the rare syphilitic diseases may be named ulceration of the bronchial tubes, with the symptoms of chronic bronchitis, and of the lungs, with symptoms simulating phthisis. A very clear decription of these lesions is given by Aitkin, which I quote.

1007. "The following are the kinds of lesions which predominate:

1. "*Evidences of Inflammation of the Mucous Membrane of the Bronchial Tubes.*—In such cases bronchial irritation, with fever in many cases, precedes the skin lesions, and may disappear wholly or partially when the skin lesions are established. On the other hand, if the syphilitic eruption suddenly disappears, bronchitis may ensue. Walshe records well-marked instances of this; and it is a circumstance to be looked for amongst soldiers especially, who, having recovered from a primary syphilitic sore, are apt to be exposed to the risk of bronchitis when mounting guard soon after being discharged to duty. Secondary symptoms and pulmonic lesions are then apt to date their commencement; and all the general symptoms of phthisis may supervene, and yet no tubercle in the lung may be developed; but chronic bronchitis remains persistent. On this point Dr. Walshe observes, that in the persistence of the general symptoms there 'is assuredly enough to create a strong suspicion of the existence of tubercle in the lungs, taken in conjunction with the indubitable tendency of syphilis *plus* Mercury to induce the outbreak of phthisis in a person having the requisite constitutional aptitude. How are the cases to be distinguished? By the total want of accordance between the physical signs and the constitutional symptoms: the patient with syphilitic bronchitis has neither consolidation signs nor, *a fortiori*, the evidences of excavation. But there is a curious source of difficulty which sometimes starts up in these cases, and renders doubt imperative,—the infra-clavicular ribs and clavicle thicken from periostitis, and produce

dullness under percussion, which can not with positiveness be distinguished from that of tubercle within the lung. Here the observer must wait for events to clear up the diagnosis.' (*Diseases of the Lungs*, p. 233.)

2. "*The Occurrence of Gummatous Nodules in the Pulmonary Substance.*—These are, in the first instance, of the same histological constitution as the well-known node of the shin, or the subcutaneous product described by Ricord, Barensprung, Virchow, and McCarthy. They form especially toward the periphery and bases of the lungs. In the former site they resemble nodules of lobular pneumonia. They may soften and be eliminated much in the manner of tubercle, although they may have at first a consistence like scirrhus. It is concerning those which soften in this way that Ricord gives the warning 'not to confound suppuration of a few syphilitic nodules of the lungs with phthisis.' Regarding those gummatous nodules Dr. Walshe observes: 'I can find no positive answer to the query, Do these gummata ever form independently of other tertiary evidences of syphilis in the bones and cellular tissue? If they do, their diagnosis must be infinitely difficult—difficult, indeed, under all circumstances; for the physical signs can be none other than those of solidification, followed by softening and excavation, while the local and general symptoms closely simulate those of phthisis.' (*Diseases of the Lungs*, p. 431).

3. "*The Occurrence of Gummatous Nodules in various Stages of Growth and Degeneration, associated with the Miliary Deposit of Tubercle.*—In such cases the history of events in the illnesses of the patient may be found to correspond more or less closely with the appearances seen in the lungs—appearances which distinctly indicate the formation of lesions commenced at different dates—appearances which denote the occurrence of lesions in crops, or as a succession of events which may be illustrated by the history of the symptoms during life.

"The minute structure of these *gummatous nodules* has been closely examined by many observers. They consist of a growth of elements which leads to the development of an elastic tumor composed of a well-defined tissue, and the elements of which are extremely minute. The tumor takes origin from the connective tissue, or the analogues of such; and hence the universality of the site of syphilitic lesions. When these are sufficiently large to attract attention—as in the form of a node on the shin-bone, or on some part of the true skin—they are small, solid, pale knots, like a hard kernel, about the size of a pea. They are generally first seen on some part of the true skin or subcutaneous or submucous tissue; and when the tissue in which they happen to grow is sufficiently lax, they grow to a considerable size, and convey to the touch a sensation as if they were filled with gum. Repeated examinations of this growth show that in its gelatinous or soft state it arises from a proliferation of nuclei amongst the elements of the connective tissue, not unlike the formation of granulations in a wound. The component cell-elements appear as round, oval, or oat-shaped particles imbedded in a matrix of fine connective tissue of a granular character, and tending to fibrillation. The cell-elements are a little larger than blood-globules, and are distinctly granular in their interior when mature. In the growing part of the node, and immediately in its vicinity, where growth is abnormally active, the minute cell-elements are seen to be developed in groups within the elongated and enlarged corpuscles of the connective tissue. In form, therefore, the node or gummatous nodule resembles a tubercle; and by fatty degeneration or tuberculization may not be capable eventually of being distinguished from tubercular deposit. How, then, are we to recognize the specific nature of such gummatous nodules? There is nothing in them so specifically and anatomically distinct that, apart from their history, they can be recognized. The history of the syphilitic case during life is the great guide. The nodes on the shin-bone, or clavicles, have long been recognized as the product of syphilis. It may almost be said that they have been seen to grow under the eyes of the patient and the observer; and their anatomical characters are found to be such as compose the gummatous nodules just described. In a case of inveterate syphilis, therefore, whose history is fully known, in whom the node on the shin or other bones is characteristic, and has been seen to grow, and in whom also we find similar nodules in the lungs, or in the liver, or in the testicles—symmetrically growing in these latter organs, and consisting of minute cell-elements exactly the same as the node on the shin—it is impossible to overlook the fact, or not to be impressed with the belief, that all of these lesions acknowledge one and the same cause of development—namely, the syphilitic poison—of which they are the expression. The progress of the node is also characteristic and suggestive. Growths of a similar form which result from idiopathic inflammation generally proceed to the formation of an abscess, or to the hypertrophy of fibrous tissue. Abscesses are recognized by their pus; fibrous tumors or hypertrophies, by the fibre-elements which compose them.

"Growths of a form similar to the node, which result from cancer, are in general to be recognized by the juice expressed from them. In the gummatous nodule we have no juice, and the cell-elements seen in cancer are generally so diversified in their form and mode of growth as not to be easily mistaken. The gummatous nodule is uniform as to the size and form of its cell-elements, and forms a growth less highly supplied with bloodvessels than a cancer. Cancers tend to infiltrate and involve neighboring textures; the gummatous nodule remains isolated and distinct.

"By way of elimination, therefore, and by duly observing the history of the case, we are generally able to recognize the nature of such growths, and to assign to them their proper place in pathology.

"The gummatous nodule has now been recognized and described in almost all the solid viscera of the body. Symmetrical development is a most constant characteristic. If a node grows on one shin, it is probably also to be found advancing on the other; if found in one testicle, it is extremely probable that it will be seen in the same relative spot in the other. Numerous examples of this symmetrical development may be seen preserved in the Pathological Museum of the Army Medical Department at Netley. During the growth of the nodule, proliferation advances slowly, and gluey-like material forms, which constitutes the inner cell-material of the nodule. If near the surface, such a nodule is apt to melt down, soften, open, and ulcerate; and such a result seems to be associated with other evidence of active constitutional disease, such as exists with a predisposition to tubercle, or with its actual existence. The tumor, however, continues gelatinous and coherent if it is inclosed in a dense part, or is deeply seated, as in gummata of the periosteum, scalp, brain, liver, testicle, lungs, and heart, if constitutional disease remains latent or inactive. Fatty degeneration may also eventually occur in the gummatous nodule, and eventually lead to its absorption; or its absorption takes place as a natural process of cure, the changes of which are not exactly known. We know only that the node on the shin-bone not seldom disappears from view, and does not return.

"For reasons already stated, phthisis must be regarded in many cases as the product of syphilis; and I would fully indorse the statement of Dr. Balfour, from what I have seen in the *post-mortem* rooms, when he says that a great cause of pulmonary disease among the Guards is the amount of syphilis which prevails amongst the men, which he has not the least doubt is a very fertile cause of its being called into active operation. The influence of syphilis on the health of the soldier is indeed powerful for evil throughout the whole army."

1008. The treatment of these lesions will require much care, and should be carefully directed to conserve vital power. It would be difficult here, without occupying too much space, to give the means in detail, but they may be classed in three groups—1st, those that influence the respiratory apparatus, removing irritation, giving rest, and stimulating the impaired mucous membranes; 2d, those that improve the vegetative function, increasing digestion, blood-making, and nutrition; 3d, those directed to the removal of the specific disease.

1009. Among the first, I may call attention to Veratrum, Sanguinaria and Lobelia. The first is *par excellence* the remedy to relieve irritation of the circulatory and respiratory apparatus, and we employ it quite frequently in the treatment of all forms of syphilitic disease. It may be associated with Cod-Oil, Arsenic, the Iodides, or other means, and in proportion as it gives a better circulation of blood it will be found beneficial. I like the action of *small* doses of Sanguinaria upon the respiratory mucous passages, and in the single case of syphilitic disease of these structures that I have seen, marked benefit attended its use. I prefer the Nitrate of Sanguinaria, grs. ij. to Syrup, ℥iv.; in doses of half to one teaspoonful four times a day. Lobelia is also used in small doses, gtts. x. of the Tincture to Water, ℥iv.; a teaspoonful every three or four hours.

1010. Much will depend upon the proper selection and use of the second class. In the rarer cases, the Bitter Tonics will prove useful. In a larger number, the bitter will take the form of a nerve stimulant, as in the Triple Phosphates of Quinine, Strychnine and Iron. In some cases Nitric Acid; in some the Hypophosphites; but in the larger number more benefit will be had from the use of Cod-Oil, and small doses of Arsenic.

The third class of remedies will be selected as in other syphilitic manifestations.

SYPHILITIC AFFECTIONS OF THE DIGESTIVE ORGANS.

AFFECTIONS OF THE MOUTH AND THROAT.

1011. Erythema of the throat is an early symptom, as we have already noticed. It may pass away soon, or re-appear several times, before the parts become permanently diseased. The disease makes its appearance in the mouth, in the form of small ulcers, usually situated on the edges of the tongue, inside of the lips, or upon the cheeks. The parts adjacent to the inflammation are reddened and tender, while the ulcer is more or less painful. It will vary in size from a grain of wheat to the size of a dime, rounded, oval, or irregular in form, with sharply cut edges, and its base covered with a coppery-yellow or gray material. Sometimes they remain stationary, but at others they manifest a tendency to spread and involve adjacent parts. We will occasionally find them remaining unchanged in size and appearance for months. When healed a cicatrix is left, and the part retains a peculiar hardness for some time.

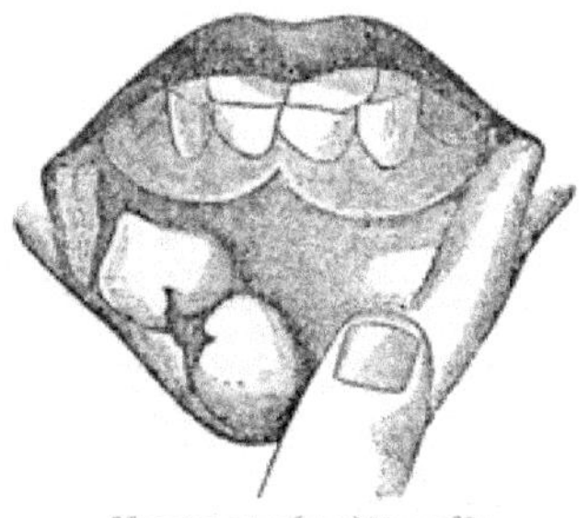

Mucous papulæ of lower lip.

1012. Ulceration of the throat commences in a similar manner, in many cases, the ulcer being the cause of the soreness. At others, the throat becomes inflamed, giving rise to uneasiness and pain in deglutition. On examination it is found of a dusky red, the mucous membrane thickened, and the follicles enlarged. The ulcers are usually of a circular form, the edges well defined, and covered with a dirty yellow or white, pultaceous material. As in the mouth, they manifest a tendency to enlarge, but at other times attaining the size of a three or five cent piece they remain stationary.

1013. In addition to the general treatment heretofore described, we may use the following local means: Frequently the ulcers of the mouth are benefited, or heal rapidly by free cauterization with Nitrate of Silver, a mouth wash of a strong decoction of Hydrastis or Baptisia being employed. Hydrastin one part, to Chlorate of Potash five parts, is sometimes a very good application, as is a solution of Permanganate of Potash, one or two grains to the ounce of water.

1014. For the disease of the throat we employ a gargle of a decoction of Baptisia with Chlorate of Potash, or instead a lotion of Iodide of Ammonium in Glycerine and water. The solution of Permanganate of Potash will be found an excelcellent remedy, using it three or four times a day. The ulcers may be touched occasionally with Muriated Tincture of Iron, or with Nitrate of Silver, which assists in removing them.

TUBERCLE OF THE TONGUE.

1015. In the advanced stages of syphilis we sometimes find well defined nodules of aplastic material deposited in the tongue. This may be a cause of soreness, usually of difficult movement, but sometimes will continue for a long time without suffering. Finally this material breaks down, ulcers are formed, and it is discharged. This is usually associated with a low grade of inflammatory action.

1016. Fissures of the tongue are usually symptomatic of inflammatory lesions of the kidneys, and will always suggest great care in the use of remedies. The deep fissures, with ulceration, observed in old cases of syphilitic disease, may be dependent upon the deposit of tubercle.

GUMMATA.

1017. The gummy deposit (aplastic) of syphilis, presents itself in the pillars of the fauces, the soft palate, and adjacent structures, and is frequently the origin of the destructive ulceration of these parts.

1018. The first symptoms are of soreness, and uneasiness in deglutition, with a feeling of fullness or constriction of the parts. A careful examination shows at first a discoloration and localized engorgement, which after a time gives evidence of a low grade of inflammation terminating in ulceration. These ulcers are remarkable for their depth, and in many cases soon perforate the structures. Thus we will find them perforating the pillars of the fauces, sometimes showing the ulceration in front, but in others upon the posterior surface. A very common and unpleasant location is about the middle of the soft palate, which may be first noticed as an elongated ovoid ulcer, covered with a grayish-yellow slough. This thrown off, and the perforating character of the ulcer is clearly seen, and sometimes passes through the tissues in a few days. Similar points of ulceration, evidently from gummy deposit, may be seen at the point of attachment between the soft and hard palates, and in the roof of the mouth, at any point between this and the alveolar process. It is singular that they appear so constantly on the mesial line, and retain the ovoid character.

1019. These points of ulceration may progress only to the size, and for the removal of the deposit, and will then heal kindly. But in other cases the ulcerative process once set up, seems to grow in intensity as it progresses, until the tissues seem to soften and break down before it. Or possibly the majority of these would be better described by saying, that the inflammation which attends them causes a continuous infiltration of adjacent tissue with aplastic material, destroying the resisting power of the structures.

1020. This destructive process once set up, and all tissues yield before it, mucous membrane, connective tissue, fibrous tissue, muscles, cartilage and bone. It may perforate and destroy the soft palate, the hard palate, the roof of the mouth, or the structures of the fauces. Commencing in these parts it may progress upwards, attacking the structures of the nasal cavities, destroying structure after structure, until mouth, throat and nose become one cavity, or the drain upon the economy is so severe that life is lost.

1021. The general treatment of these lesions will not differ from that heretofore named. The reader will see the importance of conserving the life of the patient, and the life of the tissues affected, and as far as possible making the treatment restorative. This is one of the cases in which Cod-Oil and Arsenic come into promiuence as restoratives, and may arrest the local destruction.

1022. In the early stage of ulceration, I would advise the local use of Nitric Acid with the pine pencil, and the usual local applications. The use of Sulphurous Acid, with the spray apparatus, may be suggested, as giving excellent results in some of these cases. Of the vegetable remedies I have obtained better results from the Alnus, Scrofularia and Rumex, than any others. I employ them in infusion, both internally and as a local application.

1023. All operative interference with the bones of mouth or nose should be avoided. Even when a sequestrum seems loose, much force should not be used in taking it away. As a local application to diseased parts, to facilitate the removal of that which is dead, and to stimulate the tissues against the destructive process, I know of nothing so good as our old-fashioned Sesquicarbonate of Potash.

1024. The *œsophagus* is rarely the seat of syphilitic disease, though sometimes the ulcerative process extends to it from the pharynx. Cases are on record, in which the cicatrization of such ulcers produced permanent stricture and death. In the majority of cases, *dysphagia* is nervous, and does not ensue from stricture. In some it is due to irritation of the nerves of the œsophagus, from ulceration of the throat. In others it is a symptom of disease of the brain, and probably one of the most common and distinctive symptoms we meet with.

1025. Nervous dysphagia is treated with Pulsatilla, Bromide of Ammonium, or Lobelia, as may be indicated. The first is especially useful, when there is dizziness, want of power to control the voluntary muscles, and fear of impending danger. The second, when the attacks are epiliptiform. And the third where there is præcordial oppression.

1026. The *stomach* shows the influence of the syphilitic poison upon its function, as we have already noticed in "syphilitic fever," and we will find cases in which this impairment is very marked and persistent. But this functional wrong is about the only one we have to notice, as this viscus seems to be exempt from the specific ulcerative process, or the deposit of aplastic material.

1027. The *liver* has been found diseased in secondary syphilis, but it is difficult to determine whether this is to be attributed to the syphilitic virus or to the over-stimulation of mercurials given for its cure. In my opinion the latter is best supported by evidence.

1028. We can see how this organ, directly and continuously influenced by mercurials, with its circulation deranged, and its function interfered with, should suffer from low grades of inflammation, and be the seat of tubercular or gummy deposits. So far as my experience goes, and so far as I can trace the history of the *non-mercurial* treatment, no such lesions attend it.

1029. The *intestinal canal* suffers from over-medication and the abuse of cathartics, but until we reach the rectum, we find little evidence of the specific disease. Lanceaux says: "That the facts seem to prove that the intestines are not always exempt from the attacks of syphilis, for although the cases are rare in which this canal is affected, it is none the less true that the multiple and rounded ulcerations, penetrating to a greater or less depth and circumscribed by fibrous tissue, of which it is sometimes the seat, are probably only the sequence of gummy deposits, or, in other words, the result of the degeneration which these deposits have undergone."

1030. The *rectum* suffers from syphilitic disease more rarely than we would suppose. Even ulceration just within the sphincter though occasionally met with, is a rare form of the disease. Syphilitic fissures have been spoken of, but these are probably simple, and the result of other causes, in the majority of cases.

1031. *Mucous tubercle* of the anus is quite common, probably the most frequent seat of the lesion, and is sometimes very unpleasant. The patient thinks, probably, that he is troubled with hemorrhoids, and frequently is treated for this disease. Finally an examination reveals the mucous tubercles, and the treatment heretofore named soon removes them.

DISEASES OF THE NERVOUS SYSTEM.

MUSCULAR PAINS.

1032. Muscular pains frequently accompany the earlier symptoms, though they may attend all stages of the disease. These pains are sometimes attended with a sense of stiffness and soreness, as if caused by over exertion, but at others they are more of the nature of cramp, and are relived by pressure. The addition of Conium to the remedies employed is usually required to remove them. If they are located in the fibrous structures near the joints, Macrotys will also prove useful; if there is œdema, give Apocynum.

NEURALGIA.

1033. Among the later symptoms of syphilis is a most intense and persistent neuralgia, not associated with nodes, or other structural lesions. Intense pain may, in some cases, be dependent upon disease in the course of the nerves, as in a case of ulnar neuralgia I witnessed from disease of the humerus, but this will be readily detected. The disease we wish to describe is associated with marked impairment of the vegetative functions, and some of the lesions classed as tertiary.

1034. In the majority of cases the pain is of the extremities, and seems to be in or about the denser fibrous tissues, and in these situations is sometimes most intense. In a recent case it was located in the feet, seemingly in the plantar fasciæ, and for six weeks the patient suffered beyond all description. It was associated here with a very sore mouth, the tongue being fissured, and bleeding on the slightest pressure. Both hands had been badly diseased for some months, with syphilitic psoriasis, so that the patient was incapacitated from work. The sore mouth and skin disease were cured with Rhus, the neuralgia yielded to Iodide of Potassium as soon as the digestive organs would tolerate the drug in sufficient quantities.

DISEASES OF THE BRAIN.

1035. Syphilitic lesions of the brain are also among the later symptoms, and though very serious and frequently fatal, are often overlooked. The lesions shown after death are very distinct, and it is a wonder sometimes, not that death should have resulted, but that life was maintained so long.

1036. Gummata of the brain is probably the most common lesion. Obscure in its course, there is a slow deposit of imperfect albuminoid material in the substance of the brain, or its meninges, or sometimes in the connective tissue between the dura-mater and bones of the cranium. For a time the organism accommodates itself to the changed condition and process, with the development of one after the other of the symptoms hereafter described, until finally death results from compression, or from the breaking down of the deposit. This condition is described by Ricord, as syphilitic tubercle of the brain.

1037. Degeneration of the nerve substance may result from impaired nutrition without any syphilitic deposit, presenting the ordinary symptoms of cerebral softening. In other cases the cerebral vessels suffer from syphilitic disease, and atheromatous patches, aneurismal dilatations, and the presence of a loose cicatrical tissue, are the evidences of its progress.

1038. Wilks remarks, with reference to some of these cases, that, "a quantity of tough, yellow, fibrous tissue unites together the surface of the brain with the adjacent membrane, and this again is adherent to the bone. The cortical substance of the brain at the affected spot is often partly destroyed, and the adventitious material occupies its place. The question has still to be solved as to what structure is primarily affected. Many have given the authority of their names to the opinion that the disease commences first in the bone, but simply for the reason that the osseous system is that which has so long been recognized as liable to be affected. But since we now know that other structures may be similarly attacked, we are prepared to look for its commencement in other parts, and even in the brain structure itself. . . The cases which are so frequently met with are those where the deposit involves both sides of the *dura mater*, and includes in it the bone on one side and the brain on the other. The probabilities are in favor of its occurring in the *dura mater* first, as it arises in the periosteum on the exterior of the cranium." (Wilks in *Med· Times and Gaz.*, Oct. 25, 1862.)

1039. The symptoms in these cases, at first obscure, become gradually more pronounced. In many cases, the patient will first complain of a sense of fullness or sometimes lightness of the head, with dizziness and want of command over the voluntary muscles. There may be impairment of hearing, with tinnitus aurium, impairment of vision with muscæ volitantes, ptosis, or other local lesion depending upon the situation of the lesion in the brain. A very common symptom is an impediment in walking, a "dragging gait," usually more marked in one side than the other.

3040. Following these symptoms, the patient will sometimes suffer acute pain in the head, which may continue in rare cases for days or weeks. This is the precursor of paralysis in some of its forms, or sometimes of the softening and breaking down of the gummatous or tubercular deposit.

1041. The situation and degree of paralysis vary greatly in different cases. In the majority it is never complete, and is not constant, being now better, now worse, for months or even years.

1042. The treatment of these lesions is sometimes quite successful, but only when the right antisyphilitic is selected. If Iodide of Potassium is *the* remedy, we will find that pain, dizziness, paralysis, and the series of symptoms will rapidly fade out before it, and this is the case with other remedies employed in the disease. If we do not find such remedy, the disease will run its course, and we can only palliate the symptoms.

IRITIS.

1043. Inflammation of the iris is one of the most serious lesions of syphilis, involving as it does so important an organ, and if not arrested, causing the destruction of the eye. It most generally makes its appearance from six to fourteen months after the primary disease, being associated with papulæ, alopecia, and sore throat. It does not differ materially in its symptoms from non-syphilitic iritis, and can only be diagnosed from it by its association with other lesions.

1044. Dimness of sight and fatigue in using the eye is usually the first symptom, and may continue for several days before the disease is developed. Soon the globe becomes sore when pressed upon or when moved, and injection of the circum-corneal vessels is noticed. The pain soon becomes severe, with a feeling of extreme distension of the eyeball, and dull pain extending to the orbit and forehead. There is much intolerance of light, with increased secretion of tears, when the eye is exposed, and dimness of vision and haziness become prominent at this time. If we examine the eye, we will notice a redness situated beneath the conjunctiva, which is formed by vessels passing in radii toward the cornea. The pupil is contracted and looks dull, and the motion of the iris is impaired. Its color is also changed, becoming yellowish-green if the person had blue eyes, and dusky red if they were dark. Some writers base a distinction between common and syphilitic iritis, by the scattered and furuncular appearance of the redness for some time, and upon the rusty color of the iris near its pupillary margin which is observed in the last.

1045. If the disease is allowed to progress, the iris bulges forward toward the cornea, the pupil is irregular in form, and at last becomes obliterated, and the exterior half of the eye and cornea become more convex; myopia, hardness of the eye and amaurosis follow more or less promptly.

1046. Though a severe affection, the treatment is comparatively simple, and very successful. Open the patient's bowels and keep them regular with the Podophyllin pill heretofore named, and give a solution of Iodide of Ammonium in ordinary doses. Keep the stomach and digestive organs in good condition by the use of tonics and small portions of Quinine. At first use the spirit vapor bath, with cold sponging daily, afterward a simple bath will be sufficient.

1047. The most important part of the treatment is to keep the pupil dilated with Belladonna. If this is done, impairment of the structure of the eye need not be feared. I prefer a solution of Atropia, from one to five grains, to the ounce of distilled water, and dropped into the eye every four to six hours. The same object may be accomplished by the use of the Extract of Belladonna around the eye and to the lids, or by a collyrium of: ℞ Fluid Extract of Belladonna, ʒj.; Water, ℥j. No other local means should be employed, as it would interfere with the above and lead to bad results. Keep the patient quiet, in a darkened but well ventilated room, until the pain and intolerance of light has entirely disappeared.

SYPHILITIC DISEASE OF THE BONES.

1048. Disease of the bones is among the latest symptoms of constitutional syphilis, and is included in the *tertiary* form of the disease, when this division is made. It is very difficult at this day to determine what part in the causation of these affections the virus of syphilis plays, as it is well known and now admitted by most writers, that Mercury will give rise to all the phases of them noticed. It is my belief that they are wholly due to mercurialization, and that syphilis has nothing to do with them. We will notice some authorities upon this subject.

1049. Mr. Parker writes, "We may naturally inquire whether Mercury has anything to do with the production of nodes. I confess that I am disposed to think that a great deal of mischief is due to a mercurial cure." "It is a fact," says Mr. Carmichæl, "that in those cases of syphilis treated without Mercury, the secondary symptoms are particularly mild, and the bones are seldom or never affected." Dr. Chas. A. Lee, in a note to Copland's Dictionary of Medicine, remarks: "The symptoms following mercurial treatment are more severe and difficult to remove than those following primary sores not treated with Mercury; and when relapses do occur in the secondary stage, they are far more readily removed in those cases where no Mercury has been given. Mercury, when given incautiously, or in too large quantities, especially in syphilitic diseases, tends to undermine the constitution, to predispose to and aggravate constitutional affections, to increase general irritability, to induce inflammation and ulceration in, and destroy the mucous textures, to promote morbid absorption and removal of the fatty, fibrinous and osseous substance of the system, and to induce synovial, albuminous, and serous accumulations. The extent and injury to the soft and bony parts of the system produced by Mercury, are more to be dreaded than any primary or secondary effects of venereal poisons."

NODES.

1050. Nodes are hardened elevations upon the bones, caused by exudation between the periosteum and bone, the result of a low grade of inflammation. In other cases the material thrown out resembles the provisional cartilage in fracture, and occasionally deposits of bony material takes place within it, giving it almost an ivory hardness. In some cases this growth progresses to considerable size without any unpleasant symptoms, but in others there is more or less pain, usually deep-seated, tensive and aching.

1051. Nodes may form upon any of the bones, but are more frequently met with where they are superficial. The tibia is a favorite location, as is the bones of the cranium, and in these situations they are always unpleasant and painful. In some cases nodes of the cranial bones give rise to excessive pain, which is not relieved until suppuration occurs, or the tension is removed by the use of the knife.

1052. Nodes terminate in a variety of ways. Resolution frequently results under appropriate internal treatment, the enlargement gradually passing away, though almost always leaving a roughness or unevenness that remains for life. In other cases, inflammation of the bones occurs, followed by suppuration and caries.

1053. In addition to the general means, which should be carefully selected, we sometimes employ local applications with advantage. Penciling the surface with Collodion will sometimes relieve pain, and by its contraction cause absorption of the effused material. A saturated solution of Iodide of Ammonium is a favorite local application. It may be improved by combining equal parts of a strong Tincture of Iodine and Aqua Ammonia; if allowed to stand for a few days it is decolorized. Conium, Aconite, Veratrum and Belladonna have been employed in some cases with advantage, but unless specially indicated they frequently fail.

1054. If the pain is excessive, and is not relieved by the local means named, and the internal treatment is slow in its influence, we may employ the hypodermic injection, or resort to free incision. We use the common solution of Morphia, (grs. x. to ℥j.) with or without the solution of Atropia (grs. j. to ℥j.) throwing it under the skin as near the point of disease as possible. This always gives temporary relief, and will sometimes be followed by the disappearance of the node. It is bad treatment, however, to persist in the use of Morphia hypodermically, merely for temporary relief. A better practice is, to make a free incision through the distended periosteum to the bone, giving exit to the glairy deposit underneath. This is almost always followed by relief, and the disappearance of the disease at this point.

NOCTURNAL PAINS.

1055. Are almost always associated with nodes, and are sometimes so severe that they prevent sleep and cause much nervous exhaustion. These pains may also occur without apparent disease of the bones, in each case being deep-seated and aching, or as if there was a foreign body in the part that should be removed.

1056. In some cases the suffering is most intense, preventing rest, and finally impairing the nutritive processes. The patient may suffer but very little if any during the day, and examination shows no structural cause for the severe pain, yet as soon as he lies down, the pain commences, or he is awakened out of his sleep by the pain.

1057. We may employ the usual means for temporary relief, but no permanent benefit need be expected except from the general antisyphilitic treatment. The administration of Opiates either by mouth or hypodermic injection, will generally interfere with, or may wholly prevent the action of proper remedies.

SYPHILITIC PERIOSTITIS.

1058. The superficial bones are those most commonly affected, though once in a while the deeper seated will suffer. Commencing as a node, the periosteum and adjacent bone become more vascular, a peculiar viscid material is deposited, and finally inflammation results. This runs a variable course, sometimes acute, at others very slow, not unfrequently terminating in suppuration, and caries of the bone.

1059. The disease of the bones thus set up is in some cases very destructive. As we have already seen, it may destroy the bones of the nose, and those forming the roof of the mouth, producing great deformity. Commencing in the bones of the legs, especially the tibia, it may continue for months or years, each succeeding outbreak confining the patient to his room for days or weeks. Affecting the bones of the feet, the disease is very painful, and is frequently prolonged, and results in permanent disability. Affecting the former, the inflammation is deep seated, and involves the

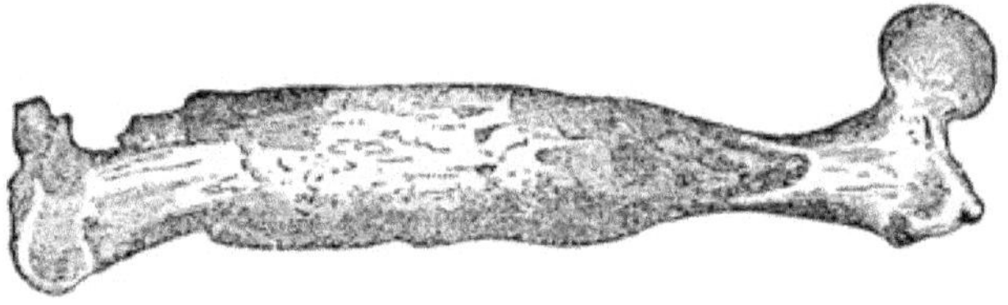

Syphilitic Hypertrophy.

superimposed parts, producing extensive abscess and great exhaustion. In the bones of the cranium, the disease is especially painful, as we have already seen, and frequently groes on to the destruction of the external table of the skull, and in some rare cases to the entire destruction of the bones, and exposure of the brain.

1060. The upper extremities suffer like the lower. The disease may attack the clavicles, and be followed by caries or necrosis, and by contiguity the deeper structures, and even the lungs may be implicated. Disease of the arm or forearm is almost always followed by deformity, and impaired function. The ribs and the cartilages suffer, and disease of the sternum has been observed, going on to its destruction and the exposure of the organs beneath.

1061. As no part of the osseous system is exempt, so we will find every form of bone disease, from the simple osteoperiostitis, which terminates in resolution, to caries and extensive necrosis.

1062. Permanent cures may be expected in many cases, but in some, the bones once affected there is successive outbreaks as long as the patient lives. In these the bones become thickened and rough; the tissues above show abundant cicatrices of former ulcerations; sinuses leading to diseased bones persist, and discharge continuously, and sometimes sequestra are carried for years.

1063. The treatment of these cases will be the same as in simple periostitis and osteitis, except in so far as it is directed against the syphilitic poison. A cure is always slow, and if we can make it permanent, it is with months of careful attention.

SYPHILITIC ORCHITIS.

1064. Syphilitic orchitis has been classed by some writers with the secondary symptoms, by others with the tertiary. It rarely comes during the first year, yet it has been seen as early as the sixth month. In some cases it is purely inflammatory, in others the enlargement is from gummy deposit, and there may be but little inflammatory action.

1065. In the majority of cases the enlargement is quite slow, and the patient is only aware that there is disease of the testes by the dragging sensation upon the cord. As the enlargement continues, there is occasionally tensive pain, associated with a feeling of great weight and dragging upon the cord, when the organs are not supported. Exercise will frequently increase this so much, that the sufferer is forced to keep quiet.

1066. In some cases there is never any pain, and the organ is not sensitive to pressure, the only discomfort the patient experiences being from the increased weight of the testes. These are said to be the typical cases, and that when we find the enlarged organs, without pain or even ordinary sensitiveness, the patient having had syphilis, we may conclude it is syphilitic orchitis. This, however, has not been my experience.

1067. The treatment will not differ from other similar lesions. In many cases Iodide of Potassium will be found the internal remedy, as a solution of Iodide of Ammonium is the best external application. But in this as in other cases, the treatment must be adapted to the case in hand. A friend of mine suffered from syphilitic orchitis for many months, and after exhausting all the common means, cured himself with small doses of Proto-Iodide of Mercury, and the use of electricity. It was suggested that probably the galvanic current might have removed the disease alone (?) I think in many of these cases it will be found a useful remedy.

1068. The Phytolacca will prove a good remedy when the disease is acute, and may be employed as a local application as well as internally. The Iris Versicolor has also given good results, using a Tincture of the fresh root.

INFANTILE SYPHILIS.

1069. Secondary syphilis may be transmitted from either parent to the child, which will be born impregnated with the poison. The disease either shows itself at birth or a few months after, though in rare cases several years may elapse. The most common affections of the child is the squamæ, and pustular skin diseases, though occasionally the mucous membranes are affected. There is almost always contraction of the jaws, and deformity of the teeth, and this is looked upon as evidence of syphilitic parentage, even when no other symptoms present. The following are the propositions laid down by M. Ricord regarding the transmission of syphilis:

"1. The father and mother may transmit the disease to their child indifferently, if either or both of them be affected.

"2. Transmission may occur from the parents to the child, when they are affected with constitutional symptoms, or when a concealed syphilitic diathesis exists in them.

"3. The absence or existence of constitutional symptoms in parents at the moment of impregnation and conception exerts no influence on the form of the disease, which may afterward appear in the child. The distinction established by M

Cazenave between congenital and hereditary syphilis, and which is based on the absence of constitutional symptoms in the parents at the moment of generation, or which have been developed in the mother during gestation, is totally erroneous; and indeed M. Cazenave confesses that his opportunities of observing have not been ample.

"4. The character and period of the manifestation of the symptoms in the child are governed by the stage to which the disease had advanced in the parents at the moment of generation. The treatment to which the parents were subjected may also retard, prevent, or modify its appearance in the child.

"5. If the parents are both healthy at the time of generation, and the mother contracts syphilis during gestation, she may transmit the disease to her child. Of this I have seen several examples at various periods of pregnancy, even to the seventh month inclusive.

"6. When the venereal poison is transmitted from the mother to the child during pregnancy, infection takes place through the medium of the placenta, and in this case, appears to occur after the fourth month of utero-gestation.

"If the father alone be diseased at the moment of generation, an abortion may occur at any period of pregnancy. If the mother alone be diseased at the time of conception, the abortion will not take place until after the fourth month.

"7. Children born of a father or mother affected with syphilis may escape infection; for a certain disposition to receive constitutional disease is necessary for the child as well as the adult, and this may be absent.

"8. Observations made as accurately as possible seem to prove that constitutional syphilis may be transmitted from the child to the mother during utero-gestation."

SYPHILIZATION.

1070. The minds of syphilographers are now agitated with the question, can the constitutional disposition to syphilis be so entirely removed that the person will be no more affected by it than he would be by smallpox, if he had previously had the disease? This question is not only answered in the affirmative, but Prof. Boeck, of Christiana, Sweden, claims that continued inoculation will also remove the constitutional disease when all other means fail. Other surgeons have tested his views with favorable results. As it is a new subject, it will be better to let Prof. Boeck speak for himself, and I will quote from a lecture delivered before the physicians of Dublin:

"By syphilization I understand the mode of treatment by which, by repeated inoculations of syphilitic matter, taken from primary sores, I bring the body into the condition that it is no longer susceptible of the action of the syphilitic virus.

"It will, perhaps, be agreeable to you, gentlemen, before I proceed further, that I should lay before you a short *resume* of the history of this mode of treatment. Auzias-Turenne, of Paris, performed inoculations of syphilitic matter upon animals in order to see whether this virus could be transferred to them, which up to that time had been denied. In this he was at length successful, and it was chiefly apes which could with the greatest facility be inoculated. After chancres had been repeatedly produced in the same ape, a great many skeptical physicians wished to see his inoculation, and a meeting was appointed in the *Jardin des Plantes;* the old ape was inoculated, and a still greater crowd assembled a few days later to see the result. But when the ape was brought in nothing was to be seen. It may easily be imagined how the result was received, and that Auzias-Turenne was ridiculed, but he did not on that account give up the method;

he continued his inoculations, found that the old ape was not susceptible of fresh inoculations, but that a second ape after inoculation got chancres, though this ape also, after a series of inoculations, became unsusceptible.

"Auzias-Turenne now saw clearly that he had here a natural law, in itself resembling that which your immortal Jenner had discovered in the inoculation of vaccine matter, and we shall not upbraid him now that his French blood carried him away, and that his first idea was to employ the inoculation of syphilitic matter like that of vaccine matter—as a prophylactic. We can not gainsay him that his train of ideas is logically correct, but it is not practically correct, for the great rule is, that he only gets syphilis who himself will have it.

"As the result of this idea of employing syphilization as a prophylactic, my friend Auzias wished at the time to syphilize all public girls, seamen, and soldiers, and he would willingly have syphilized us all. No wonder, then, that such an idea met with all the opposition it deserved; but it was not long until Auzias renounced his error, and at the same time there appeared an Italian, Sperino, of Turin, who showed, by a series of experiments, that the syphilitic disease was cured during these inoculations, which Auzias, too, at the same time demonstrated. Still, this failed to reconcile physicians to the new method; such a prejudice had been raised against it, that both the Academie de Medicine of Paris and the Academy of Turin condemned it without having the necessary materials before them for passing any judgment; the paradox involved in this method appeared to all so enormous as to render proofs of its absurdity unnecessary.

"Lecturing in the University of Christiana upon syphilis, and having a section of the hospital devoted to this disease, I carefully investigated all that was advanced upon this subject, and ascertained that there must be some truth in it. I had, through a period of very many years, found that our treatment with Mercury is highly unsatisfactory; I therefore considered that, from my position, it was my duty to give a trial to this new method, although it appeared to me as paradoxical as it did to all the world, and notwithstanding that it had been condemned by two academies. But before I began, I laid down for myself certain limits, to which I still adhere. It will be at once observed that I will not speak of the method as a prophylactic: this would be immoral; but neither am I at liberty to employ it in every case of syphilis; it is only when syphilis has become constitutional—when the syphilitic virus flows with every drop of blood through the system—that I allow myself also to inoculate it upon the skin.

"The next question is, whether I shall employ syphilization in every case of constitutional syphilis?

"By a fortunate coincidence it happened that of the two individuals whom I first took under treatment by syphilization, the one had not been treated for syphilis, while the other had been the subject of all the resources of our art. In the first the inoculations proceeded without difficulty, the symptoms gradually disappeared—in a word, I found myself upon the beaten path. In the other case all was irregular. I could effect no order at all, and when my first patient was well, the phenomena in the second were still in full bloom. I immediately began to suspect that it was to the medicines previously given that this result was attributable, and on subsequently investigating this opinion, its truth has been most completely confirmed, so that I have made it a general rule to syphilize only those who have not previously been treated with Mercury, whether this has been employed for primary or constitutional symptoms. But if I be asked whether syphilization has not some effect in these cases, I can answer decidedly in the affirmative—it often acts incredibly. Dr. Simpson, of Edinburgh, has recently described two such cases, which were sent over to me by Prof. Simpson; what is there stated corresponds precisely to what I have myself noted, and of which any one may satisfy himself. But the reason why I do not undertake the treatment of such individuals is to avoid having relapses, which in these cases are apt to occur.

"Now, in order to make my usual mode of proceeding as plain as possible, I shall suppose that a person laboring under primary syphilis consults me. In this case I treat the primary sore as a simple ulcer—I prescribe a weak solution of Sulphate of Zinc or such like, and occasionally employ a slight cauterization of Nitrate of Silver. I give no internal medicine, but make the patient come to me once or twice a week, that I may observe when the constitutional symptoms break out, for the earlier syphilization can be commenced the better. So soon as I perceive the first constitutional signs, I commence the treatment by taking matter from an indurated chancre or from an artificial pustule in a patient under treatment by syphilization. I inoculate first on both sides of the chest, and make three punctures with a lancet, precisely in the mode adopted in vaccinating. After three days pustules are developed, and then I inoculate again in the sides, taking the matter from the pustules produced by the first inoculation, observing carefully to make the second inoculation at a distance from the first, so that the sores may not become confluent. At the end of three days I make the third inoculation, taking the matter from the pustules of the second inoculation; and I now continue to inoculate on both sides every third day, always taking the matter for the fresh inoculation from the pustules last formed, so long as this matter continues to afford a positive result. When it no longer takes, I procure new matter in the same mode as for the first inoculation, and continue with this as with the first. This second matter will yield smaller sores and a shorter series than the first, and when it no longer takes I procure a third and proceed in the same manner. This third matter will produce very little effect, and I therefore pass to the upper arm, where I proceed in precisely the same mode as in the sides; and when no effect is any longer visible in the upper arm I remove to the thighs, and continue there in the same way as in the two preceding places. By the time the inoculations are here brought to an end, from three to three and a half or four months have probably elapsed; the symptoms which manifested themselves from the commencement have disappeared, or if some slight symptom has remained this disappears spontaneously. It often happens that during the treatment a fresh outbreak takes place, and he who is not acquainted with the method believes that some other plan must now be adopted; another infers that syphilization is of no avail. But, let them not be deterred by any symptom, not even by the most severe iritis, which never requires anything but the instillation of a little Atropia. But, happen what may, let them shut their eyes to it, and continue the inoculations. The patient who, during the whole treatment can attend to his business, feels, after it is completed, perfectly well, and may immediately expose himself to any hardships. He can endure wet, cold—in a word, everything which after mercurial treatment would render him liable to life-long illness. It is probable that I may now be asked as to the result at a later period for these individuals, and I shall speak first of the relapses. On the whole, I have treated 429 individuals, and of these 45 have come back, making about 10½ per cent.; but, as we may calculate that some of those treated during the last year will return, I will assume that the relapses will amount to 12 or 13 per cent. But, let us now examine more closely what is called a relapse after syphilization. In many instances a single mucous tubercle, a small white spot on the tongue or in the throat—symptoms for which nothing more than external means is employed, and for which the patients are treated only for a few days in hospital. So far as I at this moment remember, thirteen were taken again under treatment with syphilization, and two with Iodide of Potassium.

"You will next ask whether tertiary symptoms have been developed in any of them. This has been the case, I believe, with three; but at the same time these individuals have been perfectly well — their general health has not, as so often happens after mercurial treatment, been broken down, and in those who have had relapses it has been good, as it is evident that in those who have had no relapse it has been particularly good.

"We come now to the children of those who have been syphilized. Here we are not much better off than after the mercurial treatment; we see the same rule to prevail as after this last method, namely—that when the mother has been syphilitic, the first child or children is or are syphilitic; that they are healthy is the exception. If the father has been syphilitic, the children are, in general, healthy; that they are syphilitic is the exception.

"You will next propose to me the question how I treat syphilitic children. I treat them precisely as I do adults; and it is interesting to see that the sores in these little ones bear in size a proportion to that of the child, and that the patients suffer less, and not more, than adults. The results of syphilization in children with hereditary syphilis have not been brilliant; of forty-two children, twenty-two died, but I have taken under treatment every case that I have met with, and every one knows that in such children there are very often affections of the internal organs which lie beyond our power to cure. I can not at this moment say how many little children with acquired syphilis I have syphilized, but they are not few, and of these only one died, the cause of death in that instance being croup after I had performed tracheotomy. Of adults, two died—an old woman of dysentery, and a young woman of puerperal fever. This latter case I forgot to include in the *résume* I have given in the *British Medical Journal.*

"Now, in order to give you a definite idea of the confidence I have in this method after having practiced it daily for thirteen years, I shall say only that if I myself, or any of mine, were so unfortunate as to get syphilis, I should employ no other means than syphilization.

"Still, a few words in conclusion, gentlemen. Vaccination has for many years stood alone; syphilization now comes to join it. Shall we stop here? I believe not. Vaccine and the syphilitic matter are both animal viruses; we see them contained under a similar law. May not also the other animal poisons be referred to a similar law? We see that nature is simple in her diversity: should this not also here be the case? Should not glanders, hydrophobia, etc., some time be curable? Let us all seek to clear up this dark point in our science, and let us not, as hitherto, with respect to syphilization, seek only to extinguish the rising gleam."

The majority of observers now unite in condemning the practice of syphilization. It not only requires a long period of time, but is as unpleasant and disgusting as it is tedious. And as the old methods are dispensed with, the disease is found more tractable, and even if syphilization was successful, it will be found unnecessary.

EXPLANATION OF PLATE I.

Fig. 1.—Shows the result of the inoculation two hours after the matter was inserted by the lancet; already may be marked a tumefaction of the tissues, and in the center is seen the puncture made by the lancet, surrounded by a reddish areola of small extent, almost confined to the projecting parts.

Fig. 2.—Drawing six hours and a half after inoculation. The inoculation is still more elevated. The areola is of a deeper color.

Fig. 3.—Drawing twenty-four hours after inoculation. The projecting parts appear clearly defined, and their base is of a deep-red hue. On the summit is seen a grayish point, corresponding to the incision of the lancet. The inflammatory areola has comparatively greatly extended.

Fig. 4.—Drawing in thirty-one hours. The pustule is formed. The grayish point of the morning has become completely black, and forms a small gangrenous eschar, around which the epidermis is elevated by the pus.

Fig. 5.—Drawing forty-eight hours after inoculation. All the elements of the pustule are progressing.

FIG. 6.—Drawing three days after inoculation. General progress. We remark an irregularity in the periphery of the pustule, which during the night discharged some pus, and in the center of which the gangrenous eschar is depressed, and appears to be adherent to the subjacent parts.

FIG. 7.—Drawing four days after inoculation. General progress. The pustule is lacerated at several points, and appears to be free from pus.

FIG. 8.—Drawing five days after inoculation. General progress with the exception of the inflammatory areola, which appears less intense. The irregular eschar, covering the wound made by inoculation, was removed, and beneath it is seen a roseate base studded with yellow spots. On the edges which are scarcely separated, is seen a whitish border formed by the epidermis.

FIG. 9.—Chancroid of posterior lip of the cervix. It has assumed a slight phagedenic character, and has lost its circular appearance.

Plate II

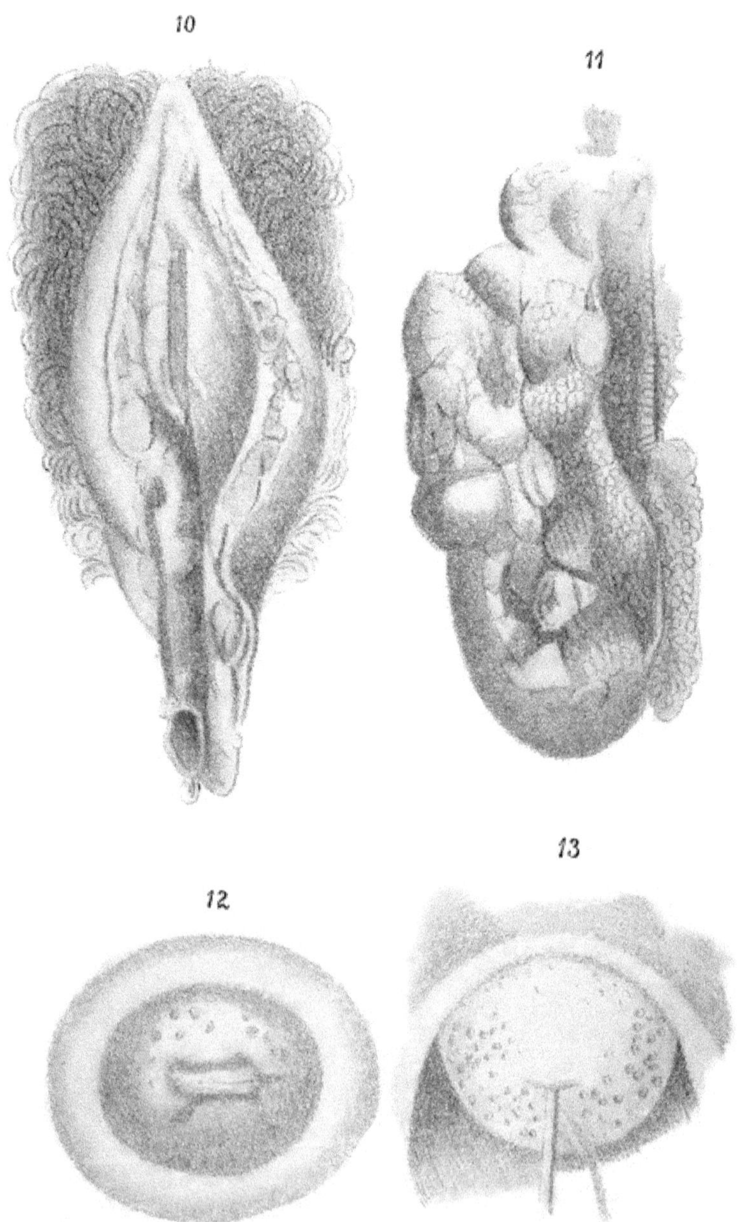

EXPLANATION OF PLATE II.

FIG. 10. Mucous papulæ of the vulva. Secondary symptoms in the third month from single ulcer—chancre.

FIG. 11.—Polymorphous vegetations.

FIG. 12.—Secondary syphilitic ulceration of os uteri, with rose-colored granulations of anterior lip.

FIG. 13.—Secondary syphilitic granulations of cervix, with chronic inflammation.

Plate III

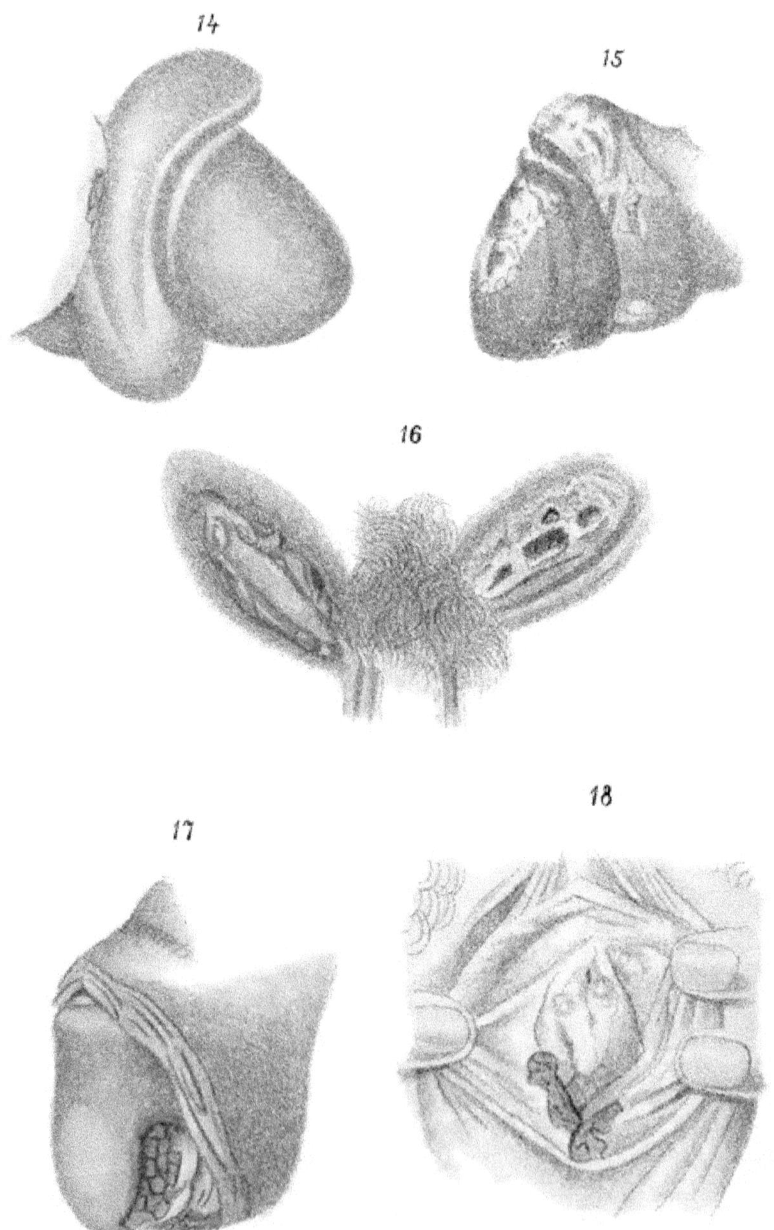

EXPLANATION OF PLATE III.

Fig. 14.—Swelling of the prepuce attending chancroid—paraphimosis.

Fig. 15.—Chancroid, with paraphimosis.

Fig. 16.—Suppurating bubo, following chancroid.

Fig. 17.—Single chancroid, which has destroyed a portion of the glans, prepuce and frænum. Circumcision has been performed, and the sore is healing.

Fig. 18.—Chancroid of vulva.

Plate IV

19

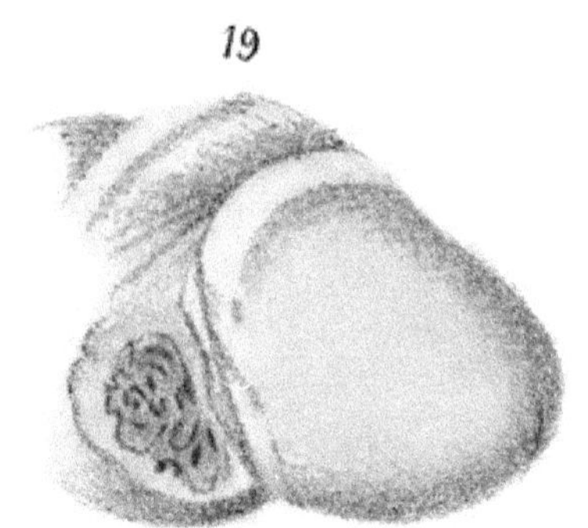

20

21

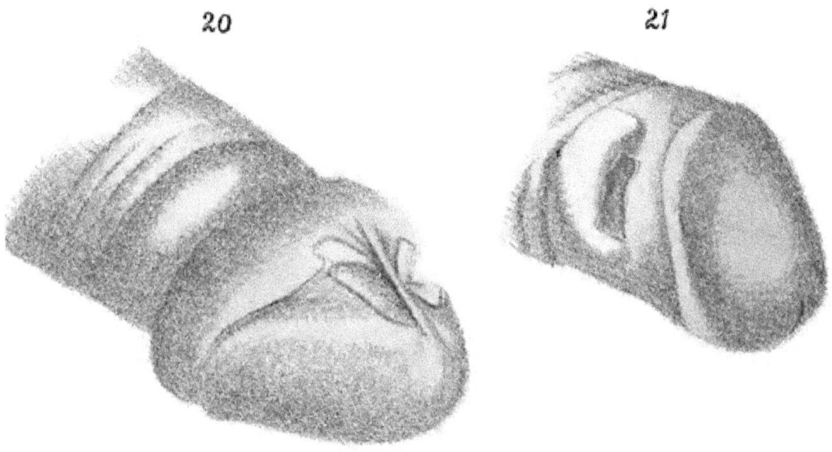

22

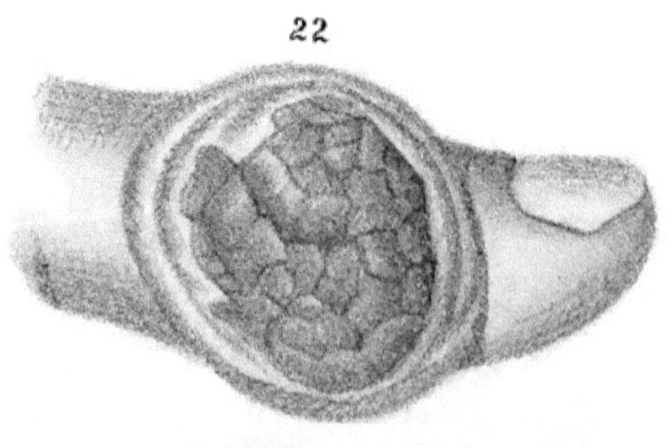

EXPLANATION OF PLATE IV.

Fig. 19.—Chancre of the prepuce just behind the glans.

Fig. 20.—Non-indurated ulcer of the frænum—perforating, (chancroid). It was followed by suppurating buboes—virulent; no constitutional infection.

Fig. 21.—Chancre of the frænum—the sore healing.

Fig. 22.—Chancre of the thumb. This was associated with the ulcers on the penis, all indurated. The disease was followed by constitutional infection.

23

24

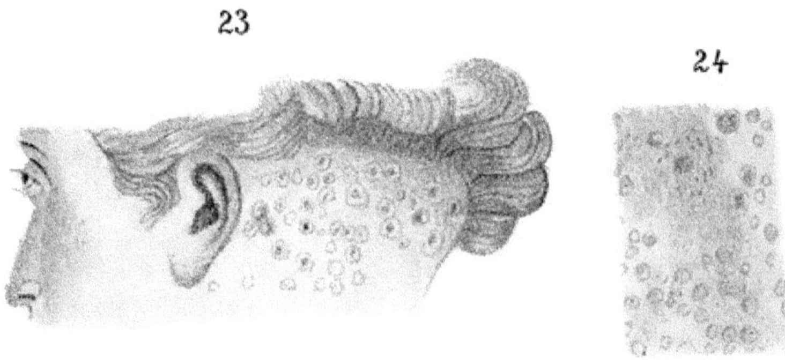

25

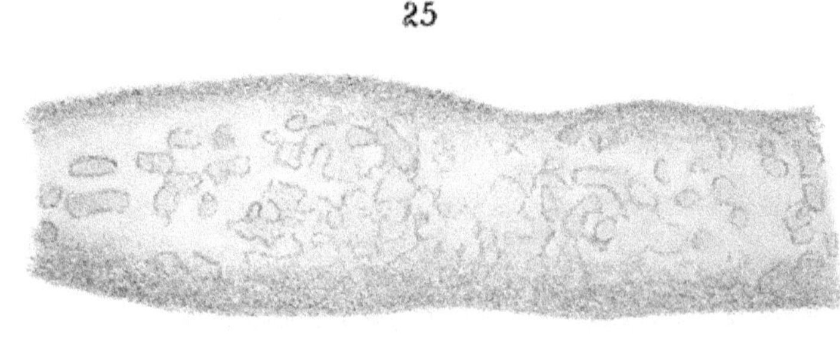

26

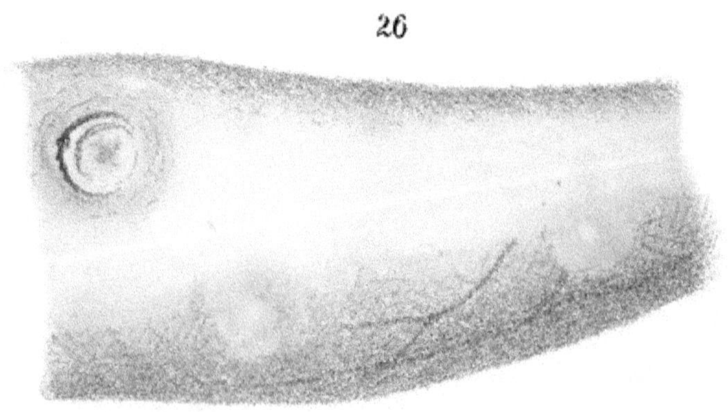

EXPLANATION OF PLATE V.

Fig. 23.—Pustular syphilide—impetigo.

Fig. 24.—Papular syphilide.

Fig. 25.—Syphilitic litchen.

Fig. 26.—Gummata of the forearm. In one ulceration has occurred.

Plate VI

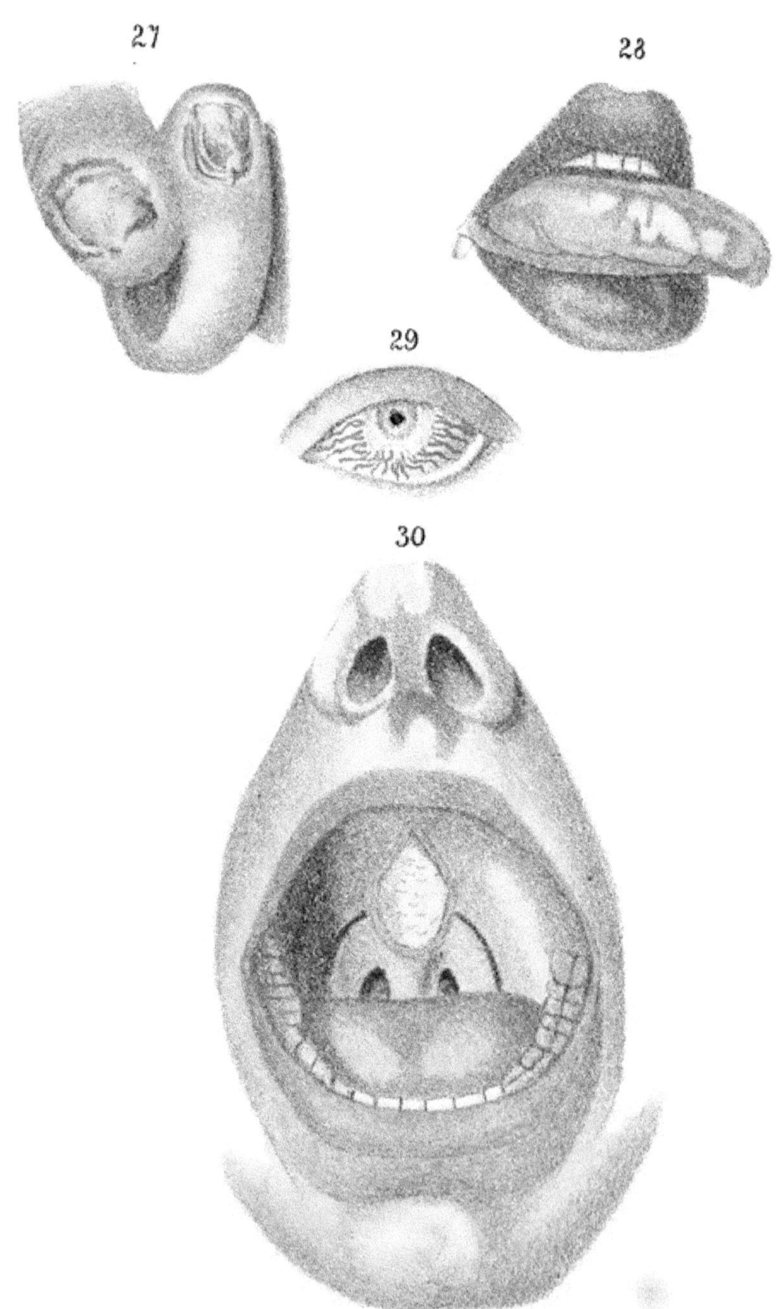

EXPLANATION OF PLATE VI.

Fig. 27.—Onychia of thumb and forefinger, in the form ot mucous patches affecting the matrix of the nails.

Fig. 28.—Syphilitic ulceration of the tongue.

Fig. 29.—Syphilitic iritis.

Fig. 30.—Syphilitic ulcer of the soft palate.

INDEX.

A

B

C

J

L

M

N

O

P

R

T

U

V

W

www.ingramcontent.com/pod-product-compliance
Lightning Source LLC
Chambersburg PA
CBHW031351290326
41932CB00044B/880

* 9 7 8 3 3 3 7 7 3 3 4 9 0 *